Advances in Antiarrhythmic Drug Therapy

Guest Editors

PETER R. KOWEY, MD, FACC, FHRS, FAHA

GERALD V. NACCARELLI, MD, FACC, FHRS, FAHA

CARDIAC ELECTROPHYSIOLOGY CLINICS

www.cardiacEP.theclinics.com

Consulting Editors

RANJAN K. THAKUR, MD, MPH, MBA, FHRS

ANDREA NATALE, MD, FACC, FHRS

September 2010 • Volume 2 • Number 3

SAUNDERS an imprint of ELSEVIER, Inc.

W.B. SAUNDERS COMPANY
A Division of Elsevier Inc.

1600 John F. Kennedy Boulevard ● Suite 1800 ● Philadelphia, Pennsylvania 19103-2899

http://www.theclinics.com

CARDIAC ELECTROPHYSIOLOGY CLINICS Volume 2, Number 3
September 2010 ISSN 1877-9182, ISBN-13: 978-1-4377-2429-5

Editor: Barbara Cohen-Kligerman
Developmental Editor: Donald Mumford

Cardiac Electrophysiology Clinics (ISSN 1877-9182) is published quarterly by Elsevier Inc., 360 Park Avenue South, New York, NY 10010-1710. Months of issue are March, June, September, and December. Subscription prices are $167.00 per year for US individuals, $250.00 per year for US institutions, $84.00 per year for US students and residents, $187.00 per year for Canadian individuals, $299.00 per year for Canadian institutions, $239.00 per year for international individuals, $299.00 per year for international institutions and $120.00 per year for Canadian and foreign students/residents. To receive student/resident rate, orders must be accompanied by name of affiliated institution, date of term, and the signature of program/residency coordinator on institution letterhead. Orders will be billed at individual rate until proof of status is received. Foreign air speed delivery is included in all Clinics subscription prices. All prices are subject to change without notice. **POSTMASTER:** Send address changes to Cardiac Electrophysiology Clinics, Elsevier Health Sciences Division, Subscription Customer Service, 3251 Riverport Lane, Maryland Heights, MO 63043. **Customer Service: 1-800-654-2452 (US and Canada). From outside of the US and Canada, call 314-477-8871. Fax: 314-447-8029. E-mail: JournalsCustomerService-usa@elsevier.com (for print support); JournalsOnlineSupport-usa@elsevier.com (for online support).**

Reprints. For copies of 100 or more of articles in this publication, please contact the Commercial Reprints Department, Elsevier Inc., 360 Park Avenue South, New York, NY 10010-1710. Tel.: 212-633-3812; Fax: 212-462-1935; E-mail: reprints@elsevier.com.

Printed and bound by CPI Group (UK) Ltd, Croydon, CR0 4YY

Transferred to Digital Print 2011

Cover photo courtesy of Rodrigo Senna. Chart shows action potential.

Contributors

CONSULTING EDITORS

RANJAN K. THAKUR, MD, MPH, MBA, FHRS
Professor of Medicine and Director, Arrhythmia
Service, Thoracic and Cardiovascular Institute,
Sparrow Health System, Michigan State
University, Lansing, Michigan

ANDREA NATALE, MD, FACC, FHRS
Executive Medical Director of the Texas
Cardiac Arrhythmia Institute at St David's
Medical Center, Austin, Texas; Consulting
Professor, Division of Cardiology, Stanford
University, Palo Alto, California; Clinical
Associate Professor of Medicine, Case
Western Reserve University, Cleveland,
Ohio; Senior Clinical Director, EP Services,
California Pacific Medical Center, San
Francisco, California; Department
of Biomedical Engineering, University
of Texas, Austin, Texas

GUEST EDITORS

PETER R. KOWEY, MD
William Wikoff Smith Chair, CV Research,
Lankenau Institute for Medical Research;
Chief of Cardiology, Main Line Health System;
Professor of Medicine and Clinical
Pharmacology, Jefferson Medical College,
Wynnewood, Pennsylvania

GERALD V. NACCARELLI, MD
Bernard Trabin Chair of Cardiology;
Professor of Medicine; Chief, Division
of Cardiology, Penn State University
College of Medicine, Hershey,
Pennsylvania

AUTHORS

ALESSANDRO CAPUCCI, MD
Professor of Cardiology, Università
Politecnica delle Marche; Director,
Clinica di Cardiologia, Ospedali Riuniti di
Ancona, Ancona, Italy

PAUL DORIAN, MD, MSc
Professor of Medicine, Division of Cardiology,
St Michael's Hospital, University of Toronto,
Toronto, Ontario, Canada

**MICHAEL D. EZEKOWITZ, MB,
ChB, DPhil, FRCP**
Vice President, Lankenau Institute for
Medical Research, Clinical Research Center,
Wynnewood, Pennsylvania

PAMELA S.N. GOLDMAN, DO
Lankenau Institute for Medical Research,
Clinical Research Center, Wynnewood,
Pennsylvania

AUGUSTUS O. GRANT, MB, ChB, PhD
Professor of Medicine and Vice Dean,
Cardiovascular Division, Duke University
School of Medicine, Durham,
North Carolina

HESSEL F. GROENVELD, MD
Research Fellow, Department of Cardiology,
University Medical Center Groningen,
University of Groningen, Groningen,
The Netherlands

JULIA H. INDIK, MD, PhD
Associate Professor of Medicine,
Sarver Heart Center, University of Arizona
College of Medicine, Tucson, Arizona

ALESSANDRO MARINELLI, MD
Medical Doctor and Research Fellow,
Università Politecnica delle Marche,
Clinica di Cardiologia, Ospedali Riuniti di
Ancona, Ancona, Italy

JOHN P. MORROW, MD
Assistant Professor, Division of Cardiology,
Department of Medicine, Columbia
University Medical Center, New York,
New York

KATHERINE T. MURRAY, MD
Associate Professor, Division of Clinical
Pharmacology, Departments of Medicine
and Pharmacology, Vanderbilt University
School of Medicine, Nashville, Tennessee

RICHARD L. PAGE, MD, FACC, FAHA, FHRS
George R. and Elaine Love Professor, and
Chair, Department of Medicine, University of
Wisconsin, School of Medicine and Public
Health, Madison, Wisconsin

ARNOLD PINTER, MD
Assistant Professor of Medicine, Division
of Cardiology, St Michael's Hospital,
University of Toronto, Toronto, Ontario,
Canada

PHILIP J. PODRID, MD
Professor of Medicine, Professor
of Pharmacology and Experimental
Therapeutics, Boston University
School of Medicine; Lecturer,
Harvard Medical School; Associate Chief,
Section of Cardiology, West Roxbury
Veterans Administration Hospital,
West Roxbury, Massachusetts

JAMES A. REIFFEL, MD
Professor of Clinical Medicine, Division of
Cardiology, Department of Medicine; Director
of Electrocardiography, Columbia University
Medical Center, New York, New York

STEVEN A. ROTHMAN, MD
Clinical Associate Professor, Lankenau
Institute for Medical Research; Chief,
Cardiovascular Disease, Lankenau Hospital,
Wynnewood, Pennsylvania

BRUCE S. STAMBLER, MD
Professor of Medicine, Division
of Cardiology, Cardiac Electrophysiology,
University Hospitals Case Medical Center,
Cleveland, Ohio

ISABELLE C. VAN GELDER, MD, FESC
Professor, Department of Cardiology,
University Medical Center Groningen,
University of Groningen, Groningen;
Interuniversity Cardiology Institute
Netherlands, Utrecht, The Netherlands

MOHAN N. VISWANATHAN, MD
Assistant Professor of Medicine, Division
of Cardiology/Cardiac Electrophysiology,
University of Washington, Seattle, Washington

DEBORAH WOLBRETTE, MD
Professor of Medicine, Penn State Heart
and Vascular Institute, Penn State College
of Medicine, Penn State Milton S. Hershey
Medical Center, Hershey, Pennsylvania

RAYMOND L. WOOSLEY, MD, PhD
Professor of Medicine and Pharmacology,
Sarver Heart Center, University of Arizona
College of Medicine; The Critical Path
Institute, Tucson, Arizona

MICHAEL S. ZAWANEH, MD
Fellow, Cardiac Electrophysiology,
Department of Cardiovascular Medicine,
Cleveland Clinic, Cleveland, Ohio; Arizona
Arrhythmia Consultants, Scottsdale, Arizona

Contents

> Available evidence suggests that the ion channels that generate the normal action potential are also the basis for the arrhythmias that occur in disease states. Therefore, a thorough understanding of the function of the ion channels that generate the action potential is an important foundation for understanding the bases of arrhythmias and their treatment. This need is made all the more pressing by the discoveries in molecular genetics and membrane biophysics that have elucidated the fundamental mechanisms of a broad range of cardiac arrhythmias.

> This article describes the pharmacology of antiarrhythmic medications. Although these medications are broadly considered in terms of their blockade of either sodium or potassium channels, they act by a variety of pharmacodynamic mechanisms. Elimination may be via hepatic metabolism or renal mechanisms, or a combination. In particular, interactions between antiarrhythmic medications and other drugs that interfere with hepatic metabolism by P450 enzymes is a source for toxicity.

> Recent progress in genomic sequencing has begun to elucidate the basic mechanisms for several adverse responses, as well as the clinical efficacy, for antiarrhythmic drugs. DNA variants in drug metabolizing enzymes have been implicated in excessive drug accumulation, and genetic variability in drug targets can identify individuals at increased risk for serious side effects, in particular proarrhythmia. It is hoped that future advances in the area of genomic medicine will lead to more individually tailored or personalized pharmacologic therapy in the management of cardiac arrhythmias.

> Women have a higher risk of developing torsade de pointes when taking QT-prolonging antiarrhythmic drugs. Elderly women with heart failure may have the highest risk of proarrhythmia. Greater caution should be used when treating women with these drugs, especially when additional risk factors for developing proarrhythmia

are present. Women with congenital heart disease frequently experience arrhythmias during pregnancy, and use of antiarrhythmic drugs in this setting poses a special challenge. In the elderly population, the risk of antiarrhythmic drug use may outweigh the benefit, especially in individuals with asymptomatic arrhythmias. Limited data suggest potential ethnic differences in arrhythmic substrates and in proarrhythmic response to antiarrhythmic drugs.

Pharmacologic therapy is commonly used for the acute treatment and termination of paroxysmal supraventricular tachycardia (SVT) and continues to be an important long-term option for some patients. Drug choice depends on the correct diagnosis of the arrhythmia and an understanding of its mechanism. Pharmacologic agents commonly used in the acute and chronic treatment of SVT are reviewed along with their effect on the various types of SVT. Drugs that are well tolerated with minimal side effects are preferred over agents with perhaps more efficacy but higher risk of toxicity.

Atrial fibrillation and atrial flutter are common arrhythmias in everyday clinical settings. Pharmacologic cardioversion (CV) is a simple and widely used strategy for the treatment of these arrhythmias, and many drugs are currently available. The choice of drug is strongly influenced by the time elapsed from atrial fibrillation onset and by a patient's clinical subset. Electrical direct-current CV is the treatment of choice in long-lasting forms; nevertheless, some agents also show efficacy in this setting. In addition, promising results come from studies on the efficacy and safety of new antiarrhythmic drugs and from therapeutic approaches that reduce the need for hospitalization and improve quality of life.

Atrial fibrillation (AF) is a growing public health concern. For most patients the treatment of AF involves antiarrhythmic drugs. Despite the widespread use of antiarrhythmic drugs for the conversion of AF and maintenance of normal sinus rhythm, their use is limited by modest efficacy, frequent intolerance, and the potential for serious ventricular proarrhythmia and organ toxicity. Better medications are urgently needed. Optimizing the way current agents are used is vital in the interim. This article discusses such issues.

Rate control may now be adopted as a first-choice therapy in a variety of patients, especially older relatively asymptomatic patients with hypertension or other underlying heart diseases. The goal of rate control therapy is to minimize symptoms, improve quality of life, decrease the risk of development of heart failure, and prevent thromboembolic complications. A lenient rate control approach may be the initial therapeutic strategy. If symptoms persist, a stricter rate control approach may be adopted. Although long-term randomized studies are lacking, the evidence available suggests that a β-blocker with or without digoxin is the first-choice rate control therapy.

Mohan N. Viswanathan and Richard L. Page

Ventricular arrhythmias (ventricular tachycardia and ventricular fibrillation) are often associated with underlying structural heart disease and require prompt assessment and treatment. Acute treatment involves initial hemodynamic stabilization of the patient followed by suppressive treatment with pharmacologic and nonpharmacologic approaches for reducing the risk of recurrence of ventricular arrhythmias and potential development of sudden cardiac death. This article reviews acute antiarrhythmic drug therapy for ventricular arrhythmias based on the clinical presentation.

Michael S. Zawaneh and Bruce S. Stambler

In this review, we examine the data evaluating the role of adjuvant therapy with antiarrthymic drugs (AADs) in chronic suppression of ventricular tachyarrhythmias in the patient with an ICD. It must be noted that all uses of AADs for this indication represent "off-label" prescription. No AAD is approved by the Food and Drug Administration (FDA) specifically as a therapy to reduce ICD shocks.

Philip J. Podrid

Arrhythmia aggravation by antiarrhythmic drugs (proarrhythmia) can be caused by worsening or a change of a preexisting arrhythmia, development of a new arrhythmia, or development of a bradyarrhythmia. Aggravation of arrhythmia usually occurs within several days of beginning an antiarrhythmic drug or increasing the dose of the drug. The time of occurrence is based on the particular drug and its pharmacokinetic properties. Although there are no ways to predict the patient at risk for developing arrhythmia aggravation with any specific agents, risk factors include QT interval prolongation, elevated serum levels of the drug, electrolyte abnormalities, presence of heart failure, a history of a sustained ventricular tachyarrhythmia, and underlying myocardial ischemia.

Arnold Pinter and Paul Dorian

Despite major advances in the nonpharmacologic therapy for arrhythmias in the past decades, there is still a substantial role for antiarrhythmic drugs especially in the treatment of atrial fibrillation and ventricular tachycardia, the most effective of which is amiodarone. Dronedarone has been developed by modifying the amiodarone molecule, thus retaining its multichannel blocking action while still reducing its toxicity. New potassium channel blockers such as vernakalant are currently under development for the treatment of atrial fibrillation and flutter. So-called upstream therapies such as renin-angiotension system antagonists, statins, and n-3 polyunsaturated fatty acids offer promise for the treatment of antiarrhythmia. This article reviews dronedarone, which is already approved and available; antiarrhythmic agents that are the most advanced in development; and upstream therapy for atrial fibrillation.

Anticoagulation is required in cardiac arrhythmias, specifically atrial fibrillation (AF) and atrial flutter, to reduce the risk of thromboembolism. Principles of anticoagulation of both AF and atrial flutter are similar because the location and nature of the arrhythmias are similar. Approximately 2 million people in the United States are affected by AF, and the prevalence is expected to exceed 10 million by the year 2050. Warfarin is known to reduce stroke risk by 68% in patients with AF and is the most effective agent for this indication, although it is not without risk. Antithrombotic therapy with antiplatelets or anticoagulants is recommended for most patients with AF. This review discusses the principles of anticoagulation and the mechanism of action, pharmacologic profile, and phase of development of the therapeutic agents used as anticoagulants.

Cardiac Electrophysiology Clinics

READ THE CLINICS ONLINE!

Access your subscription at:
www.theclinics.com

Foreword
Contemporary Issues in Antiarrhythmic Drug Therapy

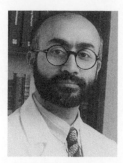
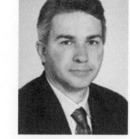

Ranjan K. Thakur, MD, MPH, MBA, FHRS   Andrea Natale, MD, FHRS
Consulting Editors

Antiarrhythmic drugs continue to play an important role in the management of cardiac arrhythmias. This issue of *Cardiac Electrophysiology Clinics*, edited by Drs Peter Kowey and Gerald Naccarelli focuses our attention on this important issue in cardiac electrophysiology today. Drs Kowey and Naccarelli have each been leaders in this field for over 25 years and bring their collective experience to bear.

Readers will find a broad-spectrum coverage of contemporary issues, from cellular mechanisms of drug action, all the way to clinical efficacy. This issue of the *Clinics* provides a modern framework for understanding mechanisms of drug action; clinically relevant pharmacokinetic concepts; genetic determinants of drug safety and efficacy; proarrhythmia; the role of age, gender, and race on antiarrhythmic drug efficacy; and a review of current thinking on the uses of antiarrhythmic drugs for atrial and ventricular arrhythmias. The editors have assembled thought leaders in each area to update readers, and the authors have been true to the mission of the *Clinics*, which is to provide clinically relevant dissertations. We have learned much from these pages and we sincerely hope that readers will find this issue of the *Clinics* illuminating.

Ranjan K. Thakur, MD, MPH, MBA, FHRS
Thoracic and Cardiovascular Institute
Sparrow Health System
Michigan State University
405 West Greenlawn, Suite 400
Lansing, MI 48910, USA

Andrea Natale, MD, FHRS
Texas Cardiac Arrhythmia Institute
Center for Atrial Fibrillation at St David's Medical
Center, 1015 East 32nd Street
Suite 516, Austin, TX 78705, USA

E-mail addresses:
Thakur@msu.edu (R.K. Thakur)
Andrea.natale@stdavids.com (A. Natale)

doi:10.1016/j.ccep.2010.08.001

Preface
Advances in Antiarrhythmic Drug Therapy

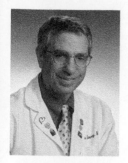 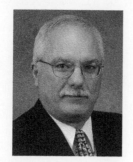

Peter R. Kowey, MD   Gerald V. Naccarelli, MD
Guest Editors

In this issue of *Cardiac Electrophysiology Clinics* entitled "Advances in Antiarrhythmic Drug Therapy," our role as Guest Editors was to invite an impressive group of experts to review a broad spectrum of contemporary topics. Dr Grant starts with a masterful review of the basic electrophysiology of antiarrhythmic drugs. Information from this article will help the practitioner understand the complex action of drugs used on a daily basis. Drs Indik and Woosley follow with an important discussion of the pharmacokinetics and pharmacodynamics of antiarrhythmic drugs. Understanding these concepts is a requirement for the proper use of all drugs. Dr Murray adds to these keystone articles by explaining how genetics influence antiarrhythmic drug pharmacokinetics and pharmacodynamics. Dr Wolbrette nicely details how age, race, and gender modulate the safety and efficacy of these drugs. This is followed by an article on the use of antiarrhythmic drugs for supraventricular tachycardia by Dr Rothman and a summary of data supporting pharmacologic conversion of atrial fibrillation/flutter by Drs Marinelli and Capucci.

Drs Morrow and Reiffel review established antiarrhythmic drugs for sinus rhythm maintenance, and this fine summary is followed by an overview of rate control therapy for atrial fibrillation by Drs Van Gelder and Groenveld. Drs Viswanathan and Page critique acute antiarrhythmic therapy for suppression of sustained ventricular tachycardia/fibrillation, and this is followed by a discussion of the role of oral antiarrhythmics for arrhythmia suppression in patients with implantable defibrillators by Drs Zawaneh and Stambler.

To put the risks of antiarrhythmic therapy in perspective, Dr Podrid reviews the incidence of and risk factors for proarrhythmia. Drs Pinter and Dorian discuss new and emerging antiarrhythmic drug therapies followed by the review from Drs Goldman and Ezekowitz of new anticoagulant therapies as they compare to vitamin K antagonists for the prevention of thromboembolic events in patients with atrial fibrillation.

Our goal is to bring readers of this issue of *Cardiac Electrophysiology Clinics* up to date with regard to existing and emerging therapies in the dynamic field of antiarrhythmic and anticoagulant therapy.

Peter R. Kowey, MD
Division of Cardiovascular Diseases
Main Line Heart Center
556 Medical Office Building East
100 Lancaster Avenue
Wynnewood, PA 19096, USA

Gerald V. Naccarelli, MD
MSHMC Cardiology
500 University Drive
Hershey, PA 17033-0850, USA

E-mail addresses:
koweyp@mlhs.org (P.R. Kowey)
gnaccarelli@hmc.psu.edu (G.V. Naccarelli)

Basic Electrophysiology

Augustus O. Grant, MB, ChB, PhD

KEYWORDS
- Electrophysiology • Arrhythmias • Ion channels
- Action potential

The available evidence suggests that the ion channels that generate the normal.action potential are also the basis for the arrhythmias that occur in disease states. Therefore, a thorough understanding of the function of the ion channels that generate the action potential is an important foundation for understanding the bases of arrhythmias and their treatment. This need is made all the more pressing by the discoveries in molecular genetics and membrane biophysics that have elucidated the fundamental mechanisms of a broad range of cardiac arrhythmias.

The normal action potential is the membrane-voltage time relationship and is the unit of information that is transmitted between cardiac cells.

Fig. 1 illustrates the five phases of the normal action potential:

1. Phase 4, or the resting potential, is stable at approximately −90 mV in working myocardial cells. The resting membrane is predominantly permeable to potassium ions. Variation in $[K^+]_o$ modulates the resting potential.
2. Phase zero is the period of rapid depolarization (up to 1000 V/s). The membrane permeability to sodium increases dramatically and forces the membrane potential into the positive voltage range. This phase of the action potential is central to the rapid propagation of the cardiac impulse (1 m/s in Purkinje and myocardial cells).
3. Phase 1 is the initial repolarization phase of the action potential. It is the result of a rapid decline of the sodium permeability and an increase in permeability to potassium and chloride ions.
4. Phase 2 is the plateau phase of the action potential. This is the longest phase of the action potential and distinguishes the cardiac action potential from that of nerve and skeletal muscle. This phase is the result of a delicate balance of residual inward sodium and calcium currents and outward components of current carried by potassium ions.
5. Phase 3 is the phase of rapid repolarization. It restores the membrane potential to its resting value. This phase is primarily the result of a sustained increase in potassium permeability.[1]

The action potential of pacemaker cells in the sinoatrial (SA) and atrioventricular (AV) nodes are significantly different from that of working myocardial cells (**Fig. 2**). The membrane potential at the outset of phase 4 is depolarized (−50 to −60 mV) and undergoes slow diastolic depolarization and gradually merges into phase zero. The diastolic depolarization is the aggregate effect of a decline in potassium permeability, a steady background current, and the hyperpolarization-activated current, I_F. The rate of depolarization is much slower than in working myocardial cells and results in the slow propagation velocity of 0.1 to 0.2 m/s characteristic of these cells. Calcium ions are the principal charge carriers during phase zero of the action potential of the SA and AV nodes.

The characteristics of the action potential change across the myocardial wall from endocardium to midmyocardium to epicardium. Epicardial cells have a prominent phase 1 and the shortest action potential. The action potential duration is longest in the midmyocardial regions. The variation in the action potential duration across the myocardial wall contributes to the differences in the direction of depolarization, endo- to epicardium, and repolarization, epi- to endocardium.

Disclosures: Dr Grant has received honoraria from Boston Scientific Co, Medtronic Co, and St Jude Medical and Sanofi Aventis.
Cardiovascular Division, Duke University School of Medicine, Box 3504, Durham, NC, USA
E-mail address: grant007@mc.duke.edu

Card Electrophysiol Clin 2 (2010) 325–340
doi:10.1016/j.ccep.2010.07.002

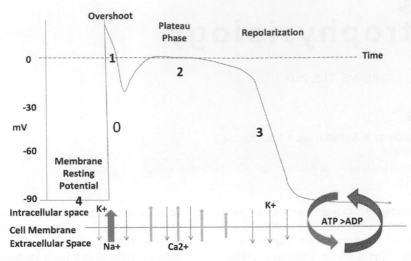

Fig. 1. Facsimile of the action potential in a working myocardial cell. The resting potential is approximately −90 mV. Phase 4 abruptly transitions to the rising phase (zero) of the action potential. Phase 1 is the initial period of rapid repolarization. Phase 2 is the plateau phase. The terminal phase of repolarization is marked phase 3. The membrane currents controlling the action potential are shown in the lower segment of the figure. Downward arrows mark outward current; upward arrows mark inward current.

The average duration of the ventricular action potential is reflected in the QT interval on the surface electrocardiogram (ECG). This relationship is important in identifying the factors that produce QT interval prolongation and an important class of arrhythmias, torsades de pointes. A decrease in the outward potassium current, an increase in the late component of sodium current, or the L-type calcium current during phase 2 prolongs the action potential duration (APD) and hence the QT interval on the ECG. The QT interval of males and females is equal during early childhood. Shortening of the QT interval of males at puberty, however, accounts for the gender differences in QT in adults (QT females > QT males). Unfortunately most studies of the gender differences in QT interval have focused on the longer interval in females.

ACTION POTENTIAL INITIATION, CONDUCTION, AND EXCITABILITY

Cardiac cells generate action potential either as a response to external stimulation or as a result of inherent automaticity. The underpinnings of excitation in response to external stimulation are important in pacemaker technology and arrhythmia analysis in the clinical electrophysiology laboratory (**Fig. 3A**). Applied current must displace the membrane potential from its resting or maximum diastolic value to a level that results in the regenerative increase in sodium or calcium

Membrane currents during the pacemaker action potential

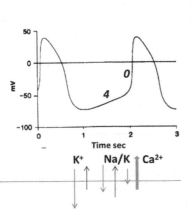

- Outward K+ Current I_{Kr}; declines during phase 4
- Inward I_f current (Na/K)
- Inward calcium current ($I_{Ca}L$, I_{CaT})
- Background inward current, I_B (not shown)

Fig. 2. Action potential and underlying currents in pacemaker cells. The maximum diastolic potential is relatively depolarized. Slow diastolic depolarization occurs during phase 4 and transitions smoothly into phase zero. The major underlying currents are shown in the right.

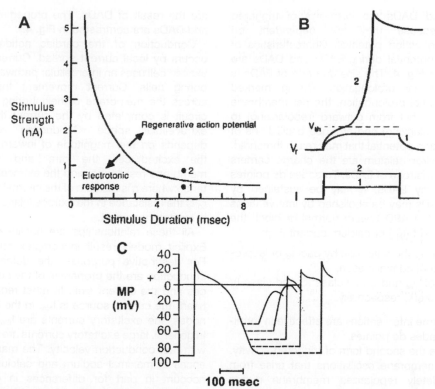

Fig. 3. Membrane response to stimulation. (*A*) The relationship between stimulus strength and stimulus duration. Because excitation requires a certain amount of charge, a low-amplitude stimulus has a long duration. (*B*) The membrane response to stimulation. A subthreshold stimulus results in a local response. A stronger stimulus results in a propagated action potential. (*C*) Contrasts the response to stimulation during phase 3 of the action potential. Action potential elicited early in phase 3 has a slow upstroke and low amplitude. The amplitude of the premature response approaches normal response during phase 4.

current. A certain amount of charge Q must be applied to the cell membrane to attain the threshold potential (V_{TH}),

$$Q\alpha(V_{TH} - V_r)$$

where V_{TH} is threshold potential and V_r is resting potential.

The charge is the time integral of the stimulating current:

Cells maybe excited either by a small current over a long time period or a large current over a brief period. These relationships are the basis of the stimulus strength-duration relationship (see **Fig. 3**A). In general, brief stimuli of large amplitude are more effective for excitation.

Re-excitation of a cell before full repolarization entails other considerations (see **Fig.** 3B). The membrane potential most repolarize to a potential at which a sufficient number of sodium channels have recovered from inactivation to generate another action potential. Recovery from inactivation is also time dependent; time must be spent at a given potential for recovery to assume its steady-state value. At short coupling intervals,

a sufficient number of channels have not recovered and no stimulus, however strong, can result in re-excitation. The cell is absolutely refractory. At later time, a stimulus greater than the diastolic value is enough to initiate re-excitation, defined as the relative refractory period. Because fewer channels are available during the relative refractory period, action potential upstroke and conduction velocity are slow and more susceptible to block.

Action potentials may be initiated within cells or groups of cells that have the property of automaticity. Diastolic depolarization during phase 4 of the action potential is the basis for automaticity in the SA and AV nodes and in Purkinje cells. SA node cells have the highest intrinsic rate, so function as the dominant pacemaker. Automaticity is abnormal when it arises outside the nodes and Purkinje cells. Abnormal automaticity may take the following forms:

1. Early afterdepolarizations (EADs)
2. Delayed afterdepolarizations (DADs)
3. Depolarization-induced automaticity.

EADs and DADs are examples of triggered activity because they are dependent on a preceding action potential. Characteristics of the action potential during EADs and DADs are illustrated in **Fig. 4**. The sine qua non of EADs is action potential prolongation. During marked action potential prolongation, the net membrane current may shift from outward (repolarizing) to inward (depolarizing) and produce oscillations of the membrane potential that may reach threshold. Sodium and/or calcium are the charge carriers during the upstroke of EADs. Torsades de pointes is initiated by EADs. It may be sustained by re-entry. EADs may be abolished by interventions that return the APD toward normal or block the sodium current (I_{Na}) or calcium current (I_{Ca}):

> Increasing the heart rate by pacing or isoproterenol administration.
> Block of I_{Na} and I_{Ca} by class IC and class IV blockers, respectively.

These same interventions are effective in terminating torsades de pointes.

DADs are the second form of triggered activity. They are membrane oscillations that arise from the completely repolarized membrane during phase 4. The amplitude of the oscillations is enhanced by increasing the rate of stimulation. If the oscillations are large enough to reach threshold, they result in repetitive activity. DADs are characteristic of conditions that lead to Ca^{2+} overload. Oscillatory release of calcium from the sarcoplasmic reticulum, activity of the Na^{+}/Ca^{2+} exchanger, and a Ca^{2+}-activated nonspecific channel all play a role in the genesis of DADs. They are blocked by Ca^{2+} antagonists. The tachyarrhythmias associated with digitalis intoxication

are the result of DADs. The properties of EADs and DADs are contrasted in **Fig. 4**.

Conduction of the cardiac action potential occurs by local current spread. Current from an excited cell uses an intercellular pathway to neighboring cells. Current movement then occurs across the membrane of neighboring cells. The circuit is completed by the current through the extracellular space. Conduction velocity (θ) depends on the magnitude of inward current in the excited cell, the intra- and intercellular membrane resistance, and the extracellular resistance:where r_i is the sum of the internal resistance, r_o is the resistance in the extracellular space, and I is excitatory current.

All these relationships are nonlinear function. Explicit models result in complex relationships. For descriptive purposes, the determinants of conduction are the properties of the current sources and the current sink. In most regions of the heart, the current source is I_{Na}. In the SA and AV nodes, the excitatory currents are I_{CaL} and I_{CaT}. In general, large excitatory currents are associated with fast conduction velocity. The marked differences in maximal sodium and calcium currents account in part for differences in conduction velocity in the nodes and in the ventricular conduction system.

The current sink is composed of three major elements: the resistance of the myoplasm, the intercellular resistance, and the sarcolemma (**Fig. 5**). The intercellular resistance is the most important element. Gap junctions are the relatively low resistance intercellular connection. They are formed by a family of specialized proteins, the connexins, connexin-43 being the most abundant in the heart. Gap junctions are not uniformly

EADs and DADs

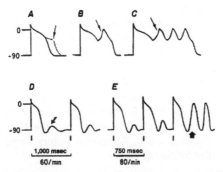

Comparison of the modulation of EADs and DADs

	EADs	DADs
Slow heart rate	↑↑	↓↓
Low K+	↑	↑
High Ca2+	↑↓	↑↑
βadrenergic agonist	↑	↑↑
Caffeine	↑	
Ischemic metabolites		↑↑
Digitalis		↑↑

Fig. 4. Triggered activity as a basis for action potential generation. Progressive prolongation of the action potential eventually results in oscillations at the plateau level of membrane potential (*A–C*). The action potentials arising at the plateau level are examples of EADs. Oscillations arising from action potentials of normal duration during phase 4 are examples of DADs (*D, E*).

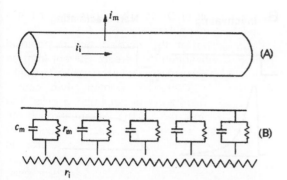

Fig. 5. Conduction in cardiac muscle. The cell membrane is modeled as a parallel combination of a capacitor and resistor. Stimulus current travels along the internal resistance (r_1) across the membrane (r_m) and the circuit is completed by a return pathway into the cell.

distributed over the surface of cells; the density is higher in the longitudinal direction compared with the transverse direction. This anisotropy has important implications for conduction. Conduction velocity is fast in the longitudinal direction and slow in the transverse direction and more likely to fail in that direction. The conductance of gap function channels is dynamic. It is reduced by low intracellular pH and high $[Ca^{2+}]_i$.

Slow conduction is the basis for re-entry and may also be analyzed in terms of abnormalities of current sources and sinks. Conduction is slowed by marked reductions in the sodium current. The reduction in sodium currents in disease states is usually the result of membrane depolarization. Acute ischemia results in the rapid efflux of potassium ions into the narrow extracellular space and causes prompt membrane depolarization. The depolarization results in partial or complete inactivation of the sodium channels. With marked depolarization, the calcium current may be the principal current during phase zero of the action potential. Because of its small amplitude, Ca-dependent action potentials are conducted slowly and susceptible to block.

Changes in the current sink also play an important role in re-entry. Several mechanisms contribute to an increase in coupling resistance between cardiac cells. The fall in intracellular pH and the rise in $[Ca^{2+}]_i$ that occurs in ischemia decrease the conductance of gap junction channels. Hypertension and aging are associated with a loss of the side-to-side connections between cardiac cells and the laying down of connective tissue septa. Transverse conductance is decreased to a greater extent than longitudinal conductance. These changes set up a mechanism for re-entry based on structure. With premature stimulation, conduction block occurs in the longitudinal direction (large current sink) whereas very slow conduction occurs in the transverse direction because of the low coupling conductance. The slow conductance provides enough time for recovery of excitability at distal sites. Retrograde excitation of the initial sites of block results in re-entry.

GENERAL PROPERTIES OF ION CHANNELS

The generation of the action potential and the regional differences that are observed throughout the heart are the result of the selective permeability of ion channels distributed on the cell membrane. The ion channels reduce the activation energy required for ion movement across the lipophilic cell membrane. During the action potential, the permeability of ion channels changes and each ion (eg, X) moves passively down its electrochemical gradients ($\Delta V = [Vm-Vx]$, where Vm is the membrane potential and Vx is the reversal potential of ion X) to change the membrane potential of the cell. The electrochemical gradient determines whether or not an ion moves into the cell (depolarizing current for cations) or out of the cell (repolarizing current for cations). Homeostasis of the intracellular ion concentrations is maintained by active and coupled transport processes that are linked directly or indirectly to ATP hydrolysis. The sodium-potassium pump is the most thoroughly studied active transport process. The movement of three sodium ions out of the cell is coupled to the inward movement of two potassium ions and the hydrolysis of ATP. Because of the unequal stiochiometry of sodium to potassium movement across the cell membrane, the pump is electrogenic.

Ion channels have two fundamental properties, ion permeation and gating[2] (**Fig. 6A**). Ion permeation describes the movement through the open channel. The selective permeability of ion channels to specific ions is a basis of classification of ion channels (eg, Ca^{2+}, K^+, and Ca^{2+} channels). Size, valency, and hydration energy are important determinants of selectivity. The selectivity ratio of the biologically important alkali cations is high. Ion channels do not function as simple fluid-filled pores but provide multiple binding sites for ions as they traverse the membrane. Ions become dehydrated as they cross the membrane as ion-binding site interaction is favored over ion-water interaction. Like an enzyme-substrate interaction, the binding of the permeating ion is saturable. The equivalent circuit model of an ion channel is that of a resistor. The electrochemical potential, ΔV, is the driving force for ion movement across the cell membrane. Simple resistors have a linear

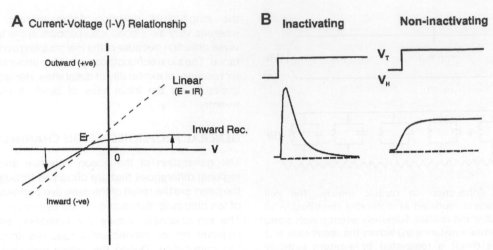

A Current-Voltage (I-V) Relationship

B Inactivating   Non-inactivating

Fig. 6. (*A*) The current-voltage relationship of ion channels is illustrated. The simplest pattern of conduction is a linear relationship (*broken line*) described by Ohms law, E = 1R. Many ion channels have a nonlinear current voltage relationship (*solid line*); inward current (*downward arrow*) is larger than outward current (*upward arrow*) is larger than outward current (*upward arrow*). E_r, reversal potential. (*B*) Patterns of response of membrane channels to a step change in voltage. Most channels open in response to depolarization. Despite the fact that depolarization is maintained, some channels, however (eg, the sodium channel) close by inactivation. Other channels remain open during sustained depolarization (eg, the delayed rectifier channels).

relationship between ΔV and current I (Ohm's law, $I = \Delta V/R = \Delta Vg$, where g is the channel conductance). Most ion channels have a nonlinear current-voltage relationship (see **Fig. 6A**). For the same absolute value of ΔV, the magnitude of the current depends on the direction of ion movement into or out of the cells. This property is termed, *rectification*, and is an important property of K$^+$ channels; they pass little outward current at positive (depolarized) potentials. Block by internal Mg$^+$ and polyvalent cations is the mechanism of the strong inward rectification observed in many K$^+$ channels.[3]

Gating is the mechanism of opening and closing of ion channels and is their second major property. Ion channels demonstrate three mechanisms of gating: voltage-dependent, ligand-dependent, and mechano-sensitive gating. Voltage-gated ion channels change their conductance in response variations in membrane potential. Voltage-dependent gating is the commonest mechanism of gating observed in ion channels. A majority of ion channels open in response to depolarization. The pacemaker current channel (I_f channel) opens in response to membrane hyperpolarization.

Ion channels have two mechanisms of closure. Certain channels, such as the Na$^+$ and Ca^{2+} channels, enter a closed inactivated state during maintained depolarization (see **Fig. 6B**). To regain their ability to open, the channel must undergo a recovery process at hyperpolarized potentials. The inactivated state may also be accessed from the closed states. Inactivation is the basis for

refractoriness in cardiac muscle and is fundamental for the prevention of premature re-excitation. The multiple mechanisms of inactivation are discussed later. If the membrane potential is abruptly returned to its hyperpolarized (resting) value while the channel is open, it closes by deactivation, a reversal of the normal activation process. These transitions are summarized in **Fig. 7** (as proposed for the Na$^+$ channel)[4]: where C_1 is the initial closed state, C_N is the closed state before the O state, O is the open state, and I is the inactivated state. The C → I transition may occur from multiple closed states. Because these states are nonconducting, however, the kinetics of transition between them is difficult to resolve with certainty.

Ligand-dependent gating is the second major gating mechanism of cardiac ion channels. The acetylcholine-activated K$^+$ channel is the most thoroughly studied channel of this class. Acetylcholine binds to the M2 muscarinic receptor and

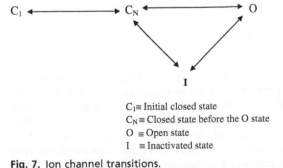

$C_1 \longleftrightarrow C_N \longleftrightarrow O$

I

$C_1 \equiv$ Initial closed state
$C_N \equiv$ Closed state before the O state
$O \equiv$ Open state
$I \equiv$ Inactivated state

Fig. 7. Ion channel transitions.

activates a G-protein signaling pathway, culminating in the release of the subunits, Gαi and Gβγ. The Gβγ subunit activates an inward-rectifying K$^+$ channel, I$_{Kach}$, that abbreviates the action potential and decreases the slope of diastolic depolarization in pacemaker cells. I$_{KAch}$ channels are most abundant in the atria and the SA and AV nodes. I$_{KAch}$ activation is a part of the mechanism of the vagal control of the heart. The ATP-sensitive K$^+$ channel, also termed the *ADP-activated K$^+$ channel*, is a ligand-gated channel distributed abundantly in all regions of the heart. The open probability of this channel is proportional to the adenosine diphosphate [ADP]/adenosine triphosphate [ATP] ratio. This channel couples the shape of the action potential to the metabolic state of the cell. Energy depletion during ischemia increases the [ADP]/[ATP] ratio, activates I$_{K ATP}$, and abbreviates the action potential. The abbreviated action potential results in less force generation and may be cardioprotective. This channel also plays a central role in ischemic preconditioning.

The mechano-sensitive or stretch-activated channels are the least studied. They belong to a class of ion channels that can transduce a physical input such as stretch into an electrical signal through a change in channel conductance. Acute cardiac dilatation is a well-recognized cause of cardiac arrhythmias. Stretch-activated channels

are central to the mechanism of these arrhythmias. Blunt chest wall impact at appropriately timed portions of the cardiac cycle may also result in PVCs or ventricular fibrillation (the VF of commotio-cordis). The channels that transduce the impact into an electrical event are unknown.

The major ion channels that shape the action potential have been cloned and sequenced. **Tables 1** and **2** list the clones of the primary α-subunits of the major ion channels. Over the past two decades, the focus of research has been the relationship between channel structure and function, including the molecular underpinnings of the permeation and gating processes. Recent studies have focused on molecular suprastructures of which ion channels are a part.[5,6] The channels are not randomly distributed in the membrane but tend to cluster at the intercalated disc in association with modulatory subunits. The sodium channel has a binding site for the structural protein ankyrin and mutations that affect its binding site result in long QT syndrome (LQTS) or Brugada syndrome.[7]

PROPERTIES OF SPECIFIC ION CHANNELS

I review the properties of the sodium channel in detail because it is the arch-type of a voltage-gated channel.

Table 1
Membrane current controlling the action potential: working myocardial cells

Action Potential Phase	Current	Description	Activation Mechanism	Clone
Phase 4	I$_{K1}$	Inward rectifier	Depolarization	Kir 2.2/2.2
Phase zero	I$_{Na}$	Sodium current	Depolarization	Nav1.5
Phase 1	I$_{to,f}$	Transient outward current, fast	Depolarization	Kv 4.2/4.3
	I$_{to,s}$	Transient outward current, slow	Depolarization	KV1.4/1.7/3.4
	I$_{Kur}$	Delayed rectifier, ultrarapid	Depolarization	KV11.5/3.1
Phase 2	I$_{CaL}$	Calcium current, L type	Depolarization	CaV 1.2
	I$_{Na}$	Sodium current, late component	Depolarization	NaV 1.5
Phase 3	I$_{Kr}$	Delayed rectifier, rapid	Depolarization	HERG
	I$_{Ks}$	Delayed rectifier, slow	Depolarization	KVLQT1
	I$_{K1}$	Inward rectifier	Depolarization	Kir 2.1/2,2
Multiple phases	I$_B$	Background current	Metabolism, stretch	TWK-1/2 TASK-1 TRAK
	I$_{KATP}$	ADP activated K$^+$ current	[ADP]/[ATP]	Kir6.2, SURA
	Na-K, NCX	Pump currents	Ionic concentrations	

Table 2
Membrane current controlling the action potential: pacemaker cells

Action Potential Phase	Current	Description	Activation Mechanism	Clone
Phase 4	I_f	Hyperpolarization-activated current	Membrane hyperpolarization	HCN2/4
	I_{KAch}	Muscarinic-gated K^+ current	Acetylcholine	Kir 3.1/3.4
Phase zero	I_{Ca-L}	Calcium current, L type	Depolarization	Cav 1.2
	I_{Ca-T}	Calcium current, T type	Depolarization	CaV 3.1/3.2

The Sodium Channel

Each sodium channel opens very briefly (<1 ms) during more than 99% of depolarizations.[8,9] The channel occasionally shows alternative gating modes consisting of isolated brief openings occurring after variable and prolonged latencies and bursts of openings during which the channel opens repetitively for hundreds of milliseconds. The patterns of opening are reflections of the inactivation processes.[10] The isolated brief openings are the result of occasional return from the inactivated state. The bursts of openings are the result of occasional failure of inactivation.[8,11] Sodium channel inactivation is a multifaceted process.[10] Fast, intermediate, and slow inactivation develop during depolarization lasting milliseconds, seconds, and tens of seconds, respectively. The trains of action potential that occurs in the course of the normal heartbeat result in all three types of inactivation.

A major focus of research on the sodium channel is the relationship between channel structure and function. The sodium channel consists of four homologous domains, DI–DIV[12,13] arranged in a 4-fold circular symmetry to form the channel (**Fig. 8**). Each domain consists of six membrane-spanning segments, S1–S6. The membrane-spanning segments are joined by alternating intra- and extracellular loops. The loops between S5 and S6 of each domain, termed the *pore loops (P loops)*, curve back into the membrane to form the pore. Residues D, E, K, and A of domains 1–IV, respectively, are critical for ion permeation. Each S4 segment has a positively charged amino acid at every third or fourth position and acts as the sensor of the transmembrane voltage. The structural basis of fast sodium channel inactivation resides in the interdomain linker between DIII and DIV (ID111/IV). The primary amino acid sequence of this region is highly conserved between species and sodium channel subtypes. The amino acid triplet, isoleucine, phenylalanine, methionine (IFM), is crucial for inactivation; the mutation IFM → QQQ abolishes inactivation.[14] The receptor site to which the triplet

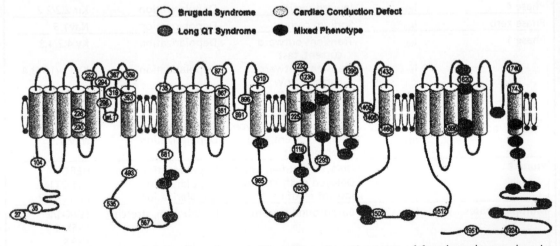

Fig. 8. Putative structure of the sodium channel. The sodium channel consists of four homologous domains, D1–D1V. Domains are joined by intracellular loops. Each domain consists of six membrane-spinning segments. Sites of mutations associated with Brugada syndrome, LQTS, conduction system defect, and mixed phenotype are highlighted.

binds has not been identified. The carboxyl terminus also plays an important role in sodium channel inactivation.

The cardiac sodium channel is modulated by protein kinase A (PKA), protein kinase C (PKC), and Ca-calmodulin kinase. Data on the effects of PKA on the I_{Na} are controversial, with some studies reporting a decrease in current whereas others report an increase.[15–17] Phosphorylation of the channel by PKC results in a decrease in I_{Na}. The [NAD+]/[NADH] ratio modulate I_{Na}.[18] An increase in NADH reduces I_{Na}. The discovery of a family with Brugada syndrome and a mutation in glycerol-3 phosphate dehydrogenase—like 1

kinase led to the discovery of the modulation of I by the [NAD+]/[NADH] ratio.[19] Reactive oxygen species enhance the late component of sodium current and may be arrhythmogenic.

Mutations in cardiac sodium channel gene, SCN5A, have been associated with LQTS, Brugada syndrome, primary cardiac conduction system disease, and dilated cardiomyopathy (**Table 3**).[20] LQTS is the result of defects in inactivation that enhance the late component of sodium current. The late component of current is more sensitive to block by class 1 antiarrhythmic drug than the peak current. Mexiletine and flecainide decrease the late component of sodium current and restore

Table 3
The genetic basis of inherited arrhythmias

Type	Gene	Protein	Functional Alteration
Long QT syndrome			
LQT1	$KCNQ_1$	I_{Ks} potassium channel α-subunit	Loss of function
LQT2	$KCNH_2$	I_{Kr} potassium channel α-subunit	Loss of function
LQT3	SCN_5A	I_{Na} cardiac sodium channel α-subunit	Gain of function
LQT4	ANK_2	Ankyrin-B	Loss of function
LQT5	$KCNE_1$	I_{Ks} potassium channel β-subunit	Loss of function
LQT6	$KCNE_2$	I_{Kr} potassium channel β-subunit	Loss of function
LQT7	$KCNJ_2$	I_{K1} potassium channel subunit	Loss of function
LQT8	$CACNA_1C$	Calcium channel α-subunit	Gain of function
Short QT syndrome			
S4T1	$KCNH_2$	I_{Kr} potassium channel α-subunit	Gain of function
S4T2	$KCNQ_1$	I_{Ks} potassium channel α-subunit	Gain of function
S4T3	$KCNJ_2$	I_{K1} potassium channel subunit	Gain of function
Brugada syndrome			
BrS1	SCN_5A	I_{Na} sodium channel α-subunit	Loss of function
BrS2	*GPD1L*	G-3PD 1–	Altered function
BrS3	*CACNA1C*	I_{Ca} calcium channel α-subunit	Loss of function
BrS4	*CACNB2b*	I_{Ca} Calcium channel β-subunit	Loss of function
BrS-other	*ANKRYN-B*	Ankryin-B	Altered function
Catecholaminergic polymorphic VT			
	RYR_2	Cardiac ryanodine receptor	Gain of function
	$CASQ_2$	Calsequestrin	Gain of function
Idiopathic sick sinus syndrome			
	HCN_4	I_f pacemaker channel subunit	Loss of function
	SCN_5A	I_{Na} cardiac sodium channel α-subunit	Loss of function
Cardiac conduction disease			
	SCN_5A	I_{Na} cardiac sodium channel α-subunit	Loss of function
Familial atrial fibrillation			
	$KCNQ_1$	I_{Ks} potassium channel α-subunit	Gain of function
	$KCNE_2$	I_{Kr} potassium channel β-subunit	Gain of function
	$KCNJ_2$	I_{K1} potassium channel subunit	Gain of function
	$KCNH_2$	I_{Kr} potassium channel α-subunit	Gain of function

the QT interval toward normal.[21,22] They have been used to treat patients with LQT3, particularly in the neonatal period, and in children when ICD implantation may prove technically challenging. Sodium channel mutations have been described in 20% of patients with Brugada syndrome.[23] The mutations reduce the Na^+ current as a result of synthesis of nonfunctional proteins, failure of the protein to be targeted to the cell membrane, or accelerated inactivation of the channel. As a subgroup, the patients with Na^+ channel mutations that produce Brugada syndrome have HV interval prolongation on electrophysiology study. The mechanism of ST-segment elevation and T-wave inversion in the syndrome is controversial. One group views the syndrome as primarily a repolarization abnormality[24]; others view the Na^+ channel variant as a conduction defect.[25] Slow conduction from endocardium to epicardium results in delayed epicardial activation. The sequence of transmural repolarization is reversed, resulting in the ST–T-wave changes. The mutations associated with primary cardiac conduction disease also reduce the Na^+ current.[26] The clinical syndromes include sinus node dysfunction, atrial standstill, AV block, and fascicular (infra-Hisian) block. Overlap syndromes of LQT3, Brugada syndrome, and PCCD may occur in the same kindred or individual.[27] The mechanisms by which Na^+ defects result in dilated cardiomyopathy are not well understood.[28] Longstanding conduction delay and asynchronous contraction may be contributory.

The cardiac sodium channel is the substrate for the action of class 1 antiarrhythmic drugs (**Table 4**). Open and inactivated channels are more susceptible to block than resting channels. The differential block may be the result of a difference in binding affinity or state-dependent access to the binding site.[29,30] Binding of antiarrhythmic drug occurs primarily during the action potential. This block is dissipated in the interval between action potentials. Because a fast heart rate is associated with abbreviation of the diastolic period and insufficient time for recovery, block accumulates (ie, it is use dependent). Class 1 antiarrhythmic drugs may be classified according to the kinetics of unbinding, with various drugs showing fast, intermediate, or slow unbinding kinetics.[31]

Calcium Channels

Calcium ions are the principal intracellular signaling ions. They regulate excitation–contraction coupling, secretion, and the activity of many enzymes and ion channels. $[Ca^{2+}]_i$ is highly regulated despite its marked fluctuation between systole and diastole. Calcium channels are the principal portal of entry of calcium into the cells; a system of intracellular storage sites and transporters, such as the sodium-calcium exchanger (NCX), also plays important roles in $[Ca^{2+}]_i$ regulation. In cardiac muscle, two types of Ca^{2+} channels, the low threshold type (L type) and transient type (T type), transport Ca^{2+} into the cells. The L-type channel is found in all cardiac cell types. The T-type channel is found principally in pacemaker, atrial, and Purkinje cells. The unqualified descriptor, Ca^{2+} channel, refers to the L-type channel. **Table 5** contrasts the properties of the two types of channels.

The complement of subunits of the native L-type Ca^{2+} channel is more complex than the Na^+ channel. A combination of as many as five subunits, α_1, α_2, β, γ, and δ, may unite to form the channel in its native state. The α_{1c} subunit, $Ca_v1.2$, is the cardiac-specific subunit. The β-subunit increases channel expression approximately 10-fold and accelerates the activation and inactivation kinetics. Ca^{2+} channels have a similar structure to the sodium channel: four homologous domains each consisting of six membrane spanning segments. The P loop of each domain contributes a glutamate residue to the pore structure. Several molecular mechanisms contribute to a complex system of inactivation. Like the sodium channels, a major component of inactivation is

Table 4
Classification of antiarrhythmic drug actions

Class	Unbinding Kinetics	Effect on APD	Example
1A	Intermediate	APD↑	Procainamide
1B	Fast	APD→	Lidocaine
1C	Slow	APD↓, →	Flecainide
II (β-blocker)		APD	Metoprolol
III (K^+ channel blocker)		APD↑	Dofetelide, Ibutilide
IV (Ca^+ channel blocker)	Slow	APD↑, →	Verapamil

Table 5
Comparison of the L-type and T-type Ca^{2+} channels

	L type	T type
Activation Range	Low Em (~ −30 mV)	High Em (~ −60 mV)
Inactivation Range	Low Em (~ −40 mV)	Hyperpolarized
	Slow	Fast
Voltage dependence	Yes	No
[Ca^{2+}]$_i$ dependent		
Pharmacologic sensitivity	Yes	No
Dihydropyridnes Cd N$_i$	High	Low
Isoproternol	Low	High
	Yes	No

Abbreviation: Em, membrane potential.

voltage dependent; membrane depolarization decreases the fraction of channels available for opening. The fraction of channels available for opening d$_\infty$ varies from 1 at approximately −45 mV to 0 at zero mV (compared with the sodium channel range of −90 to −55 mV). An analogous role of the III/IV interdomain linker in the inactivation has not been resolved. The carboxyl terminus has multiple Ca^{2+}-binding sites and Ca-calmodulin−dependent kinase activity. Ca^{2+} in the immediate vicinity of the channel and phosphorylation also plays roles in the inactivation of the channel. Reuptake of Ca^{2+} by the sarcoplasmic reticulum during prolonged depolarization can result in the recovery from Ca^{2+}-dependent inactivation and enable secondary depolarization. This may be the basis for EADs that triggers polymorphic VT in LQTS. The overall kinetics of the Ca channel is important in controlling contractility in response to various patterns of stimulation. At low (depolarized) membrane potentials, recovery of I$_{Ca}$ from inactivation between action potentials is slow; I$_{Ca}$ declines in response to repetitive stimulation and a negative staircase of contractility is observed. At normal resting potentials, recovery of I$_{Ca}$ from inactivation is fast and I$_{Ca}$ may increase progressively during repetitive stimulation. This positive staircase or rate-dependent potentiation of contractility is Ca^{2+} dependent. It is the result of enhanced loading of the sarcoplasmic reticulum and may be facilitated by calmodulin kinase II−dependent phosphorylation.

Arrhythmia-inducing mutations of the cardiac Ca^{2+} channel gene that are compatible with life are rare.[32] Timothy syndrome is the result of mutations of Ca$_V$1.2. It is a multisystem disease with LQTS, cognitive abnormalities, immune deficiency, hypoglycemia, and syndactyly.[32] The mutation of glycine to arginine converts a neighboring serine to a consensus site for phosphorylation by calmodulin kinase. The phosphorylation of this site promotes a slow gating mode of the calcium channel, increasing Ca^{2+} entry and resulting in cytotoxicity.[33] A sudden death syndrome has been recently described that combines the features of Brugada syndrome, including the characteristic ECG pattern, and a short QT interval.[34] The syndrome results from a loss of function of the α$_1$ or β$_{2b}$ subunit of the L-type Ca^{2+} channel.

The Ca^{2+} channel is the target for the interaction with class IV antiarrhythmic drugs. The principal class IV drugs are the phenylalkylamine, verapamil, and the benzothiazepine, diltiazem. Both drugs block open and inactivated Ca^{2+} channels. Therefore, they cause use-dependent block of conduction in cells with Ca^{2+}-dependent action potentials, such those in the SA and AV nodes, and slow the sinus node rate. The hypotensive effects of verapamil, however, may cause an increase in sympathetic tone and increase the heart rate. A third class of Ca^{2+} channel blockers, the dihydropyridines, block open Ca^{2+} channels. The kinetics of recovery from block, however, are sufficiently fast that they produce no significant cardiac effect but effectively block the smooth muscle Ca^{2+} channel because of its low resting potential.

Potassium Channels

Cardiac K$^+$ channels fall into three broad categories: voltage gated (I$_{to}$, I$_{Kur}$, I$_{Kr}$, and I$_{Ks}$), inward rectifier channels (I$_{K1}$, I$_{Kach}$, and I$_{KATP}$), and the background K$^+$ currents, TASK-1 and TWIK-1/2. It is the variation in the level of expression of these channels that accounts for regional differences of the action potential configuration in the atria, ventricles, and across the myocardial wall (endocardium, midmyocardium, and epicardium). K$^+$ channels are also highly regulated and are the basis for the change in action potential configuration in response to variation in heart rate.

Like the Na^+ and Ca^{2+} channels, voltage-gated K^+ channels consist of principal α- subunits and multiple β-subunits. The channel functional units also include the complementary proteins, K_V-channel associated protein, KChAP, and the K_V channel interacting protein, KChIP. The major subfamilies of α-subunits include $K_VN.x$ (N = 1–4), the HERG channel (gene *KCNH2*), and KvLQT1 (gene *KCNQ1*). They are important in generating outward current in the heart. Members of the $K_VN.x$ subfamily may coassemble to form heteromultimers through conserved amino terminal domains. In contrast, members of the HERG and K_VLQT1 subfamilies assemble as homotetramers. The α-subunits that coassemble to form the various types of K^+ channels and their role in the generation of the action potential are summarized in **Table 2**. Most β-subunits have been cloned and sequenced. They have oxioreductase activity. The α-subunits can generate voltage-dependent K^+ current when expressed in heterogonous systems. The accessory subunits, however, are required to recapitulate the K^+ currents seen in native cells. KChAP (*KCHAP*) and KChIP (*KCNIP2*) may increase channel activity independent of transcription and alter channel kinetics. The structure of voltage-gated K^+ channels is similar to one of the four domains of voltage-gated Na^+ and Ca^{2+} channels (ie, six membrane-spanning segments [S1–S6] and intracytoplasmic amino and carboxyl termini). S4 retains the structure of charged amino acid in every third position. A portion of S3 (S3-b) and S4 forms the activation gate. The amino acid sequence, glycine-tyrosine-glycine, is the sequence requirement for K^+ selectivity.

The transient outward current is composed of a K^+ current, I_{to1}, and a Ca^{2+}-activated chloride current, I_{to2}. The former has fast and slow components, $I_{to, f}$ and $I_{to s}$. $I_{to f}$ is the principal subtype expressed in human atrium; $I_{to, f}$ and $I_{to s}$ are expressed in the ventricle. Myocardial regions with relatively short action potentials, such as the epicardium, right ventricle, and the septum, have higher levels of I_{to} expression. Compared with other voltage-gated K^+ channels, activation of I_{to} is fast (activation time constant <10 ms). The rate of inactivation is variable and highly voltage dependent. α-Adrenergic stimulation reduces I_{to} in human myocytes through PKA-dependent phosphorylation. Chronic α-adrenergic stimulation and angiotensin II also reduce channel expression. The influence of a reduction of I_{to} on the action potential duration varies with species; in rodents, a reduction in I_{to} prolongs the action potential duration. In large mammals, a reduction in I_{to} shifts the plateau to more positive potentials increasing the activation of the delayed rectifier and promoting faster repolarization. In a rodent model of hypothyroidism, the action potential prolongation is associated with a reduction of I_{to}. The current is also reduced in human heart failure but is associated with a prolongation of the action potential duration. Because the level of the plateau is set by I_{to}, modulators that decrease I_{to} shift the plateau into the positive range of potentials. This decreases the electrochemical driving force for Ca^{2+} and hence I_{Ca}.

The delayed rectifier K^+ currents, I_{Kur}, I_{Kr}, and I_{Ks}, are slowly activating outward currents that play major roles in the control of repolarization. The deactivation of these channels is sufficiently slow that they contribute outward current throughout phase 3 repolarization. I_{Kur} is highly expressed in atrial myocytes and is a basis for the much shorter duration of the action potential in the atrium. I_{Kr} is differentially expressed, with high levels in the left atrium, and ventricular endocardium. I_{Ks} is expressed in all cell types but is reduced in midmyocardial myocytes. These cells have the longest action potential duration across the myocardial wall. The α-subunits that make up the delayed rectifier currents are summarized in **Table 2**. β-Subunits are associated with I_{Kr} and I_{Ks}. MinK-related peptide 1 (MiRP-1) and MinK are the most thoroughly studied. MiRP-1 and MinK are single-membrane spanning peptides with extracellular amino termini. The β-subunits are nonconducting but regulate β-subunit function, including gating, response to sympathetic stimulation, and drugs. β-Adrenergic stimulation regulates I_{Kr} through activation of PKA and elevation of cyclic adenosine monophosphate (cAMP). The former effect is inhibitory; the latter is stimulatory through binding to the cyclic nucleotide-binding domain of the channel. α-Adrenergic stimulation is inhibitory.

β-adrenergic stimulation increases I_{Ks} through PKA-dependent phosphorylation. This action involves a macromolecular complex of PKA, protein phosphatase 1, and the adaptor protein, yotaio.[5] Ion channel mutations that disrupt the function of the complex result in the action potential prolongation of LQT1. β-Adrenergic blockers indirectly regulate this complex and are important therapeutic options in LQT1.

The inward rectifier channel current, I_{k1}, sets the resting membrane potential in atrial and ventricular cells. Channel expression is much higher in the ventricle and protects the ventricular cell from pacemaker activity. The strong inward rectification of the I_{k1} channel is important for normal channel function. It limits the outward current during phases zero, 1, and 2 of the action potential. This limits the outward current during the positive phase of the action potential and confers energetic efficiency in the generation of the action potential. The block of the outward current by intracellular Mg^+ and the polyamines is relieved during repolarization. As a result, I_{k1} makes a significant contribution to phase 3 repolarization.

The acetylcholine-activated K^+ channel is a member of the G protein–coupled, inward-rectifying, potassium channels. The channel is highly expressed in the SA and AV nodes and atria but low in ventricle. Activation of I_{KAch} hyperpolarizes the membrane potential and abbreviates the action potential. Phase 4 depolarization of pacemaker cells is slowed. The channel belongs to a subgroup of inward-rectifying K^+ channels. The channel structure is similar to that of I_{K1}. The binding of acetylcholine to the M2 muscarinic receptor activates the G protein, G_i, and the release of the subunits, $G_{i\alpha}$ and $G_{\beta\gamma}$. The dissociated $G_{\beta\gamma}$ subunit binds to the channel and activities it. The binding of adenosine to the P1 receptor also results in the release of $G_{\beta\gamma}$ and activation of the channel. Methylxanthines, such as theophylline, block the P1 receptor and antagonized the effects of adenosine. Coexpression of the inward rectifier K^+ channel, Kir6.x, and sulfonylurea receptor yields channels with properties similar to the native $I_{K ATP}$.

Mutations of the genes encoding cardiac K^+ channels are the principal causes of arrhythmias that result from abnormal repolarization (see **Table 3**).[35] Mutations of KCNQ1, the gene encoding K_vLQT1, and KCNH2, the gene encoding HERG, account for more than 80% of autosomal dominant LQTS (Romano-Ward syndrome). Bilateral neurosensory deafness is a part of the autosomal recessive form (Jervell and Lange-Nielsen syndrome). Mutations of the α-subunit, KCNJ2, and the β-subunits of KVLQT1 and HERG are minor causes of LQTS. The K^+ channel mutations result in a loss of function as a result of synthesis of a nonfunctional protein, failure of the protein to traffic to the membrane, altered channel conductance, or gating. A majority of these mutations have a dominant negative effect, coassembling with normal subunits but impairing their function. Polymorphisms of the genes encoding the K^+ channels may increase susceptibility to drug-induced LQTS. Gain of function mutations of I_{Kr}, I_{Ks}, and I_{K1} cause marked acceleration of repolarization and the short QT syndrome. Mutations of these subunits have also been associated with familial atrial fibrillation.

Cardiac K^+ channels are the targets for the action of class III antiarrhythmic drugs. The HERG channel is susceptible to block by a broad range of drugs that are not primarily used to treat cardiac arrhythmias, including antipsychotics, and the macrolide antibiotics. The potent K^+ channel-blocking action of quinidine, procainamide, and disopyramide account for their QT-prolonging action and occasionally torsades de pointes. HERG blockers produce greater blockade at slow heart rates; block tends to dissipate during the rapid heart rates of a tachycardia, so-called reverse use dependence. Amiodarone is exceptional in that it produces K^+ channel blockade that shows little use dependence. Although antiarrhythmic drugs have fallen out of favor, for the management for ventricular tachycardia, they retain an important role in the prevention of recurrences of atrial fibrillation. The discovery of the atrial-specific distribution of I_{Kur} has made this channel a target for novel therapies for atrial fibrillation. The drug vernakalant is an I_{Kur}/Na channel blocker and is undergoing review by the Food and Drug Administration for the acute termination of atrial fibrillation.

Hyperpolarization-activated, Cyclic, Nucleotide-Gated Channel

Autorhythmicity is one of the most characteristic features of cardiac cells. This property resides in the pacemaker cells of the specialized conducting system, including the SA and AV nodes, and His-Purkinje system. Pacemaker activity initiates and sustains electrical activity of the heart independent of the underlying innervation. Phase 4 diastolic depolarization is characteristic of pacemaker cells. Many ion channels contribute to phase 4 depolarization, the K^+ channel current activated during the preceding action potential, a background Na^+ current, the sodium-calcium exchange, the I_f channel, and the L-type and T-type Ca^{2+} channels. The I_f current channel, however, is unique to this process. Unlike other voltage-gated channels, I_f is activated by hyperpolarization negative to approximately 40 mV. The channel is not very selective for Na^+ over K^+ and has a reversal potential (Er) of -10 to -20 mV. Therefore, it carries inward current throughout the range of pacemaker potential. The phase 4 depolarization reduces the membrane to the threshold for the regenerative activation of $I_{Ca,T}$ and I_{CaL}.

The genes encoding I_f channels have been cloned and sequenced in the past decade. I_f channels (HCNI–HCN4) are members of a family of cyclic, nucleotide-activated, voltage-gated channels. Although members of this family of channels are expressed in heart and brain, HCN2 and HCN4 are expressed in the heart. Expression is both developmentally and regionally regulated. Neonatal cardiac ventricular myocytes, which show pacemaker activity, predominantly expressed HCN2. Expression of HCN2 declines in adulthood. HCN4 is the subtype primarily expressed in the sinus node, AV node, and ventricular conducting system. Knockout of the HCN4 gene is embryonic lethal. Channels are formed by the assembly of four α-subunits, each with a structure analogous to that of the voltage-gated K^+ channels: six membrane-spanning segments (S1–S6), with S4 highly charged and a P loop connecting S5 and S6. The carboxyl terminus contains a cyclic nucleotide-binding domain. The binding of cAMP to this domain shifts the voltage dependence of I_f activation to more depolarized potentials and increases the rate of pacemaker discharge. Protons shift the activation of I_f to more hyperpolarized potentials and slow pacemaker activity. The I_f channel is the target for a new class of bradycardic agents (eg, ivabradine). They have the advantage over β-blockers in that they slow the heart rate without the disadvantage of negative inotropy or hypotension. They have proved effective in the management of patients with chronic stable angina.

Isolated reports of mutations in the HCN4 gene have appeared recently. One kindred had idiopathic sinus bradycardia and chronotrophic incompetence.[36] Severe bradycardia, QT prolongation and torsades de pointes have been described in another family. I_f expression is up-regulated in cardiac hypertrophy and congestive heart failure. This response may contribute to the arrhythmias observed in these disease states.

Gap Junction Channels

That cardiac tissues are made up of discrete cells was a seminal observation in cell biology. The rapid conduction of the cardiac impulse required the presence of low resistance connections between cardiac cells.[37] In the young, gap junctions are distributed over the surface of the cells. Cells become elongated and arranged in parallel bundles in the adult heart, and gap junctions become localized principally at the ends of cells. The density of gap junctions is lower at the lateral margins of cells, particularly conduction system myocytes. This non-uniform distribution of gap junctions changes the pattern and safety of conduction. Each of a pair of neighboring cells

contributes hemi-channels or connections to the junction. The connections are made up of six connections. These are the fundamental building blocks of the junction. Three types of connections are expressed in heart and are defined on the basis of their molecular weight: connection 40, connection 43, and connection 45 (molecular weights 40, 43, and 45 kD). Connection 43 is the principal connection expressed in the heart. Regional differences in the type and distribution of connections are important determinants of the passive spread of excitation over boundaries such as those of the SA and AV nodes. The connections may assemble as homomultimeric or heteromultimeric channels.

The conductance of gap junctional channels is regulated in health and disease states. Protein kinase A phosphorylation and low pH decrease junctional conductance. The latter may be an important contributing factor to slow conduction during acute ischemia. With aging, the density of gap junctions declines and cells become separated by connective tissue septa. This favors the occurrence of slow conduction, fractionated extracellular electrograms and block.

Gap junctions are the targets for a new class of antiarrhythmic drugs.[38] An antiarrhythmic peptide (AAP) inhibits ischemia-induced conduction slowing. An analog rotigaptide prevents ischemia-induced ventricular tachycardia.

FUTURE DIRECTIONS

The cloning and sequencing of the ion channel genes that regulate the action potential hold the promise that these genes could be manipulated to treat arrhythmias. Proof of principle has been established. The initial problem approached is the control of the ventricular response in atrial fibrillation. Beta-adrenergic blockers are the drugs most widely used to control the ventricular response in atrial fibrillation. Adrenergic inhibition decreases intracellular (cAMP) and the Ca^{2+} current. This would slow conduction over the AV node. Donahue and colleagues developed an indirect strategy to decrease sympathetic activity in AV nodal cells.[39] They inserted the inhibitory G protein $G_{\alpha i}$ into an adenoviral vector. The adenoviral vector- $G_{\alpha i}$ construct was infused in the AV nodal artery of pigs with atrial fibrillation. $G_{\alpha i}$ over-expression decreased the heart rate in atrial fibrillation by 20% compared to the drug-free state. Persistence of the effect was limited and the delivery of vector would be challenging in the clinical situation.

Sick sinus syndrome is the most common cause for permanent pacemaker implantation. A genetic strategy to treat sinus node failure would be attractive. Rosen and colleagues have provided a state of the art review on the genetic approach to the development of biological pacemakers by manipulating the HCN4 gene.[40] The biological pacemakers have relatively slow rates. The initial effort is focused on a biological pacemaker that will complement rather than replace the normal sinus node pacemaker.

REFERENCES

1. Hoffman BF, Cranefield PF. Electrophysiology of the Heart. New York: McGraw-Hill Book Company; 1960. p. 1–323.

2. Hille BF. Ionic channels of excitable membranes. Sunderland (MA): Sinauer Associates, Inc; 1984. p. 249–71.

3. Lopatin AN, Makhina EN, Nichols CG. Potassium channel block by cytoplasmic polyamines as the mechanism of intrinsic rectification. Nature 1994; 372:366–9.

4. Hodgkin AL, Huxley AF. A quantitative description of membrane current and its application to conduction and excitation in nerve. J Physiol 1952;117:500–44.

5. Marx SO, Kurokawa J, Reiken S, et al. Requirement of a macromolecular signaling complex for β adrenergic receptor modulation of the KCNQ1-KCNE1 potassium channel. Science 2002;295:496–9.

6. Gilmon AG. G Proteins: transducers of receptor-generated signals. Annu Rev Biochem. 1987;56: 615–49.

7. Mohler PJ, Splawski I, Napolitano C, et al. A cardiac arrhythmia syndrome caused by loss of ankyrin-B function. Proc Natl Acad Sci U S A 2004;101: 9137–42.

8. Patlak JB, Ortiz M. Slow currents through single sodium channels of adult rat heart. J Gen Physiol 1985;86:89–104.

9. Grant AO, Starmer CF. Mechanisms of closure of cardiac sodium channels in rabbit ventricular myocytes: single-channel analysis. Circ Res 1987;60: 897–913.

10. Richmond JE, Featherstone DE, Hartmann HA, et al. Slow inactivation in human cardiac sodium channels. Biophys J 1998;74:2945–52.

11. Zilberter YI, Starmer CF, Starobin J, et al. Late Na channels in cardiac cells: the physiological role of background Na channels. Biophys J 1994;67: 153–60.

12. Noda M, Shimizu S, Tanabe T, et al. Primary structure of electrophorus electricus sodium channel deduced from cDNA sequence. Nature 1984;312:121–7.

13. Marban E, Yamagishi T, Tomaselli GF. Structure and function of voltage-gated sodium channels. J Physiology 1998;508:647–57.

14. West JW, Patton DE, Scheuer T, et al. A cluster of hydrophobic aminoacid residues required for fast Na+-channel inactivation. Proc Natl Acad Sci U S A 1992;89:10910–4.

15. Ono K, Kiyosue T, Arita M. Isoproterenol, DBcAMP and forskolin inhibit cardiac sodium current. Am J Physiol 1989;256:C1131–7.

16. Kirstein M, Eickhorn R, Kochsiek K, et al. Dose-dependent alteration of rat cardiac sodium current by isoproterenol: results from direct measurements on multicellular preparations. Pflugers Arch 1996; 431:395–401.

17. Frohnwieser B, Chen L-Q, Schreibmayer W, et al. Modulation of the human cardiac sodium channel a-subunit by cAMP-dependent protein kinase and the responsible sequence domain. J Physiol 1997; 498:309–18.

18. Liu M, Sanyal S, Gao G, et al. Cardiac Na+ current regulation by pyridine nucleotides. Circ Res 2009; 105:737–45.

19. London B, Michalec M, Mehdi H, et al. Mutation in glycerol-3-phosphate dehydrogenase 1-like gene (GPD1-l) decreases cardiac Na+ current and causes inherited arrhythmias. Circulation 2007;116:2260–8.

20. Clancey CE, Kass RS. Inherited and acquired vulnerability to ventricular arrhythmias: cardiac Na+ and K+ channels. Physiol Rev 2005;85:33–47.

21. Schwartz PJ, Priori SG, Locati EH, et al. Long QT syndrome patients with mutations of the SCN5A and HERG genes have differential responses to Na+ channel blockade and to increases in heart rate. Circulation 1995;92:3381–6.

22. Wang DW, Yazawa K, Makita N, et al. Pharmacological targeting of long QT mutant sodium channels. J Clin Invest 1997;99:1714–20.

23. Antzelevitch C, Brugada P, Borggrefe M, et al. Brugada syndrome: report of the second consensus conference. Heart Rhythm 2005;2:429–40.

24. Yan G-X, Antzelevitch C. Cellular basis for the Brugada syndrome and other mechanisms of arrhythmogenesis associated with ST-segment elevation. Circulation 1999;100:1660–6.

25. Zhang ZS, Tranquillo J, Neplioueva V, et al. Sodium channel kinetic changes that produce Brugada syndrome or progressive cardiac conduction system disease. Am J Physiol 2007;292:H399–407.

26. Schott J-J, Alshinawi C, Kyndt F. Cardiac conduction defects associate with mutations in SCN5A. Nat Genet 1999;23:20–1.

27. Grant AO, Carboni MP, Neplioueva V, et al. Long QT syndrome, Brugada syndrome, and conduction system disease are linked to a single sodium channel mutation. J Clin Invest 2002;110:1201–9.

28. McNair WP, Ku L, Taylor MRG, et al. SCN5A mutation associated with dilated cardiomyopathy, conduction disorder, and arrhythmia. Circulation 2004;110: 2163–7.

29. Hondeghem LM, Katzung BG. Time- and voltage-dependent interactions of antiarrhythmic drugs with cardiac sodium channels. Biochim Biophys Acta 1977;472:373—98.

30. Starmer CF, Grant AO. Phasic ion channel blockade: a kinetic and parameter estimation procedure. Mol Pharmacol 1985;28:348—56.

31. Harrison DC. Is there a rational basis for the modified classification of antiarrhythmic drugs? In: Morganroth J, Moore EN, editors. New drugs and devises. Boston: Martinus Nijhoff; 1985.

32. Splawski I, Timothy KW, Decher N, et al. Severe arrhythmia disorder caused by cardiac L-type calcium channel mutations. Proc Natl Acad Sci U S A 2005;102(23):8089—96.

33. Erxleben C, Liao Y, Gentile S, et al. Cyclosporin and Timothy syndrome increase mode 2 gating of CaV1.2 calcium channels through aberrant phosphorylation of S6 helices. Proc Natl Acad Sci USA 2006;103:3932—7.

34. Antzelevitch C. Role of spatial dispersion of repolarization in inherited and acquired sudden cardiac death syndromes. Am J Physiol Heart Circ Physiol 2007;293:H2024—38.

35. Splawski I, Shen J, Timothy KW, et al. Spectrum of mutations in long-QT syndrome genes KVLQT1, HERG, SCN5A, KCNE1, and KCNE2. Circulation 2000;102:1178—85.

36. Schulze-Bahr E, Neu A, Friederich P, et al. Pacemaker channel dysfunction in a patient with sinus node disease. J Clin Invest 2003;111:1537—45.

37. Rohr S. Role of gap junctions in the propagation of the cardiac action potential. Cardiovasc Res 2004;62:309—22.

38. Nattel S, Carlsson L. Innovative approaches to antiarrhythmic drug therapy. Nat Rev Drug Discov 2006;5:1034—49.

39. Donahue JK, Heldman AW, Fraser H, et al. Focal modification of electrical conduction in the heart by viral gene transfer. Nat Med 2000;6:1395—8.

40. Rosen MR, Brink PR, Cohen IS, et al. Cardiac pacing: from biological to electronic… to biological? Circ Arrhythm Electrophysiol 2008;1:54—61.

Pharmacokinetics/ Pharmacodynamics of Antiarrhythmic Drugs

Julia H. Indik, MD, PhD[a],*, Raymond L. Woosley, MD, PhD[a,b]

KEYWORDS

- Pharmacokinetics • Pharmacodynamics
- Antiarrhythmic medications • Drug interactions

Understanding the pharmacodynamic and pharmacokinetic properties of antiarrhythmic drugs is of particular importance given the complexity of their effects and their potential for interactions with other medications. The Vaughan Williams classification remains a useful framework to describe pharmacodynamic properties of antiarrhythmic drugs, namely how a drug affects the body. The potential for toxicity of an antiarrhythmic agent itself or of another drug that it may interact with relates to pharmacokinetic properties, namely how the body affects the drug and its metabolism. Drugs may be metabolized by renal, hepatic, or other routes. Given these complexities, the opportunities for drug errors and drug toxicity increase. This article discusses the mechanisms of antiarrhythmic drug action, metabolism, and potential drug interactions.

PHARMACOKINETIC CONCEPTS OF DRUG ABSORPTION, DISTRIBUTION, AND METABOLISM

The bioavailability of an orally administered drug depends on several factors. Absorption from the intestinal tract depends on intestinal transit time and blood flow as well as the solubility of the drug. Food can decrease the absorption of a drug with poor lipid solubility. A drug may undergo extensive first-pass metabolism in the liver, further limiting its availability to the systemic circulation. Hepatic enzymes, namely the P450 enzymes, play a key role in this first-pass metabolism, and interactions with other drugs that may either promote or inhibit P450 enzymes can dramatically affect ultimate plasma levels.

Within the systemic circulation, drug distribution is described by parameters such as the volume of distribution (V_d), clearance (Cl), and elimination half-life ($t_{1/2}$). The volume of distribution refers to the apparent volume within which a drug is distributed. Drugs with a high lipid solubility have a high V_d and require a large loading dose; amiodarone is an example. Clearance refers to the volume of plasma that is cleared of a drug in a unit of time, and is a sum of clearance from all organs involved in the distribution, metabolism, and excretion of the drug (ie, liver and kidney). Drugs can be eliminated by transport into the urine, or by a hepatic route by excretion into the bile and feces either in an unchanged form or after transformation to a metabolite.

Whereas a loading dose is related to V_d, the maintenance dose of a drug is related to its clearance. Drugs that are cleared in linear proportion to the drug concentration are said to undergo first-order elimination, which results in an exponential decrease in drug concentration. Assuming first-order elimination, the $t_{1/2} = 0.693 \times V_d / Cl$ and 85% of the steady-state plasma concentration is achieved after 5 half-lives. With first-order elimination, the clearance can be found by dividing the intravenous dose by the area under the curve (AUC) of the drug concentration versus time.

The authors have nothing to disclose.

[a] Department of Medicine, Sarver Heart Center, University of Arizona College of Medicine, 1501 North Campbell Avenue, Tucson, AZ 85724-5037, USA
[b] The Critical Path Institute, 1730 East River Road, #200, Tucson, AZ 85718, USA
* Corresponding author.
E-mail address: jindik@email.arizona.edu

Card Electrophysiol Clin 2 (2010) 341–358
doi:10.1016/j.ccep.2010.06.001

A loading dose allows achievement of a target drug concentration sooner, but does not affect the time to reach steady-state concentrations.

Drugs that are distributed within only one compartment, namely plasma, with first-order elimination processes, can be easily described by the parameters outlined earlier. However, many drugs distribute differently among multiple compartments such as body fat, muscle, and plasma, and pharmacokinetic modeling of drug concentration is more complex. Amiodarone is an example of a drug that distributes differently among multiple compartments and requires more complex pharmacokinetic modeling to predict plasma concentrations.

Plasma concentration is also affected by binding to plasma proteins, which predominantly include albumin and α_1-acid glycoprotein. Although protein binding may be changed by drugs that bump other drugs off plasma proteins, this is not generally a clinically important cause for drug interaction and toxicity because the change in drug concentration is generally transient, and elimination mechanisms compensate.

Elimination of a drug proceeds by renal and hepatic routes. Drugs that are cleared by the kidney may pass into the urine by direct glomerular filtration and tubular transport by specialized proteins. In the liver, and to some extent the small intestine, the cytochrome P450 enzymes play an important role in drug metabolism. The cyctochrome P450 enzymes are part of a cascade of oxidation-reduction reactions that result in the incorporation of oxygen (such as in a hydroxyl group) into a drug. The major isoforms are CYP1A2, CYP3A, CYP2C9, CYP2C19, and CYP2D6. The expression of these enzymes is variable, and may be entirely absent or of limited function in select individuals. In addition, a specific P450 enzyme may be inhibited or induced by another drug. This is an essential mechanism for drug interaction by affecting the metabolism of any drug that is the substrate for that particular P450 enzyme.[1] If hepatic blood flow is reduced, such as in heart failure, the hepatic clearance of some drugs is also affected.

CLASSIFICATION OF ANTIARRHYTHMIC DRUGS

The Vaughan Williams classification remains the most widely used scheme to categorize antiarrhythmic medications. Any one drug may have properties that are related to more than one class. Drugs with class I properties block the inward sodium channel responsible for phase 0 of the action potential. This characteristic affects the depolarization rate and decreases intracardiac conduction. There are subclasses (IA, IB, and IC), with IC agents having the most potent blocking effects. Drugs with class III actions block potassium channels responsible for repolarization during phase 3 of the action potential. Class II drugs exert β-blockade (eg, atenolol and metoprolol), whereas class IV drugs exert calcium channel blockade (eg, verapamil and diltiazem).

Alternative classification schemes have been proposed, including the Sicilian gambit, which classifies drugs according to their multiple effects on (1) channels, (2) receptors, (3) transmembrane pumps, and (4) clinical effects.[2] The advantage of this scheme is that it specifies multichannel effects with further distinction between low, moderate, and high potency. The scheme is complex, however, and has not achieved the popularity of the Vaughan Williams classification scheme. This article discusses antiarrhythmic medications according to the Vaughan Williams scheme, which remains the most widely used in clinical practice.

VAUGHAN WILLIAMS CLASS I: SODIUM CHANNEL BLOCKADE

Class I antiarrhythmic medications block the inward current of sodium during phase 0 of the action potential, slowing the rate of depolarization (V_{max}). The Hodgkin and Huxley model[3] describes sodium channels as existing in one of 3 states (open, closed, and inactivated), and each state has a different affinity for a given drug.[4,5] This characteristic can explain the feature of use-dependence of drugs in this class, whereby block increases with increasing rate of stimulation. With increased stimulation (namely faster heart rates), more sodium channels are in an open or inactivated state. Drugs that have greater affinity for their receptor when the sodium channel is open or inactivated bind more readily at faster stimulation (pacing) rates. Drugs also show different rates for association or dissociation from its receptor. Class IB drugs associate and dissociate the fastest with their receptor, whereas class IC drugs are the slowest. **Table 1** gives pharmacokinetic properties of the class I antiarrhythmic medications, and drug interactions are in **Table 2**.

Class IA: Quinidine, Disopyramide, and Procainamide

In addition to a slowing of conduction as a result of sodium channel blockade and reducing V_{max}, the class IA drugs also decrease automaticity and excitability in the atria, ventricles, and Purkinje fibers.[6] They have an intermediate rate of

Table 1
Pharmacodynamic and pharmacokinetic properties: drugs with predominant Vaughan Williams class I actions

Drug	Effect on Ion Currents, Channels	ECG Changes	Elimination or Inactivation Route	V_D (L/kg)	Bioavailability (%)	Time to Peak Plasma Concentration After Oral Dose (h)	Elimination Half-life (h)	Usual Initial Dosage	Modification of Dose if Renal (RD), Hepatic (HD) Dysfunction, Heart Failure (CHF)
Procaineamide	INa, Ikr	↑QT	Hepatic (40%–70%) Renal (30%–60%)	2	100	1	2–4	500 mg every 6 h	↓RD
Quinidine	INa, Ikr, Ito	↑QT	Hepatic (50%–90%), Renal (10%–30%)	2.5	70	1.5–3	3–19	200 mg every 6 h	↓HD
Disopyramide	INa, Ikr, anticholinergic effects	↑QT	Hepatic (20%–30%), Renal (40%–50%)	0.6	80–90	1–2	6–8	100 mg every 6 h	↓RD ↓HD
Lidocaine	INa		Hepatic	1.1			1.5–4	Load (75–225 mg), followed by 1–4 mg/min intravenously	↓HD ↓CHF
Mexiletine	INa		Hepatic	5.5–9.5	90	2–4	8–20	200 mg every 8 h	Consider ↓HD, ↓CHF In renal failure, start with low dosage
Propafenone	INa, β-blockade	↑PR, ↑QRS,	Hepatic	3–4	10–50	2–3	2–24	150 mg every 8 h	
Flecainide	INa	↑PR, ↑QRS, slight ↑QT	Hepatic (70%), Renal (30%)	7–10	90–95	2	14–20	50–100 mg every 12 h	↓RD, ↓HD

Table 2
Antiarrhythmic drug (AAD) interactions: drugs with predominant Vaughan Williams class I Actions

AAD	Relevant P450 Enzymes	AAD Level is Increased by Interaction With	AAD Level May be Decreased by Interaction With	AAD Increases Levels of
Quinidine	Metabolized by CYP3A4 and inhibits CYP2D6	Inhibitors of CYP3A4, eg, clarithromycin, telithromycin, itraconazole, ketoconazole, indinavir, nelfinavir, ritonavir, squinavir nefazodone, verapamil, diltiazem	Inducers of CYP3A4, eg, efavirenz, nevirapine, barbiturates, phenobarbital, phenytoin	Drugs metabolized by CYP2D6 are inhibited by quinidine, eg, metoprolol, fluoxetine, amitriptyline, venlafaxine
Procaineamide		Cimetidine, ranitidine (decreases renal clearance)		
Disopyramide	Metabolized by CYP3A4		Inducers of CYP3A4, eg, efavirenz, nevirapine, barbiturates, phenobarbital, phenytoin	
Lidocaine		Cimetidine (decreased liver blood flow)		
Mexiletine	Metabolized by CYP1A2 (minor) and CYP2D6 (major)	Inhibitors of CYP1A2, eg, ciprofloxacin, amiodarone, fluvoxamine Inhibitors of CYP2D6, eg, quinidine, buproprion, fluoxetine, paroxetine	Inducers of CYP2D6: eg, rifampin	
Propafenone	Metabolized by CYP2D6 (to 5-hydroxypropafenone), and CYP3A4 and CYP1A2 (to N-depropyl-propafenone)	Inhibitors of CYP2D6, eg, quinidine, buproprion, fluoxetine, paroxetine Inhibitors of CYP1A2, eg, ciprofloxacin, amiodarone, fluvoxamine Inhibitors of CYP1A2, eg, ciprofloxacin, amiodarone, fluvoxamine	Inducers of CYP2D6: eg, rifampin	Metoprolol, propanolol, digoxin, warfarin
Flecainide	Metabolized by CYP2D6	Inhibitors of CYP2D6, eg, quinidine, buproprion, fluoxetine, paroxetine	Inducers of CYP2D6: eg, rifampin	Digoxin, propanolol

association and dissociation from sodium channels. There is also blockade of the rapidly activating potassium channel, I_{Kr}, leading to a prolongation of the action potential and QT interval. Potassium channel blockade is greater for quinidine compared with procainamide, which exerts most of its I_{Kr} blockade through its active metabolite, N-acetylprocainamide (NAPA). These drugs should be particularly avoided in patients with heart failure because of their potential for negative inotropic effects and peripheral vasodilation, resulting in hypotension when used intravenously.

Quinidine in addition decreases the potassium current during phase 1 of the action potential by blocking the I_{to} current. This effect may prevent the heterogeneity in membrane potentials during phase 2, which is believed to underlie the ST segment elevation in the right precordial leads and the initiation of ventricular fibrillation seen in Brugada syndrome.

Disopyramide also exerts anticholinergic effects, such as urinary retention, dry mouth, constipation, blurred vision, closed-angle glaucoma, and esophageal reflux. Patients with glaucoma and men with symptomatic prostatic hyperplasia should not receive this agent. The anticholinergic effects may be helpful in bradycardia-induced atrial fibrillation, as can occur in young individuals. In high dosages it can also suppress sinus node function, and therefore the drug should be avoided in patients with sinus node dysfunction. It has also been used in patients with hypertrophic cardiomyopathy for its negative inotropic effects.

Hepatic metabolism of procainamide to NAPA is variable, with about half of whites being rapid acetylators (90% of Asians). The usual effective concentration for procainamide is 4 to 8 μg/mL and NAPA 7 to 15 μg/mL.[7] Monitoring of both procainamide and NAPA levels is needed during initiation of the drug or uptitration of dosage, because each component may reach steady-state levels at different times. Because NAPA is renally excreted, excessive drug levels may be reached in patients with renal dysfunction or in patients who are rapid acetylators. Cimetidine can reduce renal clearance by 30% to 50% by blocking renal tubular secretion[8,9] and ranitidine can reduce renal clearance by 14% to 23%.[10] The QT interval should be monitored to assess risk for torsades de pointes.

Adverse reactions related to procainamide include a lupuslike syndrome, occurring in up to 20% of patients, with symptoms of athralgias, arthritis, fever, malar rash, and pleural and pericardial effusions. Positive antinuclear antibodies

develop in almost all patients treated chronically with procainamide, and are not a cause to discontinue therapy in the absence of symptoms. Procainamide therapy has also been associated with agranulocytosis, perhaps more likely to occur with sustained release preparations.[11]

Quinidine is predominantly metabolized by the P450 enzyme CYP3A4, and may require a lower dosage in patients with liver dysfunction, in whom an increase in the elimination half-life has been seen.[12] There is also decreased plasma protein binding in hepatic failure, so that toxicity can occur at lower total plasma concentrations as a result of the effect of altered protein binding.[13] Quinidine reduces the renal clearance of digoxin, and may result in digoxin toxicity. Metabolism of quinidine is inhibited by cimetidine and increased by phenytoin, phenobarbital, rifampin, and other inducers. Quinidine itself is an inhibitor of the P450 enzyme CYP2D6, and therefore there can be interactions with drugs that are metabolized by this enzyme, including β-blockers such as metoprolol and carvedilol and other class I drugs (propafenone, mexiletine, and flecainide).[1] Side effects of quinidine include hypotension and worsening of neuromuscular blockade. The drug may worsen symptoms in patients with myesthenia gravis.[14]

Disopyramide is eliminated by both renal and hepatic (N-dealkylation) routes. Disopyramide may also show saturable protein binding, which can then lead to disproportionately increased levels of the free drug. Therefore, the drug should be gradually uptitrated from low dosages. Metabolism of disopyramide is enhanced by phenytoin, rifampin, and phenobarbital.

Class IB: Lidocaine, Mexilitine

Lidocaine and mexilitine are used in the treatment of ventricular tachyarrythmias, often as adjunctive therapy to amiodarone. There is no significant effect on atrial tissue, and these drugs are not of value for supraventricular tachyarrhythmias. As class I agents, these drugs block fast sodium channels, decreasing V_{max}, the rate of depolarization during phase 0 of the action potential. Lidocaine may slightly shorten the action potential duration and effective refractory period of normal conducting tissue, but some studies have suggested a facilitation of subnodal block in patients with abnormal conduction.[15,16] Central nervous system toxicity includes tinnitus, seizures, altered mental status, and coma. Lidocaine may also suppress sinus node function.

Mexilitine is an oral analogue of lidocaine but also structurally similar to tocainide. In addition to blockade of sodium channels and reducing V_{max}, mexiletine has also been shown to shorten action potential duration in canine ventricular myocardium.[17] Mexiletine has minimal effects on hemodynamic parameters or myocardial contractility and therefore can be used safely in patients with severe systolic dysfunction.

Lidocaine if orally administered undergoes extensive first-pass hepatic metabolism, making it useful only as an intravenous agent. Lidocaine clearance is via the liver, although 2 less potent metabolites, which may be responsible for central nervous system side effects, are excreted by the kidneys.

A 2-compartment model has been used to describe the distribution of lidocaine, with the central compartment showing rapid clearance (half-life of 8 minutes). Therefore, loading doses are needed followed by maintenance infusion to achieve rapidly therapeutic plasma and tissue levels of the drug. A steady-state concentration occurs in about 8 to 10 hours, but is prolonged up to 24 hours in individuals with heart failure or hepatic disease. One described loading regimen for an average 75-kg patient[18] is an initial dose of 75 mg, followed by 50 mg every 5 minutes for 3 dosages, for a total of 225 mg. Patients must be constantly monitored for side effects because peak concentrations are variable. Maintenance infusion rates are typically in the range of 20 to 60 µg/kg/min (about 1–4 mg/min), for an expected plasma concentration of 3 µg/mL. Lidocaine has little effect at concentrations less than 1.5 µg/mL and toxicity is more likely to occur at more than 5 µg/mL. The elimination half-life is about 2 to 4 hours. In heart failure the loading dose should be halved to reflect the reduced central V_d, and the maintenance infusion should be similarly reduced. Renal dysfunction does not change recommendations for dosing.

Mexilitine has an approximate 90% bioavailability and a large V_d, with only 1% of total body content within the plasma. Steady-state concentrations are reached in about 1 to 3 days with an elimination half-life of 8 to 20 hours. Side effects of mexilitine can include tremor, blurred vision, nausea, dysphoria, and dizziness.

Both lidocaine and mexilitine are metabolized in the liver by the P450 enzyme CYP2D6, which is absent in 7% of the white population and thus clearance of these drugs may be variable. In addition, drug interactions related to this P450 enzyme must be recognized. Drugs that inhibit CYP2D6 (ie, amiodarone, quinidine, citalopram, cimetidine, and other inhibitors) increase lidocaine and mexilitine levels and the risks of toxicity. Cimetidine has also been reported to decrease the V_d of

lidocaine and to decrease hepatic blood flow, further increasing lidocaine plasma levels. Hepatic metabolism is increased by rifampin and other inducing agents, thus leading to decreased drug concentrations. Mexilitine is also partially excreted by the kidneys, and patients with renal failure should have the drug initiated at lower dosages.

Class IC: Flecainide and Propafenone

Flecainide and propafenone slow conduction velocity and V_{max} by blockade of sodium channels as class IC agents, with slow association/dissociation channel kinetics, resulting in marked use-dependent characteristics. Flecainide and propafenone both prolong the PR and QRS interval, whereas flecainide can slightly increase the QT interval.

Propafenone blocks both open and inactivated sodium channels[19] but has other pharmacodynamic effects in addition to sodium channel blockade. Propafenone also blocks both voltage-dependent calcium currents and potassium currents such that the action potential duration is essentially unchanged. It has β-blocking properties that are particularly pronounced in patients who poorly metabolize propafenone to 5-hydroxypropafenone, via CYP2D6.[20] Even patients with usual metabolism of propafenone can display marked β-blockade but at higher dosages. However, the antiarrhythmic (sodium channel blockade) effects of propafenone are similar between poor and extensive metabolizers,[20] as both 5-hydroxypropafenone and a second metabolite, N-despropyl-propafenone, block sodium channels.[19]

Flecainide slows conduction in all cardiac tissues: atria, ventricles, Purkinje fibers, and the atrioventricular (AV) node. Similar to propafenone, it has negative inotropic effects. It has also been shown in feline ventricular myocytes to block the delayed rectifier potassium channel,[21] but the clinical relevance of this effect is unclear, and risk for torsades de pointes is extremely low.

Propafenone and flecainide should not be used in patients with reduced ventricular function because of their direct negative inotropic effects, and increased mortality in such patients has been found in clinical trials, including the Cardiac Arhythmia Suppression Trial (CAST)[22] for suppression of ventricular arrhythmias in patients after myocardial infarction treated with flecainide or encainide, and the Cardiac Arrest Study Hamburg (CASH) trial[23] for the prevention of sudden cardiac death. Other adverse effects for flecainide include sinus node dysfunction. Flecainide can also increase pacing thresholds.

Propafenone reaches peak plasma concentration 2 to 3 hours after an oral dose, and absorption is increased with food. However, hepatic metabolism reduces the bioavailability of the drug, and bioavailability is therefore increased in patients with hepatic dysfunction. Plasma drug concentrations are nonlinearly related to dose. Propafenone is also highly protein bound, particularly in uremic states and is correlated with α_1-acid glycoprotein levels.[19]

Propafenone is metabolized by the hepatic enzyme CYP 2D6 to the active metabolite 5-hydroxypropafenone, and by a different hepatic pathway (CYP3A4 and CYP1A2) to a second metabolite, N-despropyl-propafenone. Patients who are deficient in CYP2D6 have increased levels of propafenone, and increased blockade of β-receptors. Inhibitors of CYP2D6 also increase this effect. Propafenone also increases levels of digoxin, metoprolol, propanolol, and warfarin.[24]

Concentrations of flecainide peak 2 hours after administration and decline with a half-life of 14 to 20 hours.[25] It is metabolized by CYP2D6 and in addition excreted by the kidneys, therefore patients with renal dysfunction who are either deficient in CYP2D6 or given medications that inhibit this enzyme are at risk for developing high levels of flecainide. In addition, flecainide can increase levels of digoxin and propanolol.

VAUGHAN WILLIAMS CLASS II: β-RECEPTOR BLOCKADE

Medications in this class include those that selectively block receptors in cardiac tissue (β_1) or nonselectively, including receptors in lung and blood vessels (β_2). These drugs competitively inhibit binding by catecholamines. Predominant actions include a reduction in automaticity in cardiac tissue, such as the sinus node, and conduction through the AV node. Medications with predominant β_1 selectivity include metoprolol, bisoprolol, and atenolol, but in higher dosages these drugs block β_2-receptors as well. Nonselective drugs that block both β_1- and β_2-receptors include propanolol, nadolol, pindolol, timolol, and carvedilol, which in addition blocks α_1-adrenergic receptors. Carvedilol and metoprolol have been shown to improve survival in patients with systolic heart failure and reduce sudden death.[26-28] Pindolol also shows intrinsic sympathomimetic activity, by paradoxically activating the β-receptor, with less of a decrease of resting heart rate. Side effects of β-blocking agents can include fatigue, worsening of depression, and hypoglycemic reactions

in diabetic patients. β_2-blockade may exacerbate asthma and claudication.

Pharmacokinetics varies among these agents. About 50% of an oral dosage of atenolol is absorbed from the gastrointestinal tract, with a peak plasma concentration reached in 2 to 4 hours. It distributes throughout the body but little penetrates into the central nervous system, unlike propanolol, which lowers sympathetic outflow from the central nervous system as well. The half-life of atenolol is 6 to 7 hours but is reduced in elderly patients and in patients with impaired renal function. Metoprolol tartrate is almost completely absorbed from the gastrointestinal tract and undergoes first-pass metabolism in the liver. The extended release formulation, metoprolol succinate, has a longer time to peak plasma concentration of about 7 hours,[29] compared with 90 minutes for metoprolol tartrate.

Metoprolol is metabolized by the P450 enzyme CYP2D6. Therefore medications that inhibit this enzyme, such as cimetidine, fluoxetine, paroxetine, propafenone, and bupropion, increase plasma concentration of metoprolol. Carvedilol is metabolized predominantly by CYP2D6 and CYP2C9. Propanolol is metabolized by CYP2D6, CYP1A2, and CYP2C19.

VAUGHAN WILLIAMS CLASS III: POTASSIUM CHANNEL BLOCKADE

Antiarrhythmic medications with class III actions block potassium channels, resulting in prolongation of the action potential. The antiarrhythmic medications in this group are sotalol, ibutilide, amiodarone, dronedarone, and dofetilide. Vernakalant is a new agent that also blocks potassium currents, selectively in atrial tissue. However, potassium channel blockade is also shared with antiarrhythmic medications in the class IA group (quinidine, disopyramide, and procainamide via its metabolite NAPA).

Agents that block the rapidly activating inwardly rectifying potassium channel, I_{Kr}, display reverse use-dependence, wherein block is greater at slower heart rates. At fast heart rates, the slowly activating channel, I_{Ks}, is active and can ensure repolarization. At slow heart rates, there is sufficient time for the I_{Ks} channel to deactivate and thus repolarization is largely handled by the I_{Kr} channel. Therefore, drugs that block I_{Kr} result in delays in repolarization and QT prolongation predominantly at slower heart rates. **Table 3** gives pharmacokinetic properties of the class I antiarrhythmic medications, and drug interactions in **Table 4**.

Table 3
Pharmacodynamic and pharmacokinetic properties: drugs with predominant Vaughan Williams class III Actions

Drug	Effect on Ion Currents, Channels	Electrocardiography Changes	Elimination or Inactivation Route	V_D (L/kg)	Bioavailability (%)	Time to Peak Plasma Concentration After Oral Dose (h)	Elimination half-life (h)	Usual Initial Dosage	Modification of Dose if Renal (RD), Hepatic (HD) Dysfunction, Heart Failure (CHF)
Amiodarone	Ikr, Iks, IKAch (minor), Ca, INa (inactivated), α and β-blockade	↑QT, ↑PR, ↑QRS	Hepatic	66	50	3–7 (onset of action may take weeks)	13–103 days	200 mg daily after loading regimen (oral) 150 mg intravenously over 10 minutes followed by 1 mg/min for 6 h, followed by 0.5 mg/min (intravenously)	
Dronedarone	Ikr, Iks, IKAch, Ca, INa, α and β-blockade	↑QT, ↑PR	Hepatic		4–15 (bioavailability increased with high fat meal)	3–6 hours	13–19	400 mg twice a day	
Dofetilide	IKr	↑QT	Renal (major) Hepatic (minor, via CYP 3A4)	3	>90	2–3	10	500 µg twice a day	↓RD
Sotalol	IKr, β-blockade	↑QT	Renal		>90	2.5–4	12	80–120 mg twice a day	↓RD
Ibutilide	IKr, and promotes slow inward Na current	↑QT	Hepatic (oxidation/hydroxylation, not by P450)	11			2–12	1 mg intravenously over 10 minutes, may repeat	None, but increased risk of torsades in CHF
Vernakalant	IKur (predominant) also It0, HERG, IKAch	↑QT↑QRS	Hepatic (via CYP2D6)	1.8 L/kg			3–8	3 mg/kg intravenously over 10 minutes, followed by 2 mg/kg	

Table 4
Drug interactions: antiarrhythmic drugs (AAD) with predominant Vaughan Williams class III Actions

AAD	Relevant P450 Enzymes	AAD Level is Increased by Interaction With	AAD Level May be Decreased by Interaction With	AAD Increases Levels of
Amiodarone	Inhibits CYP2D6 and CYP3A4			Drugs metabolized by CYP2D6, eg, metoprolol, fluoxetine, amitriptyline, venlafaxine Drugs metabolized by CYP3A4, eg, simvastatin, lovastatin In addition amiodarone increases levels of digoxin (inhibition of P-glycoprotein) and increases anticoagulant effects of warfarin
Dronedarone	Metabolized by CYP3A4 and inhibits CYP2D6	Inhibitors of CYP3A4, eg, clarithromycin, telithromycin, itraconazole, ketoconazole, indinavir, nelfinavir, ritonavir, squinavir nefazodone, verapamil, diltiazem	Inducers of CYP3A4, eg, efavirenz, nevirapine, barbiturates, phenobarbital, phenytoin	Drugs metabolized by CYP2D6, eg, metoprolol, fluoxetine, amitriptyline, venlafaxine Dronedarone increases levels of digoxin (inhibition of P-glycoprotein)
Dofetilide	Metabolized by CYP3A4	Inhibitors of CYP3A4, eg, clarithromycin, telithromycin, itraconazole, ketoconazole, indinavir, nelfinavir, ritonavir, squinavir nefazodone, verapamil, diltiazem Dofetilide levels also increased by inhibition of renal clearance by these contraindicated drugs: cimetidine, ketoconazole, trimethoprim, prochlorperazine, megestrol. Verapamil and thiazide diuretics also increase dofetilide levels and are contraindicated	Inducers of CYP3A4, eg, efavirenz, nevirapine, barbiturates, phenobarbital, phenytoin	
Vernakalant	Metabolized by CYP2D6 and moderate competitive inhibitor of CYP2D6	Clearance of vernakalant not affected by CYP2D6 inhibitors		

Amiodarone

Amiodarone is a benzofuran derivative with covalent links to 2 iodine molecules. It exerts effects across all Vaughan Williams classes. There is an increase in the action potential duration and refractory period via potassium channel blockade in a use-dependent manner, and noncompetitive inhibition of α- and β-receptors.[30] The refractory period is increased in all cardiac tissues (atria, AV node, His-Purkinje fibers, ventricles), and automaticity is reduced by slowing phase 4 depolarization. Amiodarone also increases the QT interval, but torsades de pointes is rare (<1%).[31–33] Amiodarone also possesses class I effects by blocking inactivated sodium channels,[34,35] an effect that is more pronounced for its major metabolite, desethylamiodarone.[36] Amiodarone also blocks the L-type calcium channel. With intravenous therapy there can be a hypotensive effect related to the solvents, polysorbate 80, and benzyl alcohol.[37] The US Food and Drug Administration (FDA) labeling recommends amiodarone for the treatment of recurrent ventricular fibrillation and recurrent hemodynamically unstable ventricular tachycardia.

Amiodarone is structurally similar to thyroid hormone, and has been described as causing a state of cardiac hypothyroidism by noncompetitively inhibiting the binding of thyroid hormone (T3) to nuclear receptors. T3 is transported into the cardiac myocyte and binds to a nuclear receptor, leading to the regulation of several genes, including α- and β-myosin heavy chain, sarcoplasmic reticulum Ca adenosine triphosphatase (ATPase) and phospholamban, β-adrenergic receptors, and Na-K ATPase.[38] Thus by a broad range of actions, thyroid hormone affects contractile and relaxation function. In addition to inhibiting T3 binding, amiodarone further prevents the peripheral conversion of T4 to T3 by inhibiting type I iodo-thyronine 5'-deiodinase,[39] and conversion to reverse T3 continues. Overall, there is an increase in thyroxine (T4) and reverse T3 (rT3), as well as small decreases in T3 and an initial increase then normalization of thyroid-stimulating hormone.[39]

The iodine moiety in amiodarone is responsible for hypothyroid or hyperthyroid states. Iodine released from amiodarone in its metabolism directly inhibits thyroid function and hormone synthesis, giving a state of hypothyroidism.[39,40] Hyperthyroidism can occur in up to 10%, with 2 forms described.[38] In type 1 hyperthyroidism, which occurs in populations with low iodine intake, there is an association with goiter and a resulting increase in thyroid hormone production believed to be caused by the presence of excess iodine with dysfunctional autoregulation of iodine handling in the thyroid.[39] In type 2 hyperthyroidism, there is an inflammatory thyroiditis with release of stored thyroid hormone.[38,41]

In addition to the effects of amiodarone on thyroid function, there are potential adverse effects on other organ systems. A pneumonitis may develop after several months or years with a cumulative prevalence estimated between 1% and 15% depending on daily dose.[42,43] This entity can be difficult to distinguish from interstitial pulmonary edema. Both amiodarone and its metabolite, desethylamiodarone, are toxic to the lung.[42] Pneumonitis may be triggered by exposure to increased oxygen concentrations, and there may be increased risk in patients given iodinated contrast.[42] In addition, amiodarone may cause an optic neuritis, with an incidence of 0.1% to 2%, skin discoloration (4%–9%), peripheral neuropathy (0.3%), and hepatitis and cirrhosis, with an annual incidence of 0.6%,[31] although an increase in transaminases can occur without a true hepatic toxic effect.

With oral administration, amiodarone has a bioavailability of 22 to 86%.[44] The onset of action is variable, with a range of 2 days to 3 weeks with loading dosages. The V_d is large, about 66 L/kg, as a result of accumulation in fatty tissue and in the liver, lung, and spleen. Elimination is by excretion into the bile, with a slow but variable elimination rate and a half-life of 13 to 103 days,[45] because the pharmacokinetics is complex because of the range of half-lives from multiple compartments such as fat and heart. The metabolite, desethlamiodarone, also accumulates in tissues and has a long half-life.[31]

The potentiation of amiodarone of the anticoagulant effect of warfarin is well known, and warfarin dose should be reduced, with close monitoring of the international normalized ratio. Amiodarone also increases levels of digoxin by inhibition of P-glycoprotein, and its dose should be decreased by 50%. Coadministration with fluoroquinolones or macrolides can further increase QT intervals,[31] and the risk of rhabdomyolysis is increased with amiodarone combined with statins such as simvastatin. Coadministration with β-blockers and nondihydropyridine calcium channel blockers can worsen sinus bradycardia and AV nodal conduction.

Dronedarone

The chemical structure of dronedarone is similar to amiodarone, as a noniodinated benzofuran analogue. There are effects across all 4 Vaughan

Williams classes. In vitro experiments in dog,[46] guinea pig,[47] rat,[48] rabbit,[49] and human[50] myocytes have investigated its broad effects on ionic currents. There is blockade of both rapid and slow components of the delayed rectifier potassium channels, I_{kr} and I_{ks}, as well as the acetylcholine-activated potassium current, I_{Kach},[51,52] and slow L-type calcium current. It is also a more potent blockade of sodium current compared with amiodarone, and reduces the maximal upstroke velocity (dV/dt_{max}) of the action potential to a greater degree.[50] Dronedarone also has antiadrenergic properties, blocking both α- and β-receptors and inhibiting agonist-induced adenylate cyclase activity.[53] A reduction in coronary perfusion pressure in guinea pig hearts has been described that may relate to calcium current modulation.[54] Dronedarone also decreases heart rate, increases the PR interval and corrected QT interval in a dose-dependent manner and without reverse use dependency (little or no increase in effect at slow heart rates).[51] Nonetheless, only one case of torsades de pointes was reported in 2301 patients randomized to dronedarone therapy in the Assess the Efficacy of Dronedarone for the Prevention of Cardiovascular Hospitalization or Death from Any Cause in Patients with Atrial Fibrillation/Atrial Flutter (ATHENA) trial.[55]

The clearance of creatinine is decreased by dronedarone by 18% in healthy subjects[56] and can increase serum creatinine. Creatinine is cleared by both glomerular filtration as well as by active cationic transport across renal tubular epithelial cells, and it is the latter process that is inhibited by dronedarone. There is no change in renal plasma flow or glomerular filtration rate.[56] Dronedarone, theoretically because of the lack of iodine in its structure, also has less organ toxicity (hepatic, ocular, pulmonary, and thyroid) than amiodarone.

Dronedarone is extensively absorbed (more than 75%) and absorption is improved if taken with food.[52] However, it undergoes extensive first-pass metabolism, which reduces the effective bioavailability to 15%. Steady-state levels are reached in approximately 1 week, and the terminal half-life is 24 hours. The addition of a methanesulfonyl group makes the molecule less lipophilic compared with amiodarone, thus giving a smaller V_d and a shorter half-life.[51]

Dronedarone is excreted in the feces after being metabolized by CYP3A4 and thus is subject to interactions with drugs that inhibit this enzyme. Verapamil and diltiazem are moderate inhibitors of CYP3A4 and concomitant administration may worsen bradycardia or AV block. Ketoconazole is a strong CYP3A4 inhibitor, and can increase dronedarone levels by several fold.[52]

Macrolides (eg, erythromycin, clarithromycin, but not azithromycin) also inhibit CYP3A4 and should be avoided.

Dronedarone may also increase the levels of other drugs by interacting with P-glycoprotein, which can increase levels of digoxin. Simvastatin is also metabolized by CYP3A4, and therefore there is a potential for increased levels of simvastatin and muscle injury.[52] Dronedarone itself inhibits the P450 enzyme CYP2D6, which metabolizes metoprolol, and coadministration may result in further bradycardia in patients who are extensive metabolizers of metoprolol via CYP2D6.

Dofetilide

Dofetilide blocks the fast component of the delayed rectifier potassium current, I_{kr}, resulting in prolongation of the action potential and QT interval. It does not block other potassium currents or other channels and receptors. Dofetilide displays reverse use-dependence; QT prolongation therefore is more marked at slower heart rates. There is no change in QRS width or PR interval because there is no effect on cardiac conduction velocity. In isolated atria it has been reported to prolong sinus node recovery and mildly reduce spontaneous heart rate.[57] There are no negative inotropic effects, and thus no change in hemodynamic parameters such as cardiac output, systemic vascular resistance or stroke volume. In patients with heart failure, intravenous dofetilide maintained hemodynamic indices compared with amiodarone.[58]

A series of trials established the effectiveness of dofetilde for both maintenance of sinus rhythm and cardioversion from atrial fibrillation or atrial flutter. Dofetilide achieved cardioversion of persistent atrial fibrillation or atrial flutter in 29.9% of patients receiving 500 μg twice daily compared with 1.2% for placebo.[59] In the Symptomatic Atrial Fibrillation Investigative Research on Dofetilide (SAFIRE-D) trial, dofetilide maintained sinus rhythm at 1 year in 58% of patients compared with 25% of patients receiving placebo,[59] and in the Danish Investigations of Arrhythmia and Mortality on Dofetilide (DIAMOND) substudy (DIAMOND-AF) sinus rhythm was maintained after 1 year in 79% of patients randomized to receive dofetilide compared with 42% randomized to placebo.[60]

Dofetilide was compared with sotalol and placebo in the European and Australian Multicenter Evaluative Research on Atrial Fibrillation Dofetilide (EMERALD) trial,[61] Full-dose dofetilide (500 μg twice daily) was superior to low-dose dofetilide (250 μg twice daily), low-dose sotalol (80 mg twice daily), and placebo. There was no excess mortality in patients with recent myocardial infarction, severe left ventricular (LV) dysfunction,[62] or heart failure alone.[63] Overall, the risk for torsades de pointes at dosages of 250 to 500 μg twice daily was less than 1% for patients with supraventricular arrhythmias alone, but was as high as 2.9% in the DIAMOND-MI trial[62] and 3.3% in DIAMOND-CHF.[63] Because of the potential risk for torsades de pointes, the FDA recommends that dofetilide therapy be initiated in the hospital over a period of 3 days.

Dofetilide has a greater than 90% bioavailability, reaching a maximal plasma concentration 2 to 3 hours after dosing. The elimination half-life is 8 to 10 hours, with a V_d of 3 L/kg. Steady-state concentrations are reached in 2 to 3 days. About 60% to 70% of the drug is bound to plasma proteins. Dofetilide is mainly excreted by the kidneys (80% in the urine), which occurs by both glomerular filtration and cationic renal (active tubular) secretion. The latter is inhibited by cimetidine (but not ranitidine), ketoconazole, trimethoprim, prochlorperazine, and megestrol. These drugs are therefore contraindicated in the product labeling. The C_{max} of dofetilide was increased by 53% in men and 97% in women with coadministration with ketoconazole, and dofetilide plasma concentration increased 58% after coadministration with cimetidine.[64] In addition, drugs that may compete for cationic secretion should be used cautiously (triameterene, metformin, and amiloride) because they may increase dofetilide levels. Verapamil also increased peak plasma levels of dofetilide by 42%.[64] In the DIAMOND trial coadministration with verapamil increased the risk of torsades de pointes and therefore is also contraindicated.

Because of interaction and the risk of hypokalemia exacerbating the risk of torsades de pointes, thiazide diuretics are also contraindicated. Hydrochlorothiazide (50 mg) with dofetilide 500 μg twice daily for 5 days increased the dofetilide AUC by 27% and C_{max} by 21% but further increased the QTc over time by 197%.[65] These effects may in part be caused by a lowering in serum potassium but also an increase in dofetilide exposure. Digoxin should be used cautiously as it has been associated with a higher risk of torsades de pointes in patients on dofetilide. In addition, any other drug that prolongs the QT interval or promotes hypokalemia or hypomagnesemia should be avoided.

The P450 enzyme CYP 3A4 metabolizes dofetilide but with a low affinity, and metabolites are formed by N-dealkylation and N-oxidation. Drugs that inhibit CYP3A4 could potentially raise plasma levels of dofetilide, and such drugs include macrolides, azole antifungals, protease inhibitors, serotonin reuptake inhibitors, amiodarone, diltiazem, grapefruit juice, nefazodone, norfloxacin, quinine, and zafirlukast. Dofetilide itself is not known to inhibit any P450 enzyme.

The FDA recommends that dofetilide therapy be initiated in a hospital setting over a 3-day period. Dosage is determined based on renal function as determined by calculated creatinine clearance. For normal renal function (creatinine clearance greater than 60 mL/min) the starting dose is 500 μg twice daily. For a creatinine clearance of 40 to 60 mL/min, the initial dose is 250 μg twice daily, and 125 μg twice daily is used if the creatinine clearance is 20 to 40 mL/min. Dofetilide is contraindicated if the creatinine clearance is less than 20 mL/min of if the QTc is greater than 440 milliseconds. If the QTc rises by more than 15% after drug initiation, the dose is to be decreased by 50% (the 125-μg twice-daily dose should be reduced to once daily). If the QTc exceeds 500 milliseconds after the second dose, dofetilide should be stopped entirely. Women have a higher plasma concentration than men, even after correction for weight and creatinine clearance. Dosing does not need to be adjusted based on hepatic function, but patients with severe hepatic impairment have not been studied.

Sotalol

Sotalol is prepared as a racemic mixture of d and l isomers, of which the l isomer is responsible for β-blockade, the predominate action at doses less than 160 mg daily. The d and l isomers block the rapid component of the delayed potassium rectifier channel (I_{Kr}). The Survival With Oral d-Sotalol (SWORD) trial investigated the d isomer in patients with a history of myocardial infarction and reduced LV ejection fraction, but was stopped before full enrollment because of an increase in mortality,[66] particularly in patients with remote myocardial infarction.[67] The racemic mixture of d and l isomers does not increase mortality following myocardial infarction and may produce a small reduction in mortality because of its β-blocking effects.[68]

Overall, sotalol prolongs the action potential by prolonging repolarization via its class III effects by blockade of I_{Kr} channels, in both atrial and ventricular tissues. As a result of both β-blockade (nonselective) and potassium channel blockade, there is overall slowing in heart rate, AV nodal conduction, conduction across accessory bypass tracts,[69] as well as an increase in AV nodal refractory period.[70] Class III effects are seen at more than 160 mg daily; at dosages of 160 to 640 mg/d, the QT interval is increased by 40 to 100 milliseconds and the corrected QT interval by 10 to 40 milliseconds.[71] There is no expected change in the QRS duration.

Sotalol also has hemodynamic effects. In a study of patients with moderate LV dysfunction (mean LV ejection fraction of $43 \pm 15\%$), there was a decrease in heart rate and systolic blood pressure both at rest and during exercise, although cardiac index was unchanged compared with placebo.[72] There was no change in LV ejection fraction within 1 year.[72] However, there is limited experience with sotalol in patients with severe LV dysfunction.

Because of its prolongation of the action potential by its class III effects, sotalol carries a dose-related proarrhythmic risk of torsades de pointes. This risk is increased in the setting of bradycardia, female gender, preexisting QT prolongation, history of heart failure, or hypokalemia. Torsades de pointes is estimated to occur in 4% of patients with a prior history of sustained ventricular tachycardia or ventricular fibrillation, and otherwise with an incidence of 1% to 1.4% in average- or low-risk patients.[73] The risk of torsades de pointes increases with QTc. The estimated incidence is 3.4% for a QTc between 500 and 525 milliseconds, and 10.8% for a QTc greater than 550 milliseconds.[73] Risk also increases with dose, to about 3.2% for doses greater than 320 mg per day.[73]

Sotalol is excreted unchanged by the kidneys by glomerular filtration primarily, and to a minimal degree by tubular secretion. Therefore, caution should be used in patients with renal dysfunction. It is 90% to 100% bioavailable after oral administration but absorption is decreased if sotalol is given with a meal. Antacids should be avoided within 2 hours because they may reduce peak serum concentrations and area under the plasma concentration curve.[73] There is no first-pass effect, so hepatic function does not affect plasma levels. The peak plasma concentration is reached in 2.5 to 4 hours, a steady-state level is reached after 2 to 3 days, and the mean elimination half-life is 12 hours. With twice-daily dosing, the trough concentration is one-half of peak.[73] In renal dysfunction, sotalol clearance is reduced and the drug should be dosed over a longer interval. For a creatinine clearance of 30 to 59 mL/min, sotalol should be administered at an interval of 24 hours, starting at low dose (80 mg), with cautious uptitration after a minimum of 5 to 6 dosages.[73]

Because sotalol is not metabolized by the liver, it does not have any drug interactions related to P450 metabolism. However, because of its β-blocking effects, sotalol should be used with caution in asthmatic patients, or with other drugs that have β-blocking effects or calcium channel blocking medications that may further decrease AV conduction. Sotalol should also not be used in conjunction with medications that can prolong the QT interval. There are no pharmacokinetic interactions with warfarin, digoxin, or hydrochlorothiazide.

Ibutilide

Ibutilide exerts its class III actions by a combination of both blockade of the rapid component of the delayed rectifier potassium current, Ikr, as well as by promoting the slow inward sodium current. It therefore prolongs the action potential duration and the QT interval in proportion to plasma concentration, but without reverse use-dependence. Ibutilide remains effective at fast pacing rates in vitro.[74] There is no significant effect on heart rate, PR interval, or QRS duration, and no significant change in blood pressure, cardiac output, or pulmonary capillary wedge pressure,[75] In particular, there was no change in these hemodynamic parameters in patients with LV dysfunction.[75] When administered as a 1-mg dose followed by a second dose of 0.5 or 1 mg, ibutilide converted 47% of patients compared with 2% for placebo,[74] but is more effective in converting atrial flutter than atrial fibrillation.[76] It is approved by the FDA for the conversion of recent-onset atrial fibrillation and atrial flutter.

The overall risk of torsades de pointes is about 4% to 5%,[77] and thus patients must be monitored closely following administration (4 hours is recommended). In a study of 266 patients randomized to ibutilide or placebo,[76] statistically significant factors for the development of torsades de pointes included sex (13.2% in women vs 3.8% in men), heart failure (11.4% with heart failure vs 3.6% without), and race (15.9% in nonwhite vs 3.6% white).

Ibutilide must be given intravenously because it undergoes extensive first-pass metabolism. Protein binding is minimal at approximately 40%. Ibutilide has an elimination half-life in the range of 2 to 12 hours and a clearance of 29 mL/min/kg, which parallels liver blood flow.[78] Metabolism is via hepatic oxidation and hydroxylation but not by P450 enzymes. Ibutilide is excreted predominantly in the urine (82% of a 0.01/kg dose) and the rest in feces. Ibutilide can be administered to patients receiving digoxin, calcium channel blockers, or β-blockers without interaction, but the risk for proarrhythmia is increased if concomitant medications are used that increase the QT interval.

There is no recommendation for changing dosage for renal or liver dysfunction. The increased risk of the development of torsades de pointes in patients with heart failure does not seem to be related to drug exposure, as pharmacokinetic parameters including plasma concentration, systemic clearance, volume of distribution, and area under the serum concentration versus time curve are not altered in patients with heart failure.[78]

Vernakalant

Vernakalant acts predominantly on atrial tissue and blocks the rapidly activating delayed rectifier potassium channel I_{Kur} (contributed by the Kv1.5 protein present in human atrial but not ventricular tissue).[79] To a lesser extent, it blocks other potassium currents (I_{to}, hERG, and I_{KAch}) and also exhibits rate- and voltage-dependent blockade of the fast inward sodium current (I_{Na}).[79,80] It prolongs the refractory period in the atrium but has no significant effect on ventricular refractory period.[80] In addition, the drug can minimally prolong the sinus node recovery time, and AV nodal refractoriness.[80] The intravenous formulation of this drug is awaiting approval by the FDA, and an oral form of this medication is still under investigation.

The Atrial Arrhythmia Conversion Trial (ACT) I[81] and ACT III[82] trials studied 575 patients with atrial fibrillation, randomized to vernakalant (3 mg/kg followed by 2 mg/kg if sinus rhythm was not achieved) versus placebo with a primary end point of achieving sinus rhythm for at least 1 minute within 90 minutes of start of infusion. The primary end point was analyzed for 390 patients with atrial fibrillation of short duration (3 hours to 7 days), with analyses secondarily performed on patients with atrial fibrillation of longer duration (7 to 45 days). The combined results for ACT I and ACT IIII showed a conversion to sinus rhythm in 51.1% of patients treated with vernakalant compared with 3.8% treated with placebo (P<.0001). The median time for conversion was 11 minutes. For atrial fibrillation of longer duration (7 to 45 days) there was no statistically significant difference in conversion rates compared with placebo. Vernakalant slightly prolonged the QRS duration (8 milliseconds), and the corrected QT interval (20 milliseconds for the Bazett correction and 23 milliseconds by the Fridericia correction).[82]

The AVRO trial, presented at the Scientific Sessions of the Heart Rhythm Society (2010), randomized 254 patients with short duration atrial fibrillation to vernakalant versus intravenous amiodarone with a primary end point of conversion to sinus rhythm within 90 minutes of infusion. Vernakalant was more effective than amiodarone, converting 51.7% of patients compared with 5.2% of patients given amiodarone.

In the ACT II trial,[83] performed in patients after cardiac surgery with new atrial fibrillation or atrial flutter, 47% converted to sinus rhythm with up to 2 infusions of vernakalant, compared with 14% who received placebo with a median time to conversion of 12 minutes. Vernakalant was not effective for the few patients with atrial flutter.[83]

Adverse effects were analyzed from patients in all phase 2 and phase 3 trials. Ventricular fibrillation occurred in the first 2 hours of infusion of vernakalant in 2 patients, one of which was fatal in a hypotensive patient with critical aortic stenosis, and the second related to a nonsynchronized cardioversion.[82] There were 4 events of torsades de pointes, one in a placebo patient; 3 events occurred after 24 hours and one event immediately after administration of ibutilide.[82] Side effects for vernakalant include altered taste, sneezing, paresthesias, and nausea. Hypotension was reported in 5.4% of patients who received vernakalant compared with 1.0% of placebo patients and was highest in patients with heart failure.[82]

Vernakalant is administered intravenously as 2 10-minute infusions (3 mg/kg followed by 2 mg/kg). In the ACT I trial, the median value of the maximal plasma concentration, C_{max}, after 2 infusions was 4.8 μg/mL.[84] Vernakalant is metabolized by 4-O-demethylation by the CYP2D6 enzyme to RSD 1385, and has an elimination half-life of approximately 3 hours for extensive metabolizers and 8 hours for patients who poorly metabolize the drug.[84] A second, minor metabolite is RSD1390. These metabolites are equal or less potent than vernakalant[84] but the bulk of the metabolites circulate predominantly in a glucuronide conjugated form that is inactive.

Plasma concentration maximum (C_{max}) and the AUC versus time are dose dependent and similar between patients who are extensive or poor CYP2D6 metabolizers.[84] Likewise, clearance of the drug is not affected by medications that inhibit CYP2D6. Binding to plasma proteins is between 53% and 63%.[85] It is unknown what interactions vernakalant may have with P-glycoprotein. It is a moderately potent competitive inhibitor of CYP2D6 but does not inhibit other P450 enzymes.

VAUGHAN WILLIAMS CLASS IV: CALCIUM CHANNEL BLOCKADE (NONDIHYDROPYRIDINE)

Diltiazem and verapamil block the L-type calcium channel, resulting in relaxation of arterial smooth muscle and vasodilatation, and decreased contractility in cardiac myocytes. These agents also slow AV nodal conduction and increase AV node refractoriness. Blockade is greater at faster heart rates. Verapamil also blocks sodium channels, but this is not believed to be a clinically important effect. Peripheral vasodilatation may result in hypotension, which may reflexively increase sympathetic stimulation. As a result, sinus rates are only mildly reduced, and furthermore, in the presence of an accessory bypass tract, conduction may be enhanced even although there is no direct effect on conduction or refractoriness of atrial or ventricular tissue.

Verapamil and diltiazem are both well absorbed from the gastrointestinal tract and undergo significant first-pass effects in the liver, giving a bioavailability of 20% to 35% for verapamil[86] and about 40% for diltiazem.[87] Bioavailability and elimination half-life are increased in patients with hepatic impairment. Diltiazem and verapamil are metabolized in the liver by CYP3A4[1]; therefore levels can be increased in the presence of inhibitors of this P450 enzyme such as clarithromycin, itraconazole, ketoconazole, and human immunodeficiency virus antiviral agents. Norverapamil is the predominant metabolite of verapamil, with about 20% of the cardiac activity of verapamil[86] and can reach similar plasma concentrations. Verapamil can also interact with P-glycoprotein and the renal elimination of digoxin, increasing digoxin levels by 60% to 90%.[88]

REFERENCES

1. Flockhart D. Drug interactions: cytochrome p450 drug interaction table. Available at: http://medicine.iupui.edu/clinpharm/ddis/table.asp; 2007. Accessed March 23, 2010.
2. The Sicilian gambit. A new approach to the classification of antiarrhythmic drugs based on their actions on arrhythmogenic mechanisms. Task Force of the Working Group on Arrhythmias of the European Society of Cardiology. Circulation 1991;84(4):1831–51.
3. Hodgkin AL, Huxley AF. A quantitative description of membrane current and its application to conduction and excitation in nerve. J Physiol 1952;117(4):500–44.
4. Hille B. Local anesthetics: hydrophilic and hydrophobic pathways for the drug-receptor reaction. J Gen Physiol 1977;69(4):497–515.
5. Hondeghem L, Katzung BG. Test of a model of antiarrhythmic drug action. Effects of quinidine and lidocaine on myocardial conduction. Circulation 1980;61(6):1217–24.
6. Komeichi K, Tohse N, Nakaya H, et al. Effects of N-acetylprocainamide and sotalol on ion currents in isolated guinea-pig ventricular myocytes. Eur J Pharmacol 1990;187(3):313–22.
7. Roden DM, Reele SB, Higgins SB, et al. Antiarrhythmic efficacy, pharmacokinetics and safety of N-acetylprocainamide in human subjects: comparison with procainamide. Am J Cardiol 1980;46(3):463–8.
8. Somogyi A, McLean A, Heinzow B. Cimetidine-procainamide pharmacokinetic interaction in man: evidence of competition for tubular secretion of basic drugs. Eur J Clin Pharmacol 1983;25(3):339–45.
9. Christian CD Jr, Meredith CG, Speeg KV Jr. Cimetidine inhibits renal procainamide clearance. Clin Pharmacol Ther 1984;36(2):221–7.
10. Somogyi A, Bochner F. Dose and concentration dependent effect of ranitidine on procainamide disposition and renal clearance in man. Br J Clin Pharmacol 1984;18(2):175–81.
11. Ellrodt AG, Murata GH, Riedinger MS, et al. Severe neutropenia associated with sustained-release procainamide. Ann Intern Med 1984;100(2):197–201.
12. Klotz U. Antiarrhythmics: elimination and dosage considerations in hepatic impairment. Clin Pharm 2007;46(12):985–96.
13. Ochs HR, Greenblatt DJ, Woo E. Clinical pharmacokinetics of quinidine. Clin Pharm 1980;5(2):150–68.
14. Kornfeld P, Horowitz SH, Genkins G, et al. Myasthenia gravis unmasked by antiarrhythmic agents. Mt Sinai J Med 1976;43(1):10–4.
15. Gupta PK, Lichstein E, Chadda KD. Lidocaine-induced heart block in patients with bundle branch block. Am J Cardiol 1974;33(4):487–92.
16. Aravindakshan V, Kuo CS, Gettes LS. Effect of lidocaine on escape rate in patients with complete atrioventricular block. A distal His bundle block. Am J Cardiol 1977;40(2):177–83.
17. Yamaguchi I, Singh BN, Mandel WJ. Electrophysiological actions of mexiletine on isolated rabbit atria and canine ventricular muscle and Purkinje fibres. Cardiovasc Res 1979;13(5):288–96.
18. Wyman MG, Slaughter RL, Farolino DA, et al. Multiple bolus technique for lidocaine administration in acute ischemic heart disease. II. Treatment of refractory ventricular arrhythmias and the pharmacokinetic significance of severe left ventricular failure. J Am Coll Cardiol 1983;2(4):764–9.
19. Grant AO. Propafenone: an effective agent for the management of supraventricular arrhythmias. J Cardiovasc Electrophysiol 1996;7(4):353–64.

20. Siddoway LA, Thompson KA, McAllister CB, et al. Polymorphism of propafenone metabolism and disposition in man: clinical and pharmacokinetic consequences. Circulation 1987;75(4):785–91.

21. Follmer CH, Colatsky TJ. Block of delayed rectifier potassium current, IK, by flecainide and E-4031 in cat ventricular myocytes. Circulation 1990;82(1):289–93.

22. Preliminary report: effect of encainide and flecainide on mortality in a randomized trial of arrhythmia suppression after myocardial infarction. The Cardiac Arrhythmia Suppression Trial (CAST) Investigators. N Engl J Med 1989;321(6):406–12.

23. Kuck KH, Cappato R, Siebels J, et al. Randomized comparison of antiarrhythmic drug therapy with implantable defibrillators in patients resuscitated from cardiac arrest: the Cardiac Arrest Study Hamburg (CASH). Circulation 2000;102(7):748–54.

24. Food and Drug Administration.. Label information for propafenone. Available at: http://www.accessdata.fda.gov/drugsatfda_docs/anda/2000/75203_Propafenone%20Hydrochloride_Prntlbl.pdf. Accessed May 1, 2010.

25. Furlanello F, Vergara G, Bettini R, et al. Flecainide and encainide. Eur Heart J 1987;8(Suppl A):33–40.

26. The Cardiac Insufficiency Bisoprolol Study II (CIBIS-II): a randomised trial. Lancet 1999;353(9146):9–13.

27. Effect of metoprolol CR/XL in chronic heart failure: metoprolol CR/XL Randomised Intervention Trial in Congestive Heart Failure (MERIT-HF). Lancet 1999;353(9169):2001–7.

28. Packer M, Bristow MR, Cohn JN, et al. The effect of carvedilol on morbidity and mortality in patients with chronic heart failure. U.S. Carvedilol Heart Failure Study Group. N Engl J Med 1996;334(21):1349–55.

29. Sandberg A, Blomqvist I, Jonsson UE, et al. Pharmacokinetic and pharmacodynamic properties of a new controlled-release formulation of metoprolol: a comparison with conventional tablets. Eur J Clin Pharmacol 1988;33(Suppl):S9–14.

30. Charlier R, Deltour G, Baudine A, et al. Pharmacology of amiodarone, and anti-anginal drug with a new biological profile. Arzneimittelforschung 1968;18(11):1408–17.

31. Vassallo P, Trohman RG. Prescribing amiodarone: an evidence-based review of clinical indications. JAMA 2007;298(11):1312–22.

32. Goldschlager N, Epstein AE, Naccarelli G, et al. Practical guidelines for clinicians who treat patients with amiodarone. Practice Guidelines Subcommittee, North American Society of Pacing and Electrophysiology. Arch Intern Med 2000;160(12):1741–8.

33. Vorperian VR, Havighurst TC, Miller S, et al. Adverse effects of low dose amiodarone: a meta-analysis. J Am Coll Cardiol 1997;30(3):791–8.

34. Mason JW. Amiodarone. N Engl J Med 1987;316(8):455–66.

35. Mason JW, Hondeghem LM, Katzung BG. Amiodarone blocks inactivated cardiac sodium channels. Pflugers Arch 1983;396(1):79–81.

36. Talajic M, DeRoode MR, Nattel S. Comparative electrophysiologic effects of intravenous amiodarone and desethylamiodarone in dogs: evidence for clinically relevant activity of the metabolite. Circulation 1987;75(1):265–71.

37. Cushing DJ, Kowey PR, Cooper WD, et al. PM101: a cyclodextrin-based intravenous formulation of amiodarone devoid of adverse hemodynamic effects. Eur J Pharmacol 2009;607(1-3):167–72.

38. Klein I, Danzi S. Thyroid disease and the heart. Circulation 2007;116(15):1725–35.

39. Harjai KJ, Licata AA. Effects of amiodarone on thyroid function. Ann Intern Med 1997;126(1):63–73.

40. Amico JA, Richardson V, Alpert B, et al. Clinical and chemical assessment of thyroid function during therapy with amiodarone. Arch Intern Med 1984;144(3):487–90.

41. Bogazzi F, Bartalena L, Tomisti L, et al. Glucocorticoid response in amiodarone-induced thyrotoxicosis resulting from destructive thyroiditis is predicted by thyroid volume and serum free thyroid hormone concentrations. J Clin Endocrinol Metab 2007;92(2):556–62.

42. Camus P, Martin WJ 2nd, Rosenow EC 3rd. Amiodarone pulmonary toxicity. Clin Chest Med 2004;25(1):65–75.

43. Morady F, Sauve MJ, Malone P, et al. Long-term efficacy and toxicity of high-dose amiodarone therapy for ventricular tachycardia or ventricular fibrillation. Am J Cardiol 1983;52(8):975–9.

44. Singh BN, Hein JJ, Wellens MH, et al, editors. Electropharmacologic control of cardiac arrhythmias: to delay conduction or to prolong refractoriness? New York: Futura; 1994. p. 501.

45. Holt DW, Tucker GT, Jackson PR, et al. Amiodarone pharmacokinetics. Br J Clin Pract Suppl 1986;44:109–14.

46. Varro A, Takacs J, Nemeth M, et al. Electrophysiological effects of dronedarone (SR 33589), a noniodinated amiodarone derivative in the canine heart: comparison with amiodarone. Br J Pharmacol 2001;133(5):625–34.

47. Gautier P, Guillemare E, Marion A, et al. Electrophysiologic characterization of dronedarone in guinea pig ventricular cells. J Cardiovasc Pharmacol 2003;41(2):191–202.

48. Aimond F, Beck L, Gautier P, et al. Cellular and in vivo electrophysiological effects of dronedarone in normal and postmyocardial infarcted rats. J Pharmacol Exp Ther 2000;292(1):415–24.

49. Sun W, Sarma JS, Singh BN. Electrophysiological effects of dronedarone (SR33589), a noniodinated

benzofuran derivative, in the rabbit heart: comparison with amiodarone. Circulation 1999;100(22): 2276–81.

50. Lalevee N, Nargeot J, Barrere-Lemaire S, et al. Effects of amiodarone and dronedarone on voltage-dependent sodium current in human cardiomyocytes. J Cardiovasc Electrophysiol 2003;14(8): 885–90.

51. Wegener FT, Ehrlich JR, Hohnloser SH. Dronedarone: an emerging agent with rhythm- and rate-controlling effects. J Cardiovasc Electrophysiol 2006;17(Suppl 2):S17–20.

52. Patel C, Yan GX, Kowey PR. Dronedarone. Circulation 2009;120(7):636–44.

53. Chatelain P, Meysmans L, Matteazzi JR, et al. Interaction of the antiarrhythmic agents SR 33589 and amiodarone with the beta-adrenoceptor and adenylate cyclase in rat heart. Br J Pharmacol 1995; 116(3):1949–56.

54. Guiraudou P, Pucheu SC, Gayraud R, et al. Involvement of nitric oxide in amiodarone- and dronedarone-induced coronary vasodilation in guinea pig heart. Eur J Pharmacol 2004;496(1–3): 119–27.

55. Hohnloser SH, Crijns HJ, van Eickels M, et al. Effect of dronedarone on cardiovascular events in atrial fibrillation. N Engl J Med 2009;360(7): 668–78.

56. Tschuppert Y, Buclin T, Rothuizen LE, et al. Effect of dronedarone on renal function in healthy subjects. Br J Clin Pharmacol 2007;64(6):785–91.

57. Naccarelli GV, Wolbrette DL, Khan M, et al. Old and new antiarrhythmic drugs for converting and maintaining sinus rhythm in atrial fibrillation: comparative efficacy and results of trials. Am J Cardiol 2003; 91(6A):15D–26D.

58. Rousseau MF, Massart PE, van Eyll C, et al. Cardiac and hemodynamic effects of intravenous dofetilide in patients with heart failure. Am J Cardiol 2001; 87(11):1250–4.

59. Singh S, Zoble RG, Yellen L, et al. Efficacy and safety of oral dofetilide in converting to and maintaining sinus rhythm in patients with chronic atrial fibrillation or atrial flutter: the symptomatic atrial fibrillation investigative research on dofetilide (SAFIRE-D) study. Circulation 2000;102(19): 2385–90.

60. Pedersen OD, Bagger H, Keller N, et al. Efficacy of dofetilide in the treatment of atrial fibrillation-flutter in patients with reduced left ventricular function: a Danish Investigations of Arrhythmia and Mortality on Dofetilide (DIAMOND) substudy. Circulation 2001;104(3):292–6.

61. Greenbaum RA, Channer KS, Dalrymple HW, et al. Conversion of atrial fibrillation and maintenance of sinus rhythm by dofetilide. The EMERALD (European and Australian Multicenter Evaluative Research on Atrial Fibrillation and Dofetilide) study [abstract]. Circulation 1998;98(Suppl 17):I633.

62. Kober L, Bloch Thomsen PE, Moller M, et al. Effect of dofetilide in patients with recent myocardial infarction and left-ventricular dysfunction: a randomised trial. Lancet 2000;356(9247):2052–8.

63. Torp-Pedersen C, Moller M, Bloch-Thomsen PE, et al. Dofetilide in patients with congestive heart failure and left ventricular dysfunction. Danish Investigations of Arrhythmia and Mortality on Dofetilide Study Group. N Engl J Med 1999;341(12): 857–65.

64. Food and Drug Administration. Label information for dofetilide. Available at: http://www.accessdata.fda. gov/drugsatfda_docs/label/1999/20931lbl.pdf. Accessed May 1, 2010.

65. Tikosyn US physician prescribing information. Available at: http://media.pfizer.com/files/products/uspi_ tikosyn.pdf. Accessed May 19, 2010.

66. Waldo AL, Camm AJ, deRuyter H, et al. Effect of d-sotalol on mortality in patients with left ventricular dysfunction after recent and remote myocardial infarction. The SWORD Investigators. Survival With Oral d-Sotalol. Lancet 1996;348(9019):7–12.

67. Pratt CM, Camm AJ, Cooper W, et al. Mortality in the survival with oral D-sotalol (SWORD) trial: why did patients die? Am J Cardiol 1998;81(7):869–76.

68. Julian DG, Prescott RJ, Jackson FS, et al. Controlled trial of sotalol for one year after myocardial infarction. Lancet 1982;1(8282):1142–7.

69. Kunze KP, Schluter M, Kuck KH. Sotalol in patients with Wolff-Parkinson-White syndrome. Circulation 1987;75(5):1050–7.

70. Kopelman HA, Woosley RL, Lee JT, et al. Electrophysiologic effects of intravenous and oral sotalol for sustained ventricular tachycardia secondary to coronary artery disease. Am J Cardiol 1988;61(13): 1006–11.

71. Hohnloser SH, Woosley RL. Sotalol. N Engl J Med 1994;331(1):31–8.

72. Mahmarian JJ, Verani MS, Pratt CM. Hemodynamic effects of intravenous and oral sotalol. Am J Cardiol 1990;65(2):28A–34A [discussion: 35A–6A].

73. Food and Drug Administration. Label information for sotalol. Available at: http://www.accessdata.fda.gov/ drugsatfda_docs/nda/2001/19-865S010_Betapace_ prntlbl.pdf. Accessed May 1, 2010.

74. Murray KT. Ibutilide. Circulation 1998;97(5):493–7.

75. Stambler BS, Beckman KJ, Kadish AH, et al. Acute hemodynamic effects of intravenous ibutilide in patients with or without reduced left ventricular function. Am J Cardiol 1997;80(4):458–63.

76. Stambler BS, Wood MA, Ellenbogen KA, et al. Efficacy and safety of repeated intravenous doses of ibutilide for rapid conversion of atrial flutter or fibrillation. Ibutilide Repeat Dose Study Investigators. Circulation 1996;94(7):1613–21.

77. Kowey PR, Marinchak RA, Rials SJ, et al. Pharmacologic and pharmacokinetic profile of class III antiarrhythmic drugs. Am J Cardiol 1997;80(8A):16G–23G.

78. Tisdale JE, Overholser BR, Sowinski KM, et al. Pharmacokinetics of ibutilide in patients with heart failure due to left ventricular systolic dysfunction. Pharmacotherapy 2008;28(12):1461–70.

79. Fedida D, Orth PM, Chen JY, et al. The mechanism of atrial antiarrhythmic action of RSD1235. J Cardiovasc Electrophysiol 2005;16(11):1227–38.

80. Dorian P, Pinter A, Mangat I, et al. The effect of vernakalant (RSD1235), an investigational antiarrhythmic agent, on atrial electrophysiology in humans. J Cardiovasc Pharmacol 2007;50(1):35–40.

81. Roy D, Pratt CM, Torp-Pedersen C, et al. Vernakalant hydrochloride for rapid conversion of atrial fibrillation: a phase 3, randomized, placebo-controlled trial. Circulation 2008;117(12): 1518–25.

82. Food and Drug Administration. Briefing materials for Cardiovascular and Renal Drugs Advisory Committee. Astellas Pharma US, Inc; 2007. Kynapid (vernakalant hydrochloride injection) NDA 22–034. Available at: http://www.fda.gov/ohrms/dockets/ac/ 07/briefing/2007-4327b1-01-astellas-backgrounder. pdf. Accessed May 19, 2010.

83. Kowey PR, Dorian P, Mitchell LB, et al. Vernakalant hydrochloride for the rapid conversion of atrial fibrillation after cardiac surgery: a randomized, double-blind, placebo-controlled trial. Circ Arrhythm Electrophysiol 2009;2(6):652–9.

84. Mao ZL, Wheeler JJ, Clohs L, et al. Pharmacokinetics of novel atrial-selective antiarrhythmic agent vernakalant hydrochloride injection (RSD1235): influence of CYP2D6 expression and other factors. J Clin Pharmacol 2009;49(1):17–29.

85. Lemtouni S. Clinical review. Vernakalant hydrochloride. Available at: http://www.fda.gov/ohrms/dockets/ ac/07/briefing/2007-4327b1-02-fda-backgrounder.pdf. 2006. Accessed July 9, 2010.

86. Food and Drug Administration. Label information for verapamil (Calan). Available at: http://www. accessdata.fda.gov/drugsatfda_docs/label/2010/ 018817s022lbl.pdf. Accessed May 18, 2010.

87. Food and Drug Administration. Label information for diltiazem (Cardizem LA). Available at: http://www. accessdata.fda.gov/drugsatfda_docs/label/2007/ 021392s010lbl.pdf. Accessed July 9, 2010.

88. Verschraagen M, Koks CH, Schellens JH, et al. P-glycoprotein system as a determinant of drug interactions: the case of digoxin-verapamil. Pharm Res 1999;40(4):301–6.

How Does Genetics Influence the Efficacy and Safety of Antiarrhythmic Drugs?

Katherine T. Murray, MD

KEYWORDS

- Antiarrhythmic drugs • Pharmacogenetics
- Cytochrome P450

Despite recent advances in nonpharmacologic therapy, antiarrhythmic drugs remain a cornerstone in the treatment of cardiac arrhythmias. However, a major challenge in prescribing these and many other drugs is variability in the response to therapy. The pharmacologic treatment of atrial fibrillation (AF) serves as an illustrative example; long-term suppression with antiarrhythmic drugs is achieved in a minority of patients, and it is impossible to identify which patients will respond to a specific agent. Similarly, serious adverse effects, including proarrhythmia, can occur in an unpredictable manner. In the era of modern genomics, there is increasing evidence that unusual or idiosyncratic drug responses can be genetically determined, as well as clinical benefit. This review highlights our current understanding of the role of genetics in both the safety and efficacy of antiarrhythmic drugs.

Variability in drug response can occur through 2 broad mechanisms: (1) altered *pharmacokinetics*, which describes the relationship between drug dose and the subsequent concentration achieved in plasma or tissue; and (2) altered *pharmacodynamics*, or the relationship between the concentration of a drug and its pharmacologic effects. Following oral ingestion, there are 4 main pharmacokinetic processes that determine the plasma concentration of a drug: absorption, distribution, metabolism, and elimination or excretion. Although interindividual variability can occur for each of these processes, the most striking

examples result from unusual drug metabolism/ elimination, as detailed later in this article. In addition, there are a variety of pharmacodynamic mechanisms that can modulate the effects resulting from a given drug concentration, including variability of drug uptake into tissues, variable abundance or function of a target protein, and additional factors (such as disease states, electrolyte disturbances, and concomitant drug therapy) that reflect the specific biologic milieu of individual patients. As discussed later, such modulating factors play an essential role in an individual patient's response to QT-prolonging drugs.

With the recent advances and expanding use of DNA sequencing, it is increasingly evident that genetics plays an important role in interindividual variability for both pharmacokinetic and pharmacodynamic processes (**Table 1**). The earliest reports of aberrant drug response were caused by prototypical genetic mutations (for example, the occurrence of hemolytic anemia in patients lacking glucose-6-phosphate dehydrogenase treated with antimalarial drugs).[1] In general, mutations are rare genetic variants (frequency <1%) occurring most often in regions of the DNA sequence that encode protein, which typically results in a change in the amino acid sequence, leading to altered protein function and associated disease. More common DNA variants exist in both coding and noncoding regulatory regions of a gene. These variants can cause a change in an individual base pair (single nucleotide

Financial disclosures: The author has nothing to disclose.

Division of Clinical Pharmacology, Departments of Medicine and Pharmacology, Vanderbilt University School of Medicine, Room 559 Preston Research Building, 2220 Pierce Avenue, Nashville, TN 37232-6602, USA
E-mail address: kathy.murray@vanderbilt.edu

Card Electrophysiol Clin 2 (2010) 359–367
doi:10.1016/j.ccep.2010.06.004

Table 1
Proarrhythmia with antiarrhythmic drugs: pharmacokinetic and pharmacodynamic interactions

	Pharmacokinetic		Pharmacodynamic	
	Gene	Effect	Gene	Effect
Drug-induced long QT syndrome	CYP2D6	Increased risk for PMs taking QT-prolonging antipsychotic drugs (eg, thioridazine)	KCNH2 (HERG) KCNQ1 KCNE1 SCN5A	Increased risk for proarrhythmia for subclinical mutations in the long QT syndrome
Sodium channel blocker toxicity	CYP2D6	Increased risk for PMs taking flecainide (in combination with renal insufficiency)	SCN5A	Increased risk for ventricular fibrillation for subclinical Brugada syndrome mutations

Abbreviation: PM, poor metabolizer.

Data from Roden DM. Proarrhythmia as a pharmacogenomic entity: a critical review and formulation of a unifying hypothesis. Cardiovasc Res 2005;67:419–25; with permission.

polymorphism [SNP]), or larger insertions/deletions of multiple nucleotides. Although protein function or expression can be modified as a result of some SNPs, in other cases the functional consequences remain unknown.

An emerging theme in contemporary biology is the recognition of redundancy for many physiologic processes. For example, multiple ionic currents act in concert to mediate cardiac repolarization. Similarly, most drugs are eliminated by multiple metabolic pathways. Such redundancy serves as a protective mechanism, given that individual components of a process can become deficient through genetics, disease states, or pharmacologic suppression. *Pharmacogenetics* is a term relating the effects of an individual gene variant to variable drug effects. Based on the concept of physiologic redundancy, the risk for an aberrant drug response is greatest when the elimination of a compound is dependent primarily on a single pathway. This risk is particularly true for antiarrhythmic drugs, which have a narrow therapeutic ratio or margin between plasma concentrations associated with efficacy and those causing toxicity. A simple example of this concept is the effect of kidney disease to increase plasma concentrations of sotalol and dofetilide, which are renally excreted, thereby increasing the risk for QT prolongation and torsades de pointes. This principle also applies to metabolic elimination, in which the activity of specific liver enzymes can be highly variable.

VARIABLE ANTIARRHYTHMIC DRUG RESPONSE: PHARMACOKINETIC MECHANISMS

Genetically based variability in the disposition of antiarrhythmic drugs primarily involves the process of metabolism or excretion. The metabolism of exogenous compounds generally converts drugs into water soluble forms that are more easily excreted. For a given compound, the pharmacologic effects of variable drug metabolism depend on the relative potency or toxicity of the metabolites, compared with the parent compound. Metabolic pathways are classified into 2 types.[2] Phase I enzymes render exogenous compounds more reactive through chemical reactions that involve oxidation, reduction, and hydrolysis. The most important members of this group are the cytochrome P450 (CYP) enzymes (**Fig. 1**). Phase II enzymes mediate conjugation reactions (eg, acetylation, sulfation, glucuronidation, and methylation) to increase a drug's solubility to promote its excretion. There are a variety of factors that determine the activity of specific CYP enzymes for an individual patient, including normal variability in quantity, genetic variants, and drugs that inhibit or enhance enzyme activity. For antiarrhythmic drugs and other compounds (eg, warfarin) that have a narrow therapeutic ratio, the risk for adverse events is greatest when there is a single route of elimination that is variable, thus constituting a high-risk pharmacokinetic scenario.[3]

Phase I Metabolism

CYP2D6

The CYP2D6 enzyme is responsible for the metabolism of a significant number of marketed drugs (see **Fig. 1**).[4] Genetically based variation in CYP2D6 is now recognized to cause striking differences in the clinical effects and toxicity for multiple drugs metabolized by this enzyme. A large number of loss-of-function variants for CYP2D6 have been identified, and enzyme activity is deficient in 5% to 10% of Caucasian and African American patients who are

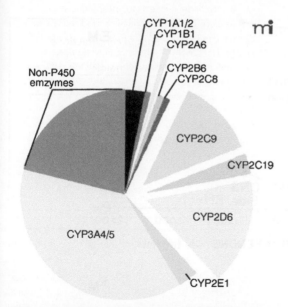

Fig. 1. Contribution of CYP enzymes to the Phase I metabolism of marketed drugs. The estimates are approximate and vary with time. Non-P450 enzymes include alcohol and aldehyde dehydrogenases. (*Reproduced from* Guengerich FP. Cytochromes P450, drugs, and diseases. Mol Interv 2003;3:194–204; with permission.)

homozygous for these alleles.[5,6] These individuals, termed poor metabolizers (PMs), have a greater likelihood of adverse reactions because of the high plasma concentrations of the affected drug (**Fig. 2**), compared to extensive metabolizers (EMs). For the class 1c drug propafenone, an important metabolic pathway is mediated by CYP2D6.[6,7] Both propafenone and its metabolites

are sodium channel blockers. On the other hand, the parent drug possesses beta-adrenergic receptor blocking activity, which is considerably weaker in the metabolites.[8] Indeed, PMs develop higher propafenone plasma concentrations compared with EMs, with an increased risk for central nervous system (CNS)-related adverse effects likely caused by beta-blockade (**Fig. 3**).[9] However, arrhythmia effect (ie, suppression of premature ventricular contractions) has been shown to be equivalent in PMs and EMs. Based on these considerations, propafenone should be used with caution in patients in whom beta-blockade would be poorly tolerated (eg, individuals with bradycardia or bronchospasm). CYP2D6 is also the primary route of metabolism for codeine, several beta-blockers (including metoprolol and timolol), and some antipsychotic drugs.[6,10] In the case of codeine, conversion to the active metabolite morphine is required for pharmacologic effect, and PMs have reduced analgesia when taking codeine.

In addition to genetic-based deficiency, several drugs inhibit CYP2D6 to mimic the PM state, including quinidine, fluoxetine, paroxetine, dronedarone, and tricyclic antidepressants.[11–13] Patients with psychiatric illnesses are often co-prescribed antipsychotics and antidepressants. However, multiple antipsychotic drugs (eg, thioridazine) prolong the QT interval,[14,15] and combination therapy with these two classes of drugs can increase the risk for marked QT prolongation and torsades de pointes (see **Table 1**). In some patients, extra copies of CYP2D6 alleles through gene duplication can lead to ultrarapid metabolism (see **Fig. 2**).

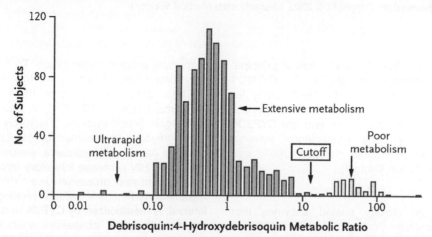

Fig. 2. Pharmacogenetics of CYP2D6. Urinary ratios of debrisoquin, a CYP2D6 substrate, and its metabolite, 4-hydroxydebrisoquin, are shown for 1011 subjects. The cutoff indicates the point of separation between poor metabolizers lacking CYP2D6 activity and extensive metabolizers. (*From* Weinshilboum R. Inheritance and drug response. N Engl J Med 2003;348:529–37; with permission. Copyright © 2003, Massachusetts Medical Society.)

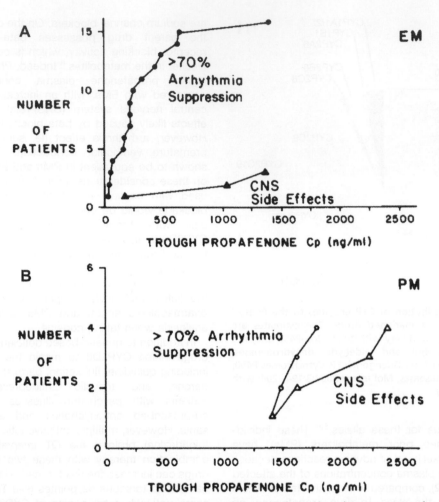

Fig. 3. CYP2D6 metabolic status and response to propafenone. Relationships between propafenone plasma concentration and the cumulative frequency of antiarrhythmic response (suppression of premature ventricular contractions), as well as CNS side effects, are shown. (*A, B*) Data are plotted with subjects separated into EM and PM groups for CYP2D6. (*From* Weinshilboum R. Inheritance and drug response. N Engl J Med 2003;348:529–37; with Murray permission. Copyright © 2003, Massachusetts Medical Society.)

The class 1c drug flecainide has 2 principal routes of elimination: metabolism by CYP2D6 and renal excretion.[6] For most patients taking flecainide, the PM status poses no clinical consequences. However, if patients who are CYP2D6 PM also develop renal insufficiency, adverse effects related to sodium channel toxicity can develop (**Fig. 4**; see **Table 1**).

CYP3A

CYP3A4/5 are closely related enzymes that together constitute the most abundant CYPs in the liver (see **Fig. 1**).[11] However, expression in humans can normally be quite variable, ranging from less than 10% to 60% of total CYP liver content. CYP3A participates in the metabolism of multiple antiarrhythmic drugs. To date, genetically based loss of activity for this enzyme has not been described. However, there are several drugs that potently inhibit CYP3A, including azole antifungals (ketoconazole), macrolide antibiotics (erythromycin, clarithromycin), calcium channel blockers (verapamil, diltiazem), amiodarone, dronedarone, HIV protease inhibitors (ritonavir), and large quantities of grapefruit juice.[11,13,16] The antihistamine terfenadine, which prolongs the QT interval, is metabolized by CYP3A to a metabolite (fexofenadine) that possesses antihistamine but no electrophysiologic properties.[17] Multiple case reports demonstrate that in the setting of co-therapy with CYP3A inhibitors, liver disease, or terfenadine overdose, subjects developed

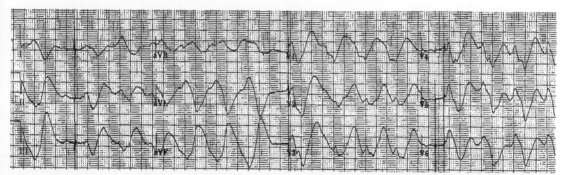

Fig. 4. Flecainide toxicity: a dual pharmacokinetic hit. The 12 lead electrocardiogram is shown for a 36-year-old woman presenting with palpitations and near syncope. She was treated chronically with flecainide for supraventricular tachycardia as well as fluoxetine (which inhibits CYP2D6), and she subsequently developed acute renal failure (serum creatinine 4.5 mg/dL, potassium 4.8 mEq/L). The ECG demonstrates marked QRS prolongation.

high plasma concentrations of terfenadine, increasing the QT interval and the risk for torsades de pointes. For both terfenadine and the antihistamine astemizole, this serious adverse response ultimately led to withdrawal of the drugs from the market. A similar pharmacokinetic scenario occurs for the prokinetic drug cisapride, which now has markedly restricted availability.[18] The macrolide antibiotic erythromycin is metabolized primarily by CYP3A, and high plasma concentrations of erythromycin (eg, with intravenous administration) can prolong the QT interval. In a pharmacoepidemiologic study using the Tennessee Medicaid database, concomitant administration of erythromycin with CYP3A inhibitors was associated with a 5- to 6-fold increased risk for sudden cardiac death, compared with erythromycin alone (2-fold increase).[19] Importantly, the class III drug dronedarone is both a substrate and inhibitor of CYP3A, and it is recommended that co-therapy with strong CYP3A inhibitors be avoided.[13,16] For example, ketoconazole causes a 9-fold increase in maximal plasma concentrations of dronedarone. For verapamil and diltiazem, dronedarone concentrations are elevated by 1.4- to 1.7 fold.

CYP2C9

CYP2C9 is responsible for the metabolic clearance of 15% to 20% of compounds undergoing phase I metabolism (see **Fig. 1**).[20] Although CYP2C9 is not a major factor in the excretion of antiarrhythmic drugs, it does mediate the metabolism of the active S-enantiomer of warfarin, which is responsible for the drug's anticoagulant effect. At least 2 loss-of-function alleles (*2 and *3) have been identified.[21,22] Very rarely, patients are homozygous for these variants, with a marked increase in warfarin plasma concentration,

international normalized ratio, and bleeding events at usual dosages. Patients heterozygous for a dysfunctional allele require less warfarin because of reduced enzyme activity. However, variants for the gene encoding the target protein for warfarin (the vitamin K epoxide reductase complex 1, or VKORC1) play a larger role than those for CYP2C9 in determining warfarin requirements.[22,23]

Phase II Metabolism

N-acetyltransferase

Genetically based variability in phase II enzymes is less common than for phase I enzymes. Nonetheless, one of the earliest examples of pharmacogenetically determined metabolism was N-acetyltransferase (NAT).[2] This enzyme acetylates multiple compounds, including procainamide, hydralazine, and isoniazid. It is now recognized that enzyme activity is controlled by 2 genes: NAT1 and NAT2.[2] Although patients normally generate sufficient quantities of NAT1, loss-of-function alleles for NAT2 lead to reduced enzyme activity and deficient metabolism (slow acetylators) of the parent compound (**Fig. 5**). During chronic oral therapy with procainamide, slow acetylators developed autoantibodies and drug-induced lupus more quickly than rapid acetylators, who had higher concentrations of N-acetyl-procainamide.[24] The NAT2 genotype also influences the risk for adverse events for other substrates (eg, increased incidence of peripheral neuropathy with isoniazid in slow acetylators).[25]

Drug Transport: P-glycoprotein

In recent years, increasing attention has focused on the role of drug transporters as a source of variable drug response. P-glycoprotein is an ATP-binding cassette protein expressed in the apical

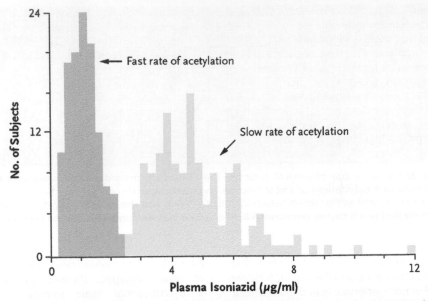

Fig. 5. Pharmacogenetics of acetylation. Isoniazid plasma concentrations were obtained in 267 subjects 6 hours after an oral dose. The bimodal distribution reflects the altered function of the N-acetyltransferase 2 (NAT2) gene in slow acetylators, compared with rapid acetylators. (*Reproduced from* Weinshilboum R. Inheritance and drug response. N Engl J Med 2003;348:529,e37; with permission.)

membrane of cells in the intestine, kidney, liver, and blood brain barrier.[26] It largely functions as an efflux pump to limit oral bioavailability and CNS accumulation of exogenous toxins and compounds by excreting them into the urine, gastrointestinal tract, and bile. It was first described in tumor cells, where it contributes to multidrug resistance (MDR) with anticancer drugs. From a cardiovascular standpoint, P-glycoprotein plays an important role to eliminate digoxin from the body. It is now recognized that variants in the gene-encoding p-glycoprotein (MDR-1) regulate its activity and appear to modulate plasma digoxin concentrations.[26] Importantly, several drugs inhibit p-glycoprotein, including quinidine, amiodarone, dronedarone, and verapamil, and this interaction is responsible for elevated digoxin plasma concentrations during concomitant therapy with these agents.[26] There is considerable overlap between substrates/inhibitors of p-glycoprotein and those of CYP3A.[27] This overlap may have developed because of the broad function of these 2 enzymes to eliminate environmental and dietary toxins.

VARIABLE DRUG RESPONSE: PHARMACODYNAMIC MECHANISMS

For patients having identical plasma concentrations of a given antiarrhythmic drug, the resultant pharmacologic effects can vary widely among individuals. Thus, pharmacodynamic variability provides another mechanism for unpredictable drug response. Proarrhythmia represents one of the most striking adverse effects of antiarrhythmic drugs, and there is now substantial evidence that pharmacodynamic factors play a major role in determining individual susceptibility.

QT Prolongation

Many antiarrhythmic drugs prolong repolarization as their major mechanism of action, usually by block of repolarizing potassium currents. However, excessive QT prolongation and ultimately torsades de pointes can develop in up to 5% of patients for some drugs.[28] More rarely, the acquired or drug-induced long QT (diLQT) syndrome can occur with a variety of noncardiac drugs, including antibiotics, antipsychotics, antihistamines, and prokinetic agents, as previously discussed.[17] The clinical and economic impact of this effect is substantial; for terfenadine and multiple other drugs, QT prolongation and associated sudden death has been a major cause for withdrawal of the drug from the United States market over the past several decades. Several clinical risk factors have been identified for the diLQT syndrome, including female gender, hypokalemia, bradycardia, underlying heart disease such as left ventricular hypertrophy, and recent conversion from AF. However, it can also occur in the absence of identifiable risk factors, strongly implying a genetic component.

Important mediators of ventricular repolarization include the rapid and slow components of the delayed rectifier potassium current (known as I_{Kr} and I_{Ks}, respectively), although additional ionic currents also contribute to this process. Virtually all drugs that cause the diLQT syndrome have been shown to block I_{Kr}.[17] The molecular basis for this current is a pore-forming alpha subunit protein encoded by KCNH2 (also known as HERG), and possibly 1 or more auxiliary channel subunits (eg, KCNE2). Thus, a primary pharmacodynamic mechanism that could increase susceptibility to the diLQT syndrome is reduced expression of the primary target protein, in this case HERG, rendering I_{Kr} blockers more potent. Alternatively, a reduction in other currents, such as I_{Ks}, that contribute to repolarization reserve would also render patients more dependent on I_{Kr}, increasing the potency of I_{Kr} block in this setting. Multiple studies have identified mutations in HERG and other ion channel genes associated with the congenital LQT syndrome in individuals and small series of subjects with the diLQT syndrome (see **Table 1**).[29–32] This finding is not surprising given that variable penetrance for the congenital LQT syndrome has been well described,[33] with an overall incidence currently estimated to be 1:3000 individuals. Patients with such mutations would have a normal QT interval at baseline, but they develop an abnormal response with drug challenge. The incidence of subclinical congenital LQT syndrome mutations in patients with the drug-induced form is 5% to 12%, indicating that it is a minor causative factor.

In addition to mutations, more common variants in congenital LQT syndrome genes have also been identified that appear to increase the risk for the drug-induced syndrome. The frequency of these polymorphisms is variable, depending upon ethnicity. The S1102Y allele in the SCN5A gene, encoding the cardiac sodium channel, is present almost exclusively in African Americans (minor allele frequency 13.2%).[34] It perturbs channel function and has been associated with increased susceptibility to sudden cardiac death and sudden infant death syndrome, as well as the diLQT syndrome. Additional variants that have been implicated include T8A and Q9E in KCNE2,[32,35,36] G643S in KCNQ1 (encoding the alpha subunit for I_{Ks}),[37] and D85 N in KCNE1 (encoding the auxiliary protein for I_{Ks}).[32]

In the diLQT syndrome, it is currently hypothesized that additional nongenetic risk factors also function to reduce repolarization reserve as a mechanism to increase arrhythmia susceptibility.[38]

Previous work has shown that hypokalemia paradoxically reduces I_{Kr} amplitude (contrary to predictions based on the Nernst equation), and this effect renders at least some I_{Kr} blockers more potent.[39]

Sodium Channel Block

Multiple lines of evidence indicate that pharmacologic or genetic suppression of cardiac sodium current can lead to proarrhythmia and sudden cardiac death.[40] Block of sodium current slows electrical impulse conduction, can promote reentry, and is associated with a variety of proarrhythmic syndromes, including 1:1 atrial flutter, incessant ventricular tachycardia in patients with poor left ventricular function, increased sudden death in patients with coronary artery disease, and exacerbation of the Brugada syndrome with ventricular fibrillation. As for the congenital LQT syndrome, genetic variants causing Brugada syndrome also demonstrate variable penetrance.[41] Thus, in an analogous manor, patients harboring mutations would demonstrate the right precordial ST elevation characteristic of this syndrome only upon exposure to a sodium channel blocker. In addition, a logical hypothesis is that subclinical Brugada syndrome mutations play a role in the increased sudden cardiac death seen with sodium channel blockers (see **Table 1**). However, this hypothesis is difficult to prove, given the challenges of ascertaining blood samples for genomic analysis from such patients. The role of genetic variants in other forms of sodium channel blocker-related proarrhythmia is currently not known.

Arrhythmia Response

Considerable progress has been made in identifying the basic mechanisms of cardiac arrhythmias, such as AF. Contemporary thinking is that AF represents a final common pathway for diverse pathophysiologic mechanisms, including genetic factors, inflammation, and neurohormonal activation, that increase arrhythmia susceptibility and fibrosis. Based on these considerations, it is reasonable to postulate that the clinical efficacy of antiarrhythmic drugs is variable because of the heterogeneous nature of the arrhythmic substrate. In the future, therapy in which causative pathways are specifically targeted offers the hope of improved efficacy and potentially reduced toxicity.

A recent study supports the concept that genetic factors involving disease pathways may be predictive of clinical response. The deletion allele (D) in the angiotensin converting enzyme gene is correlated with increased enzyme activity and adverse cardiac events. In subjects with lone

AF, the presence of 1 or 2 copies of this allele (ID or DD genotype) identified subjects less likely to respond to antiarrhythmic drugs, compared to individual homozygous for the insertion allele (II genotype).[42] Thus, increased activation of the renin-angiotensin system may outweigh the beneficial effects of antiarrhythmic drugs in these patients. These results emphasize the need for inclusion of genomic testing in antiarrhythmic drug trials, as this information may identify patients for whom alternative therapy, such as block of the renin-angiotensin system, proves to be beneficial.

SUMMARY

Recent progress in genomic sequencing has begun to elucidate the basic mechanisms for several adverse responses, as well as the clinical efficacy, for antiarrhythmic drugs. DNA variants in drug metabolizing enzymes have been implicated in excessive drug accumulation and genetic variability in drug targets can identify individuals at increased risk for serious side effects, in particular proarrhythmia. It is hoped that future advances in the area of genomic medicine will lead to more individually tailored or personalized pharmacologic therapy in the management of cardiac arrhythmias.

REFERENCES

1. Cappellini MD, Fiorelli G. Glucose-6-phosphate dehydrogenase deficiency. Lancet 2008;371: 64–74.
2. Weinshilboum R. Inheritance and drug response. N Engl J Med 2003;348:529–37.
3. Roden DM, Stein CM. Clopidogrel and the concept of high-risk pharmacokinetics. Circulation 2009; 119:2127–30.
4. Guengerich FP. Cytochromes P450, drugs, and diseases. Mol Interv 2003;3:194–204.
5. Kirchheiner J, Fuhr U, Brockmoller J. Pharmacogenetics-based therapeutic recommendations—ready for clinical practice? Nat Rev Drug Discov 2005;4: 639–47.
6. Zhou SF. Polymorphism of human cytochrome P450 2D6 and its clinical significance: part I. Clin Pharmacokinet 2009;48:689–723.
7. Funck-Brentano C, Kroemer HK, Lee JT, et al. Propafenone. N Engl J Med 1990;322:518–25.
8. Lee JT, Kroemer HK, Silberstein DJ, et al. The role of genetically determined polymorphic drug metabolism in the beta-blockade produced by propafenone. N Engl J Med 1990;322:1764–8.
9. Siddoway LA, Thompson KA, McAllister CB, et al. Polymorphism of propafenone metabolism and disposition in man: clinical and pharmacokinetic consequences. Circulation 1987;75:785–91.
10. Roden DM, Altman RB, Benowitz NL, et al. Pharmacogenomics: challenges and opportunities. Ann Intern Med 2006;145:749–57.
11. Wilkinson GR. Drug metabolism and variability among patients in drug response. N Engl J Med 2005;352:2211–21.
12. Damy T, Pousset F, Caplain H, et al. Pharmacokinetic and pharmacodynamic interactions between metoprolol and dronedarone in extensive and poor CYP2D6 metabolizers healthy subjects. Fundam Clin Pharmacol 2004;18:113–23.
13. Hoy SM, Keam SJ. Dronedarone. Drugs 2009;69: 1647–63.
14. Ray WA, Meredith S, Thapa PB, et al. Antipsychotics and the risk of sudden cardiac death. Arch Gen Psychiatry 2001;58:1161–7.
15. Ray WA, Chung CP, Murray KT, et al. Atypical antipsychotic drugs and the risk of sudden cardiac death. N Engl J Med 2009;360:225–35.
16. Dronedarone (Multaq) for atrial fibrillation. Med Lett Drugs Ther 2009;51:78–80.
17. Roden DM. Drug-induced prolongation of the QT interval. N Engl J Med 2004;350:1013–22.
18. Vitola J, Vukanovic J, Roden DM. Cisapride-induced torsades de pointes. J Cardiovasc Electrophysiol 1998;9:1109–13.
19. Ray WA, Murray KT, Meredith S, et al. Oral erythromycin and the risk of sudden death from cardiac causes. N Engl J Med 2004;351:1089–96.
20. Van BD, Marsh S, McLeod H, et al. Cytochrome P450 2C9-CYP2C9. Pharmacogenet Genomics 2010;20:277–81.
21. Kirchheiner J, Brockmoller J. Clinical consequences of cytochrome P450 2C9 polymorphisms. Clin Pharmacol Ther 2005;77:1–16.
22. Schwarz UI, Ritchie MD, Bradford Y, et al. Genetic determinants of response to warfarin during initial anticoagulation. N Engl J Med 2008;358:999–1008.
23. Rieder MJ, Reiner AP, Gage BF, et al. Effect of VKORC1 haplotypes on transcriptional regulation and warfarin dose. N Engl J Med 2005;352:2285–93.
24. Woosley RL, Drayer DE, Reidenberg MM, et al. Effect of acetylator phenotype on the rate at which procainamide induces antinuclear antibodies and the lupus syndrome. N Engl J Med 1978;298:1157–9.
25. Drayer DE, Reidenberg MM. Clinical consequences of polymorphic acetylation of basic drugs. Clin Pharmacol Ther 1977;22:251–8.
26. Marzolini C, Paus E, Buclin T, et al. Polymorphisms in human MDR1 (P-glycoprotein): recent advances and clinical relevance. Clin Pharmacol Ther 2004; 75:13–33.
27. Zhou SF. Drugs behave as substrates, inhibitors and inducers of human cytochrome P450 3A4. Curr Drug Metab 2008;9:310–22.

28. Wilke RA, Lin DW, Roden DM, et al. Identifying genetic risk factors for serious adverse drug reactions: current progress and challenges. Nat Rev Drug Discov 2007;6:904–16.

29. Donger C, Denjoy I, Berthet M, et al. KVLQT1 C-terminal missense mutation causes a forme fruste long-QT syndrome. Circulation 1997;96:2778–81.

30. Napolitano C, Schwartz PJ, Brown AM, et al. Evidence for a cardiac ion channel mutation underlying drug-induced QT prolongation and life-threatening arrhythmias. J Cardiovasc Electrophysiol 2000;11:691–6.

31. Yang P, Kanki H, Drolet B, et al. Allelic variants in long-QT disease genes in patients with drug-associated torsades de pointes. Circulation 2002;105:1943–8.

32. Paulussen AD, Gilissen RA, Armstrong M, et al. Genetic variations of KCNQ1, KCNH2, SCN5A, KCNE1, and KCNE2 in drug-induced long QT syndrome patients. J Mol Med 2004;82:182–8.

33. Priori SG, Napolitano C, Schwartz PJ. Low penetrance in the long-QT syndrome: clinical impact. Circulation 1999;99:529–33.

34. Splawski I, Timothy KW, Tateyama M, et al. Variant of SCN5A sodium channel implicated in risk of cardiac arrhythmia. Science 2002;297:1333–6.

35. Abbott GW, Sesti F, Splawski I, et al. MiRP1 forms I_{Kr} potassium channels with HERG and is associated with cardiac arrhythmia. Cell 1999;97:175–87.

36. Sesti F, Abbott GW, Wei J, et al. A common polymorphism associated with antibiotic-induced cardiac arrhythmia. Proc Natl Acad Sci U S A 2000;97:10613–8.

37. Kubota T, Horie M, Takano M, et al. Evidence for a single nucleotide polymorphism in the KCNQ1 potassium channel that underlies susceptibility to life-threatening arrhythmias. J Cardiovasc Electrophysiol 2001;12:1223–9.

38. Roden DM. Taking the "idio" out of "idiosyncratic": predicting Torsades de Pointes. Pacing Clin Electrophysiol 1998;21:1029–34.

39. Yang T, Roden DM. Extracellular potassium modulation of drug block of I_{Kr}. Implications for Torsade de Pointes and reverse use-dependence. Circulation 1996;93:407–11.

40. Knollmann BC, Roden DM. A genetic framework for improving arrhythmia therapy. Nature 2008;451:929–36.

41. Antzelevitch C, Brugada P, Borggrefe M, et al. Brugada syndrome: report of the second consensus conference. Heart Rhythm 2005;2:429–40.

42. Darbar D, Motsinger AA, Ritchie MD, et al. Polymorphism modulates symptomatic response to antiarrhythmic drug therapy in patients with lone atrial fibrillation. Heart Rhythm 2007;4:743–9.

Antiarrhythmic Drugs: Age, Race, and Gender Effects

Deborah Wolbrette, MD

KEYWORDS

- Antiarrhythmic drugs • Proarrhythmia • Atrial fibrillation
- Women • Elderly • Race • Pregnancy

Most studies of antiarrhythmic drugs in the past have comprised a fairly homogeneous male Caucasian population, which raises the question of whether data from these trials can be equally applied to women or to different ethnic groups. Elderly patients have been better represented in drug trials, but metabolic changes specific to them are not always considered when prescribing antiarrhythmic drugs. Being aware of potential differences in the response to antiarrhythmic drugs in a diverse patient population can help physicians customize arrhythmia therapy and minimize adverse effects.

GENDER DIFFERENCES IN PROARRHYTHMIA

Female gender is associated with an increased risk of torsade de pointes (TDP) in the setting of drugs that can prolong the QT interval. These drugs are all potassium channel blocking agents, and include several antiarrhythmic drugs as well as a variety of noncardiac medications. Women also have a longer baseline-corrected QT interval, and are more likely to have symptomatic congenital QT syndrome than men. The mechanism for this gender difference is unknown, but may be partly due to hormonal influences. There are data to suggest that the sex difference in the risk of TDP is not due to lengthening of the QT interval in women, but to shortening of the QT interval in men after puberty, that is, an increase in circulating androgens. This shortening of the QT interval in men is maintained at slow heart rates, and may provide a protective effect against TDP.[1] Data from the International Long QT Syndrome Registry showed the risk of cardiac events to be higher in males before puberty and higher in females during adulthood, consistent with the hormonal theory.[2]

For some years, case reports have suggested that women have a higher risk of developing TDP when taking QT-prolonging antiarrhythmic drugs. The offending agents are Vaughn Williams class IA and III antiarrhythmic drugs, which have varying degrees of potassium channel blocking effects. "Quinidine syncope" had been reported for years prior to the drug being associated with TDP. In 1968, a large study reported on patients treated with quinidine for conversion of atrial fibrillation. Of the 16 patients in this group who developed syncope on quinidine therapy, 15 were women.[3] Later, Roden's group found most cases of quinidine-induced TDP developed in the first few days of drug initiation, and could occur even at subtherapeutic concentrations.[4] The other class IA agents, procainamide and disopyramide, are also known to produce TDP. Procainamide's active metabolite, N-acetylprocainamide (NAPA), has more potent potassium channel blocking effects than its parent compound.[5] Makkar and colleagues[6] reviewed the literature and pharmaceutical databases pertaining to reported cases of cardiovascular drug-related TDP. Although women made up 70% of the 332 TDP cases reported, their proportional use of these drugs was only 44%. A greater than expected female prevalence of TDP was observed with each of the cardiovascular drugs analyzed.

Class III antiarrhythmic drugs have neutral effects on mortality in patients with structural heart

Penn State Heart & Vascular Institute, Penn State College of Medicine, Penn State Milton S. Hershey Medical Center, 500 University Drive, PO Box 850, MC H047, Hershey, PA 17033, USA
E-mail address: dwolbrette@hmc.psu.edu

Card Electrophysiol Clin 2 (2010) 369–378
doi:10.1016/j.ccep.2010.06.007
1877-9182/10/$ – see front matter © 2010 Elsevier Inc. All rights reserved.

disease, and have varying degrees of risk for causing TDP. D,L-Sotalol is a class III antiarrhythmic agent that blocks the rapid component of the delayed rectifier potassium current (I_{Kr}). In addition, it has β-blocking activity. Analysis of a database of more than 3000 patients given D,L-sotalol for treatment of atrial or ventricular arrhythmias found women to be at increased risk of developing TDP when taking this drug. Whereas only 1.0% of the men in this cohort experienced TDP, 4.1% of the women developed this proarrhythmia.[7] Similar findings were reported from a German study in which 81 patients were treated with D,L-sotalol for sustained ventricular tachycardia. Female sex and the appearance of a new U wave were found to be risks for TDP.[8] In a cohort of nearly 2000 patients treated with D,L-sotalol, women developed a greater corrected JT interval prolongation than did men. This gender difference in ventricular repolarization was not related to the dose of D,L-sotalol or to the sex difference in the baseline-corrected JT interval.[9]

The dextro-isomer of D,L-sotalol is D-sotalol, which is a pure potassium channel (I_{Kr}) antagonist, without β-blocking activity. In the Survival With ORal D-sotalol (SWORD) trial, the drug was given prophylactically to patients with left ventricular dysfunction after myocardial infarction. The study was terminated early due to increased mortality in the drug treatment group. A 4.7-fold increase in mortality was seen in women treated with D-sotalol, compared with a 1.4-fold increase in men. The fact that female sex was the major predictor of D-sotalol–induced mortality lends support to the hypothesis that TDP was the cause of death.[10]

Dofetilide is a newer class III antiarrhythmic drug, effective for the conversion of atrial fibrillation and maintenance of sinus rhythm. Dofetilide selectively inhibits I_{Kr}. In the Danish Investigations of Arrhythmias and Mortality on Dofetilide (DIAMOND CHF) trial, a significant reduction in the incidence of TDP (from 4.8% to 2.9%) was seen after adjusting the dose according to renal function and continuous cardiac monitoring during the first 3 days of therapy. Despite these precautions, female gender was found to be significantly associated with the occurrence of TDP, with an odds ratio of 3.2. Despite this increased risk of TDP in women, dofetilide had no adverse effect on mortality, regardless of sex.[11]

Amiodarone blocks not only I_{Kr} but also the slowly activating component of the delayed rectifier cardiac potassium current (I_{Ks}). Despite its marked action potential–prolonging effects, amiodarone has a very low proarrhythmic potential of less than 1%. Even so, women experience twice the expected prevalence of TDP.[6,12] No matter how low is the risk of TDP is for the total population, a gender difference remains.

Dronedarone is a class III antiarrhythmic drug recently approved by the Food and Drug Administration (FDA). It is a multichannel blocking agent with electrophysiologic properties similar to amiodarone. Dronedarone causes QT prolongation, but clinical trials have shown the drug to have a low potential to cause TDP. In the large ATHENA trial, patients with atrial fibrillation who had additional risk factors for death were randomized to receive dronedarone or placebo. Almost 50% of the study population was women. Only one person receiving dronedarone in the trial experienced TDP: a 66-year-old woman.[13] In the DIONYSOS study, 400 patients with atrial fibrillation were randomized to receive dronedarone or amiodarone. Although the median treatment duration was only 7 months, no instances of TDP were reported with either drug.[14]

Sotalol and dofetilide are associated with a higher risk of TDP than amiodarone and dronedarone. Although the reason for this proarrhythmic difference among class III agents is not entirely clear, it is likely the result of multiple mechanisms. One reason may be due to differences in QT dispersion. When amiodarone prolongs the QT interval it does so in a uniform manner, without a significant increase in the QT dispersion. On the other hand, sotalol causes a disproportionate increase in the action potential duration in M cells deep in the myocardium as opposed to the subendocardial and subepicardial cells, increasing the dispersion of ventricular recovery. M cells are thought to be responsible for the generation of U waves, which in turn are associated with TDP.[12,15] In addition, quinidine has been found to produce increased dispersion of repolarization in women.[16]

Sotalol and dofetilide also exhibit the property of reverse-use dependence, whereby their effect on the duration of the action potential becomes more pronounced at slower heart rates. This action increases the risk for early afterdepolarizations and, therefore, TDP.[12] Besides amiodarone's lack of reverse-use dependence and its decrease in dispersion of repolarization, the drug's broad range of electrophysiologic properties is another potential mechanism for its low proarrhythmic potential. Dronedarone's electrophysiologic properties are similar to that of amiodarone.[17] Amiodarone and dronedarone block both I_{Kr} and I_{Ks}, making them less selective in their potassium channel effects. This property could explain their lack of reverse-use dependent effects on the action potential duration. Dofetilide and sotalol, on the other hand, block only I_{Kr}, making them more selective potassium antagonists.

There are multiple risk factors besides female gender for the development of TDP in the setting of class IA or class III antiarrhythmic drug use. In general, they are factors that promote formation of early afterdepolarizations or prolongation of the action potential. Patients with a baseline long QT interval or with known long QT syndrome should not take any of these antiarrhythmic drugs. In the same respect, use of multiple QT-prolonging agents in any one patient increases their risk of developing TDP. In the case of amiodarone, for which the risk of proarrhythmia is very low, the few cases of documented TDP have mostly been associated with use of another potassium antagonist. Hypokalemia and hypomagnesemia facilitate the formation of early afterdepolarizations. Bradycardia or pauses prolong the action potential duration, which is particularly important in drugs such as sotalol and dofetilide because their electrophysiologic effects are more potent at slower heart rates. Sotalol and dofetilide are also renally cleared, making their risk of TDP higher in patients with renal disease.[12]

Structural heart disease can increase the risk of proarrhythmia. Left ventricular hypertrophy and cardiomyopathy can cause increased dispersion of repolarization.[18] Heart failure is an important proarrhythmic risk. The failing heart muscle is unable to maintain normal calcium homeostasis, resulting in the development of early afterdepolarizations.[19] In the setting of heart failure, perfusion of the liver and kidneys is decreased, slowing drug metabolism and clearance. The volume of distribution of drugs may also be decreased. All these factors make the pharmacokinetics of antiarrhythmic drugs unpredictable in the setting of heart failure. From a database of more than 3000 patients taking D,L-sotalol in clinical trials, the risk of TDP was 5% in those with a history of heart failure, as opposed to a lower 1.7% risk in patients without this history.[7] Women with 1 or more other risk factors for TDP are at particularly high risk of developing a proarrhythmia when taking sotalol. Further analysis of the sotalol clinical trial database found that a woman with no other risk factors taking sotalol, 320 mg/d or less, had only a 1% incidence of TDP. In contrast, a woman with heart failure taking more than 320 mg/d of sotalol had a 6% risk. When a history of sustained ventricular tachycardia was added to the mix, her risk of TDP increased to 22%.[7]

Greater caution should be used when treating women with antiarrhythmic drugs that prolong repolarization, especially when additional risk factors for developing TDP are present (**Box 1**). Patients on chronic class IA or class III drug therapy should have regular follow-up so their

---

Box 1
Checklist for minimizing torsades de pointes

1. Normal potassium level
2. Stable renal or liver function
3. Acceptable QT on ECG
4. No history of long QT syndrome
5. In-hospital initiation
6. Heart failure stabilized
7. Lowest effective dose
8. Med list reviewed

- QT-prolonging drugs
- drug interactions
- CYP3A4 inhibitors

9. Regular follow-up scheduled

---

electrocardiogram (ECG) can be checked for conduction changes or prolongation of the QT interval. Periodic monitoring of laboratory data is also important, including electrolytes, creatinine, and liver enzymes, as appropriate for the particular antiarrhythmic agent. Hypokalemia should be avoided in patients taking potassium antagonists. However, this may be difficult in patients with heart failure requiring diuretic therapy. Class 1A or class III agents should not be initiated in the setting of uncontrolled heart failure. The increased risk of TDP with sotalol use in women with heart failure has already been mentioned.[7] Dronedarone has a "box warning" in the package insert advising against use of the drug in patients with advanced heart failure. This advisory is based on the excess mortality in the ANDROMEDA trial, with heart-failure patients randomized to dronedarone therapy. There was no reported gender difference in dronedarone-related mortality in this study.[20]

Both sotalol and dofetilide are renally excreted, and their use should be carefully monitored in patients with renal disease. As mentioned previously, a significant reduction in TDP was seen after adjusting the dose of dofetilide according to renal function.[11] The package inserts for both these drugs contain instructions for calculating creatinine clearance (CrCl) and picking the appropriate drug dose. The Cockcroft-Gault formula is frequently used to determine CrCl, and there is a correction factor for use with women. The major metabolite of procainamide is NAPA. This metabolite has class III electrophysiologic properties and is renally cleared. Therefore, procainamide and NAPA drug levels should be followed, and dosing should be adjusted in patients with renal dysfunction.[21] A significant percentage of quinidine and disopyramide are also eliminated through the kidneys.

Most antiarrhythmic drugs with class III activity are hepatically metabolized (**Table 1**). Their use in patients with hepatic dysfunction should be avoided, or the dose reduced. These drugs are substrates or inhibitors of various cytochrome P450 isoenzymes, making potential adverse effects and drug interactions likely if the patient is not followed closely. Dofetilide and dronedarone are both metabolized by the CYP3A4 isoenzyme. Potent inhibitors of this isoenzyme should not be used with these drugs, as the combination could lead to high concentrations of these class III agents and result in TDP. Moderate CYP3A4 inhibitors can be used, but at lower doses.[17]

Use of the lowest effective dose of drugs with class III effects has been shown to reduce proarrhythmic risk. As noted earlier, the risk of TDP with sotalol is dose dependent, with the incidence significantly increasing at doses greater than 320 mg per day.[7] An exception to the dose dependence risk of TDP is quinidine. Because most of this drug's potassium channel blocking activity is expressed at low concentrations, TDP may occur with subtherapeutic drug levels.[22] In the case of dronedarone, only one dose (400 mg twice daily) is approved for use, and dose titration is not recommended.[17]

Due to the low risk of TDP with amiodarone and dronedarone, drug initiation in the outpatient setting is reasonable. By contrast, dofetilide, sotalol, and class IA agents should be started in a monitored hospital setting because of their higher potential for TDP. Although not all proarrhythmic events occur early, the majority of TDP events occur within the first 3 days of initiation. Monitoring allows early treatment of proarrhythmia and dose titration if QT prolongation occurs.[11,23] Women are at particularly high risk of developing TDP with antiarrhythmic drugs that prolong repolarization. Their risk is compounded when heart failure and other risks for TDP are present. Although not all proarrhythmic events can be anticipated or prevented, increased vigilance when treating women with these drugs can help minimize the potential for life-threatening proarrhythmia.

GENDER DIFFERENCES IN ATRIAL FIBRILLATION

Although atrial fibrillation is more prevalent in men of all age groups, the absolute numbers of men and women with atrial fibrillation are equal. Because the risk of atrial fibrillation increases with age, and there are almost twice the number of women as men older than 75 years, approximately 60% of people older than 75 with atrial fibrillation are women.[24] Gender differences have been found in the risk factors for atrial fibrillation. Data from the Framingham Heart Study showed that in people with atrial fibrillation, men have more ischemic heart disease and women have more valvular disease.[25] The Atrial Fibrillation Follow-up Investigation of Rhythm Management (AFFIRM) trial showed similar gender risk differences but also revealed that women with atrial fibrillation are older, and men are more likely to have abnormal left ventricular function.[26] Data from the Canadian Registry of Atrial Fibrillation (CARAF) showed women with atrial fibrillation have more hypertension and

Table 1
Pharmacokinetics of antiarrhythmic drugs

Drug	Renal Elimination of Unchanged Drug	Hepatic Metabolism	Important Metabolites
Quinidine	Yes	CYP3A4	3-Hydroxyquinidine
Procainamide	Yes	Acetylation	NAPA
Disopyramide	Yes	Yes	—
Lidocaine	No	CYP3A4	—
Mexiletine	No	CYP1A2 CYP2D6	—
Flecainide	Yes	CYP2D6	—
Propafenone	No	CYP2D6	5-Hydroxypropafenone
Amiodarone	No	CYP3A4 Others	DEA
Dronedarone	No	CYP3A4	—
Sotalol	Yes	No	—
Tikosyn	Yes	CYP3A4 (minor)	—

Abbreviations: DEA, *N*-desethylamiodarone; NAPA, *N*-acetylprocainamide.

thyroid abnormalities on presentation, whereas ischemic heart disease is more prevalent in men.[27] The women randomized in the Rate Control Versus Electrical Cardioversion (RACE) study were older than the men, and had an increased prevalence of hypertension and diabetes. The men had a higher prevalence of coronary artery disease.[28]

Several studies have shown that women with atrial fibrillation have a lower quality of life (QOL) than men with atrial fibrillation. Besides an impaired QOL, women in the CARAF trial were more likely than men to experience longer, more frequent episodes of atrial fibrillation. The women also had higher ventricular rates during episodes.[27] A post hoc analysis of the RACE trial showed women had more symptoms related to atrial fibrillation (palpitations, fatigue), and their QOL was significantly lower than the males at baseline. Over the follow-up period, QOL in women remained lower than in men, regardless of treatment strategy.[28] It should be noted that regardless of gender, the treatment strategy did not significantly influence QOL. The investigators believe this can be partly attributed to more than half the patients randomized to rhythm control actually being in permanent atrial fibrillation at the end of the follow-up.[29] However, this does not explain the persistent gender difference in QOL scores.

Analysis of the RACE trial data showed women randomized to rhythm control had 3 times greater risk of developing the end points of heart failure, thromboembolic events, and adverse effects of antiarrhythmic drugs as women assigned to rate control. This difference was not found in the male cohort. The drugs used for rhythm control in this trial were class IC agents, as well as sotalol and amiodarone. Most of the adverse drug effects were related to symptomatic sinus bradycardia and sinus nodal dysfunction. In the RACE and AFFIRM trials no gender difference in the prevalence of TDP was seen. The investigators of the post hoc RACE trial analysis suggested rate control as the preferred treatment strategy for women with atrial fibrillation. This opinion is based on the finding that rhythm control in women was associated with increased cardiovascular morbidity and mortality, without increasing QOL.[28] On the other hand, if QOL remains low in women regardless of treatment strategy, catheter ablation for a potential cure of atrial fibrillation should be considered earlier in this group.[27]

ANTIARRHYTHMIC DRUG USE DURING PREGNANCY

The need for antiarrhythmic drug use during pregnancy is rare, but when required poses a special challenge in this population. Pregnancy can be a proarrhythmic state, due to hormonal and hemodynamic changes that occur.[30] Although most arrhythmias during pregnancy are benign, in a minority of women drug therapy needs to be considered. The majority of women in this group have structural heart disease, long QT syndrome, or metabolic abnormalities such as thyroid disease or electrolyte disturbances.

Because antiarrhythmic drugs cannot be studied in pregnant women, and females of child-bearing age are not included in antiarrhythmic drug trials, there will always be the concern of possible fetal injury when these drugs are used during pregnancy. Most antiarrhythmic drugs have been given the FDA risk category C, indicating risk to the fetus cannot be ruled out. Although data are limited, sotalol has been given an FDA risk category B, with animal studies showing no fetal risk. Amiodarone is category D, with positive evidence of risk.[31] Dronedarone has recently been approved by the FDA and has been given a pregnancy category X, because it has been found to be teratogenic in animal studies. Dronedarone use is therefore contraindicated in pregnant women (**Table 2**).[32] With the exception of amiodarone and dronedarone,

Table 2
Antiarrhythmic drug risk during pregnancy

Drug	FDA Risk Category
Quinidine	C
Procainamide	C
Disopyramide	C
Lidocaine	B
Mexiletine	C
Flecainide	C
Propafenone	C
Sotalol	B
Dofetilide	C
Amiodarone	D
Dronedarone	X
Verapamil	C
Propranolol	C
Atenolol	D
Digoxin	C
Adenosine	C

Abbreviations: A, controlled studies show no risk; B, no evidence of risk in humans; C, risk cannot be ruled out; D, positive evidence of risk; X, contraindicated (teratogenic in animals).

there are no known teratogenic effects associated with antiarrhythmic drugs. However, due to the lack of study data for these drugs, chronic use should be reserved for clearly documented, hemodynamically significant arrhythmias. Because organogenesis is complete by the end of the first trimester, antiarrhythmic drug use is safer after that time. Later in pregnancy, these drugs should still be used with the utmost caution. The lowest effective drug dose and frequent ECG monitoring are advised. On the other hand, pregnancy can decrease the concentration of drugs due to an increased volume of distribution and increase in drug metabolism. Therefore, women on previous effective doses of antiarrhythmic drugs prior to pregnancy may require higher doses to prevent breakthrough arrhythmia episodes during pregnancy.[33]

Reentrant supraventricular tachycardia is the most common sustained tachycardia found in women of child-bearing age. Supraventricular tachycardia can present for the first time during pregnancy, or preexisting episodes can become more frequent.[34,35] The pregnant woman presenting to the emergency department with an acute episode of supraventricular tachycardia can be given adenosine if vagal maneuvers are not successful in terminating the tachycardia. Results of a retrospective survey suggest that adenosine use in the second and third trimesters is safe and effective.[36] Although there were insufficient data to evaluate safety in the first trimester, the short half-life of adenosine (10 seconds) should limit drug effect to the fetus. Adenosine should be given in a monitored setting with resuscitation equipment at the bedside. When possible, a fetal heart monitor should be used during administration of the drug to detect possible fetal bradycardia. Intravenous verapamil should be avoided for termination of an acute episode of supraventricular tachycardia, because of possible prolonged hypotension. Chronic antiarrhythmic drug use should be reserved for frequent episodes of supraventricular tachycardia that are hemodynamically significant. Because women should not undergo prolonged fluoroscopic procedures while pregnant, young women with known supraventricular tachycardia should be advised to undergo a curative radiofrequency ablation before planned pregnancy.

Women with long QT syndrome should continue on their β-blocker therapy throughout their pregnancy and postpartum. This recommendation is based on data from the Long QT Syndrome Registry, which revealed a significant increase in the risk for cardiac events in the 40-week period after delivery.[37] The main concern over the use of β-blockers in pregnancy has been that of fetal growth retardation. However, this adverse effect appears to be limited to atenolol use in the first trimester.[38,39] The benefit of other β-blockers to treat a potentially life-threatening arrhythmia in the mother would greatly outweigh the low risk of complications to the fetus or infant. Use of older β-blockers with a longer track record of use during pregnancy, such as propranolol or metoprolol, is advised.

Atrial fibrillation and atrial flutter are rarely seen during pregnancy, in the absence of structural heart disease or hypothyroidism. In the past, most of the cases of atrial fibrillation during pregnancy were associated with mitral stenosis secondary to rheumatic heart disease. However, in countries where medical care is easily accessed, rheumatic mitral stenosis has significantly declined. At the same time the number of pregnant women with congenital heart disease has increased. Today the majority of pregnant women with structural heart disease have some form of congenital heart defect. Women with congenital heart disease frequently develop arrhythmias during pregnancy, especially those with a history of major corrective surgery. Atrial arrhythmias are seen much more frequently than ventricular arrhythmias in this group. In the setting of mitral stenosis or significant heart disease, atrial fibrillation with rapid ventricular response will be poorly tolerated, necessitating prompt control of ventricular rate. In addition, the goal of early termination of atrial fibrillation or atrial flutter as well as prevention of recurrence is needed, because anticoagulation is problematic in these patients. For these reasons, antiarrhythmic drug therapy may be needed to accomplish these goals. For patients with structural heart disease, sotalol is a relatively safe choice. The safety of dofetilide is unknown (category C).

Ventricular tachycardia is another arrhythmia rarely seen during pregnancy. The most common ventricular tachycardia noted is benign idiopathic right ventricular outflow tract tachycardia. This tachycardia is catecholamine sensitive, and responds to β-blockade if episodes become frequent and hemodynamically significant.[40] When life-threatening ventricular tachycardia occurs during pregnancy, associated with structural heart disease, the choice for acute antiarrhythmic drug therapy should be intravenous lidocaine or amiodarone. Although an option, procainamide is associated with hypotension and is not as readily available as the aforementioned drugs. Cardioversion obviously should not be withheld when appropriate. As more young women at high risk for sudden cardiac death are receiving implantable defibrillators, and those with significant frequent arrhythmias are undergoing radiofrequency ablations, the need for antiarrhythmic therapy during pregnancy in this group may lessen.

In the past, there was a tendency to use older drugs such as digoxin and quinidine during pregnancy because they had a longer track record. Even though less data are available regarding some of the newer antiarrhythmic drugs, they are generally more effective, better tolerated, and easier to obtain than some of the older drugs. For pregnant women without structural heart disease needing antiarrhythmic drug therapy, flecainide or propafenone can be considered. For those women with structural heart disease, sotalol and, possibly, dofetilide should be tried before amiodarone, due to the latter drug's potentially significant toxic side effects to the mother and fetus.

THE RISK OF PROARRHYTHMIA IN THE ELDERLY

Earlier in the article, gender differences in the risk of proarrhythmia with class IA and class III antiarrhythmic drugs were discussed. Advanced age also increases the risk of proarrhythmia. The elderly experience a reduced volume of distribution, as well as reduced renal and hepatic function. These changes all affect drug clearance. However, even with advanced age, gender differences persist. Elderly women still generally have lower weight and volume of distribution, as well as reduced renal drug clearance when compared with elderly men. Elderly women with heart failure may have the highest risk for TDP when treated with sotalol or dofetilide. Electrolyte disturbances due to diuretics are common in this group. The importance of adjusting the dose of these drugs according to CrCl cannot be overemphasized. The package inserts for sotalol and dofetilide include instructions for calculating the starting dose based on CrCl, and decreasing the dose in response to QT prolongation. There are also important drug interactions associated with the use of amiodarone, dronedarone, and dofetilide. Physicians who prescribe these drugs should be familiar with the absolute and relative drug contraindications. Elderly women would be at the highest risk for a drug interaction. Using the lowest effective doses of antiarrhythmic drugs, while minimizing concomitant medications, may reduce adverse drug effects.[21,41]

ATRIAL FIBRILLATION IN THE ELDERLY

The elderly are well represented in clinical trials. Because the mean ages in the AFFIRM[42] and RACE[43] trials were 70 and 68 years, respectively, the results of these trials are best applied to the elderly. The subjects in these trials were also relatively asymptomatic, because they had to be willing to accept possible randomization to rate control. These trials found no significant difference in mortality between the rate and rhythm control groups. Therefore, rate control with anticoagulation is considered an appropriate treatment strategy for elderly patients without significant symptoms of atrial fibrillation. Further analysis of the AFFIRM data showed that although sinus rhythm was associated with better survival, the beneficial effect was neutralized by the adverse effects of the antiarrhythmic drugs.[44] The results of these trials may not apply to younger patients, those with lone atrial fibrillation, or those with significant symptoms of atrial fibrillation. For these patient groups, the benefit of maintaining sinus rhythm may outweigh the risk of antiarrhythmic drug use, making rhythm control the strategy of choice.

RACIAL DIFFERENCES IN ANTIARRHYTHMIC DRUG RESPONSE

The majority of subjects in clinical trials involving antiarrhythmic drug use have been white males in North America or Western Europe. Therefore, few data are available regarding possible racial differences in response to these drugs. The limited data that are available suggest potential ethnic differences in arrhythmic substrates, and proarrhythmic response to antiarrhythmic drugs.

Data were compared for 3 ethnic groups randomized in the AFFIRM study. Caucasians comprised 90% of the subjects, with African Americans 7% and Hispanics 3%. Despite the African Americans and Hispanics in the study being significantly younger than the Caucasians, they may have been a sicker group, with increased prevalence of heart failure and left ventricular dysfunction. In addition, African Americans had higher rates of hypertension and Hispanics were more likely to have cardiomyopathy. Although warfarin use and initial antiarrhythmic drug therapy were similar between the 3 ethnic groups, survival rates were different. In Caucasians, the rate control strategy resulted in improved survival over rhythm control. In African Americans, there was no difference in survival between rate and rhythm control. In the Hispanic group, rhythm control led to better survival over rate control. Although the differences in baseline characteristics between the ethnic groups may be responsible for the different survival rates, the relatively small sample sizes of the African American and Hispanic groups in this post hoc analysis prevent conclusions to be drawn from these data.[45]

Ibutilide is an intravenous class III antiarrhythmic drug approved for pharmacologic conversion of recent-onset atrial fibrillation or atrial flutter. In a study of 58 patients, in which 34% were African American, racial differences were found in the efficacy and safety of ibutilide. While significantly more African Americans were successfully converted to sinus rhythm with ibutilide, QT prolongation after drug administration was greater in African Americans than in Caucasians. Of the 4 patients who experienced TDP, 3 were African Americans. From these data, it would appear that ibutilide is more effective in African Americans, but with a higher risk of TDP. However, the study enrolled a relatively small number of patients.[46]

The Multicenter UnSustained Tachycardia Trial (MUSTT) showed that patients with coronary disease, an ejection fraction of 40% or less, and symptomatic nonsustained ventricular tachycardia benefited from implantable cardioverter-defibrillator (ICD) therapy. In this primary prevention trial, patients with inducible sustained ventricular tachycardia were randomized to standard medical therapy with β-blockers and angiotensin-converting enzyme inhibitors, or this standard regimen plus electrophysiologic (EP)-guided antiarrhythmic drug therapy. ICD therapy was offered to patients who did not respond to antiarrhythmic drugs.[47] A post hoc analysis of the MUSTT data has suggested racial differences in the benefit of EP-guided therapy. Black patients represented 11% of those studied in this trial. White patients randomized to EP-guided therapy experienced a 26% lower total mortality rate, whereas black subjects who received no EP-guided therapy survived better than those who did receive this therapy. By contrast, there was no racial difference in survival in patients assigned to standard medical therapy. Black patients had a higher rate of response to antiarrhythmic drugs at EP testing. There was no significant difference between the 2 racial groups with respect to the agents used, which included amiodarone, sotalol, propafenone, and class IA drugs. Whites were more likely to have been revascularized before enrollment, and blacks were more likely to have left ventricular hypertrophy. The investigators speculated that racial differences in the anatomic substrate could be responsible for differences in response to antiarrhythmic drugs, and possibly for more proarrhythmic effects in black subjects. The benefit of treatment in the EP-guided therapy group in MUSTT was related to ICDs. The poorer outcome for blacks in this trial was related to their lower ICD implantation rate, secondary to their higher response to antiarrhythmic drugs and their more frequent refusal of ICD implantation when it was offered.[48] Due to the low proportion of black patients in MUSTT, caution should be used when drawing conclusions from these data.

SUMMARY

Female gender is now a well-documented risk factor for proarrhythmia with potassium channel blocking agents. Advanced age also increases the chance of experiencing TDP. For both these groups, increased caution when prescribing these antiarrhythmic drugs can help reduce the risk. Just as gender differences have been found in the incidence of proarrhythmia, there may also be racial variations in response to antiarrhythmic drugs that prolong the QT interval. In future antiarrhythmic drug trials, more effort should be made to enroll a more diverse ethnic population.

REFERENCES

1. Lehmann MH, Timothy KW, Frankovich D, et al. Age-gender influence on the rate-corrected QT interval and the QT heart rate relation in families with genotypically characterized long QT syndrome. J Am Coll Cardiol 1997;29:93–9.
2. Locati EH, Zareba W, Moss AJ, et al. Age and sex related differences in clinical manifestations in patients with congenital long-QT syndrome: findings from the International LQTS Registry. Circulation 1998;97:2237–44.
3. Cramer G. Early and late results of conversion of atrial fibrillation with quinidine: a clinical and hemodynamic study. Acta Med Scand 1968; 184(Suppl):490.
4. Roden DM, Woosley RL, Primm RK. Incidence and clinical features of the quinidine-associated long QT syndrome: implications for patient care. Am Heart J 1986;111:1088–93.
5. Yang T, Snyders D, Roden DM. Drug block of I_{Kr}: model systems and relevance to human arrhythmias. J Cardiovasc Pharmacol 2001;38:737–44.
6. Makkar RR, Fromm BS, Steinman RT. Female gender as a risk factor for torsades de pointes associated with cardiovascular drugs. JAMA 1993;270: 2590–7.
7. Lehmann MH, Hardy S, Archibald D, et al. Sex difference in risk of torsades de pointes with d,l-sotalol. Circulation 1996;94:2534–41.
8. Kuhlkamp V, Mermi J, Mervis C, et al. Efficacy and proarrhythmias with the use of d,l-sotalol for sustained ventricular tachyarrhythmias. J Cardiovasc Pharmacol 1997;29:373–81.
9. Lehmann MH, Hardy S, Archibald D, et al. JTc prolongation with d,l-sotalol in women versus men. Am J Cardiol 1999;83:354–9.

10. Pratt CM, Camm AJ, Cooper W, et al. Mortality in the Survival With Oral D-sotalol (SWORD) trial: why did patients die? Am J Cardiol 1998;81:869–76.

11. Torp-Pedersen C, Moller M, Block-Momsen PE, et al. Dofetilide in patients with congestive heart failure and left ventricular dysfunction. Danish Investigations of Arrhythmia and Mortality on Dofetilide Study Group. N Engl J Med 1999;341:857–65.

12. Hohnloser SH, Singh BN. Proarrhythmia with class III antiarrhythmic drugs: definition, electrophysiologic mechanisms, incidence, predisposing factors and clinical implications. J Cardiovasc Electrophysiol 1995;6:920–36.

13. Hohnloser SH, Crijns HJ, Van Eickels M, et al. Effect of dronedarone on cardiovascular events in atrial fibrillation. N Engl J Med 2009;360:668–78.

14. Heuzey JY, DeFerrari GM, Radzik D, et al. A short-term, randomized, double-blind, parallel-group study to evaluate the efficacy and safety of dronedarone versus amiodarone in patients with persistent atrial fibrillation: the DIONYSOS study. J Cardiovasc Electrophysiol Apr 6 2010. [Published Online].

15. Prior SG, Diehl L, Schwartz PJ. Torsades de pointes. In: Podrid PJ, Kowey PR, editors. Cardiac arrhythmia: mechanisms, diagnosis, and management. Baltimore (MD): Williams and Wilkins; 1995. p. 951–63.

16. Benton RE, Sale M, Flockhart DA, et al. Greater quinidine induced QTc interval prolongation in women. Clin Pharmacol Ther 2000;67:413–8.

17. Patel C, Yan GX, Kowey PR. Dronedarone. Circulation 2009;120:636–44.

18. Reiffel JA. Impact of structural heart disease on the selection of class III antiarrhythmics for the prevention of atrial fibrillation and flutter. Am Heart J 1998;135:551–6.

19. Eckardt L, Haverkamp W, Breithardt G. Antiarrhythmic therapy in heart failure. Heart Fail Monit 2002;2:110–9.

20. Kober L, Torp-Pedersen C, McMurray JJ, et al. Increased mortality after dronedarone therapy for severe heart failure. N Engl J Med 2008;358:2678–87.

21. Reiffel JA, Appel G. Importance of QT interval determination and renal function assessment during antiarrhythmic drug therapy. J Cardiovasc Pharmacol Ther 2001;6:111–9.

22. Roden DM. Acquired long QT syndromes and the risk of proarrhythmia. J Cardiovasc Electrophysiol 2000;11:938–40.

23. Prystowsky EN. Inpatient versus outpatient initiation of antiarrhythmic drug therapy for patients with supraventricular tachycardia. Clin Cardiol 1994; 17(Suppl II):II7–10.

24. Fang MC, Singer DE, Chang Y, et al. Gender difference in the risk of ischemic stroke and peripheral embolism in atrial fibrillation: the Anticoagulation and Risk factors in Atrial Fibrillation (ATRIA) study. Circulation 2005;112:1687–91.

25. Benjamin EJ, Wolf PA, D'Agostino RB, et al. Impact of atrial fibrillation on the risk of death: the Framingham Heart Study. Circulation 1998;98:946–52.

26. Kaufman ES, Zimmermann PA, Wang T, et al. Risk of proarrhythmic events in the Atrial Fibrillation Follow-up Investigation of Rhythm Management (AFFIRM) Study: a multivariate analysis. J Am Coll Cardiol 2004;44:1276–82.

27. Kerr CR, Humphries K. Gender-related differences in atrial fibrillation. J Am Coll Cardiol 2005;46:1307–8.

28. Rienstra M, Van Veldhuisen DJ, Hagens VE, et al. Gender-related differences in rhythm control treatment in persistent atrial fibrillation. J Am Coll Cardiol 2005;46:1298–306.

29. Hagens VE, Ranchor AV, Sonderen EV, et al. Effect of rate or rhythm control on quality of life in persistent atrial fibrillation: results from the Rate Control versus Electrical Cardioversion (RACE) study. J Am Coll Cardiol 2004;43:241–7.

30. Larsen JA, Kadish AH. Effects of gender on cardiac arrhythmias. J Cardiovasc Electrophysiol 1998;9: 655–64.

31. Page RL. Treatment of arrhythmias during pregnancy. Am Heart J 1995;130:871–6.

32. Multaq [package insert]. Bridgewater (NJ), Sanofi-aventis, 2009.

33. Adamson DL, Nelson-Piercy C. Managing palpitations and arrhythmias during pregnancy. Heart 2007;93:1630–6.

34. Tawan M, Levine J, Mendelson M, et al. Effect of pregnancy on paroxysmal supraventricular tachycardia. Am J Cardiol 1993;72:838–40.

35. Lee SH, Chen SA, Wu TJ, et al. Effects of pregnancy on first onset and symptoms of paroxysmal supraventricular tachycardia. Am J Cardiol 1995;76:675–8.

36. Elkayan U, Goodwin TM. Adenosine therapy for supraventricular tachycardia during pregnancy. Am J Cardiol 1995;75:521–3.

37. Rashba EJ, Zareba W, Moss AJ, et al. Influence of pregnancy on the risk for cardiac events in patients with hereditary long QT syndrome. LQTS Investigators. Circulation 1998;97:451–6.

38. Bayliss H, Churchill D, Beevers M, et al. Antihypertensive drugs in pregnancy and fetal growth: evidence for "pharmacological programming" in the first trimester? Hypertens Pregnancy 2002;21:161–74.

39. Magee LA, Elran E, Bull SB, et al. Risks and benefits of beta-receptor blockers for pregnancy hypertension: overview of the randomized trials. Eur J Obstet Gynecol Reprod Biol 2000;88:15–26.

40. Brodsky M, Doria R, Allen B, et al. New onset ventricular tachycardia during pregnancy. Am Heart J 1992;123:933–41.

41. Schwartz JB. Gender-specific implications for cardiovascular medication use in the elderly: optimizing therapy for older women. Cardiol Rev 2003; 11:275–98.

42. Wyse DG, Waldo AL, DiMarco JP, et al. A comparison of rate control and rhythm control in patients with atrial fibrillation. N Engl J Med 2002; 347:1825–33.

43. Van Gelder IC, Hagens VE, Bosker HA, et al. A comparison of rate control and rhythm control in patients with recurrent persistent atrial fibrillation. N Engl J Med 2002;347:1834–40.

44. Corley SD, Epstein AE, DiMarco JP, et al. Relationships between sinus rhythm, treatment, and survival in the Atrial Fibrillation Follow-Up Investigation of Rhythm Management (AFFIRM) study. Circulation 2004;109:1509–13.

45. Bush D, Martin LW, Leman R, et al. Atrial fibrillation among African Americans, Hispanics and Caucasians: clinical features and outcomes from the AFFIRM trial. J Natl Med Assoc 2006;98(3):330–9.

46. Gowda RM, Punukollu G, Khan IA, et al. Ibutilide for pharmacological cardioversion of atrial fibrillation and flutter: impact of race on efficacy and safety. Am J Ther 2003;10:259–63.

47. Buxton AE, Lee KL, Fisher JD, et al. A randomized study of the prevention of sudden death in patients with coronary artery disease. Multicenter UnSustained Tachycardia Trial Investigators. N Engl J Med 1999;341:1882–90.

48. Russo AM, Hafley GE, Lee KL, et al. Racial differences in outcome in the Multicenter UnSustained Tachycardia Trial (MUSTT): a comparison of whites versus blacks. Circulation 2003;108:67–72.

Antiarrhythmic Drug Therapy of Supraventricular Tachycardia

Steven A. Rothman, MD

KEYWORDS

- Supraventricular tachycardia • Pharmacologic therapy
- Calcium channel blockers • Beta-adrenergic blockers
- Adenosine • Antiarrhythmic agents

Paroxysmal supraventricular tachycardia (SVT), excluding atrial fibrillation and flutter, typically refers to a group of arrhythmias of several different mechanisms that originate at, or above, the antrioventricular (AV) node. As a group, these arrhythmias are relatively common with a prevalence of 2.25 per 1000 persons and have a female preponderance before age 65 years.[1] About half of these arrhythmias are attributable to reentry within the AV node (AVNRT), with the remainder being atrioventricular reentrant tachycardia (AVRT) and atrial tachycardia (AT). The treatment of SVT has changed over the past couple of decades as advances in mapping techniques and catheter ablation have resulted in high cure rates for SVT. Pharmacologic therapy, however, remains the preferred therapy for the acute conversion of SVT and still has a role in the chronic treatment of some patients. Appropriate treatment, however, is dependent on the correct diagnosis of the arrhythmia and a complete understanding of the arrhythmia's mechanism.

GENERAL CONSIDERATIONS IN TREATMENT OF SVT
Mechanisms of SVT

Reentry is the most common mechanism of narrow QRS complex tachycardia[2] and requires 2 distinct pathways with different electrophysiologic properties that form an anatomic or functional circuit.[3,4] The type of arrhythmia that ensues is determined by the characteristics and location of the reentrant circuit. Reentry may use a large macroreentrant circuit (as in atrial flutter and AVRT) or smaller microreentrant circuits (as in some atrial tachycardias and AVNRT). Anatomic structures (eg, the crista terminalis and eustachian ridge in the case of typical atrial flutter) or areas of fibrosis and scar may form the boundaries of the reentrant circuit.[5] Alternatively, the circuit may result from functional electrophysiologic properties of normal or diseased tissue that create the milieu for reentry.[6]

A less common mechanism of narrow QRS complex tachycardia is automaticity. Automaticity is caused by enhanced diastolic phase 4 depolarization and when the firing rate exceeds the sinus rate, the abnormal rhythm will occur. Tissues capable of causing a narrow complex tachycardia attributable to automaticity may be found in the atria, AV junction, vena cava, and pulmonary veins. These rhythm scans can be either incessant or episodic. Triggered activity is a mechanism caused by abnormal impulse initiation and results from interruptions of the repolarization process called after-depolarizations.[7] When an after-depolarization reaches a threshold, an action potential is triggered. After-depolarizations are characterized as either "early," occurring during repolarization, or "delayed," occurring at the end

Disclosures: None
Division of Cardiovascular Medicine, Lankenau Hospital, Suite 556, MOBE, 100 East Lancaster Avenue, Wynnewood, PA 19096, USA
E-mail address: Rothmans@mlhs.org

Card Electrophysiol Clin 2 (2010) 379–391
doi:10.1016/j.ccep.2010.07.003
1877-9182/10/$ — see front matter © 2010 Published by Elsevier Inc.

of repolarization or immediately after completion of repolarization.[8] Atrial tachycardias associated with digitalis toxicity or theophylline are examples of a triggered arrhythmia.[9,10]

Management of SVT

The management of SVT is based on the clinical presentation of the arrhythmia and the patient's preferences. Patients with mild, infrequent symptoms may benefit from intermittent pharmacologic therapy (eg, "pill-in-pocket" approach), whereas patients with frequent symptomatic episodes are candidates for chronic therapy or catheter-based ablation. Patients with infrequent, but poorly tolerated arrhythmias also require a more definitive approach. An individual's lifestyle and personal preferences along with overall health and the presence of significant comorbidities should be considered when making long-term management decisions.[2] Catheter-based ablation has become the treatment of choice for many patients with paroxysmal SVT because of the high success rate and low risk of complications.[11,12] Currently, the main role of pharmacotherapy is in the acute termination of an arrhythmia or for control of the ventricular response rate during SVT episodes. The chronic use of pharmacologic agents to suppress SVT is usually reserved for patients who are not candidates for catheter-based ablation procedures or patients who prefer a pharmacologic option.

ACUTE PHARMACOTHERAPY IN THE TREATMENT OF SVT

In general, SVT is considered to be a non–life-threatening condition with a good long-term prognosis. Acute intervention, however, may be necessary in patients with prolonged episodes of SVT or in those with hemodynamic instability and severe symptoms. Although electrical cardioversion may be used in urgent, life-threatening situations, pharmacologic therapy is most often used to terminate SVT. Agents commonly used for the acute treatment of SVT are listed in **Table 1**.

Adenosine

The most commonly used agent for acute conversion of SVT is adenosine. Adenosine is a short-acting, endogenous purine nucleoside with negative dromotropic action on the AV node and negative chronotropic effect on the sinus node. It is administered as a 6-mg or 12-mg bolus followed by a saline flush and must be given rapidly, as its effects are dose dependent and it has a very short half-life of less than 10 seconds.[13] Smaller doses may be needed if a central intravenous access

site is used for administration.[14] When given to patients with paroxysmal SVT, 6 mg is effective in terminating SVT in up to 57% of subjects and 12 mg is effective in up to 93% of subjects.[15,16] The effectiveness of adenosine can be attenuated by methylxanthine derivatives, such as theophylline and caffeine, owing to competitive adenosine receptor blockade.[17] Conversely, dipyridamole inhibits the removal of adenosine and can cause a marked potentiation in its effectiveness.[18]

Adenosine exhibits its predominant effect on anterograde conduction of the AV node. In patients with typical AVNRT or AVRT, adenosine will usually cause termination of the tachycardia in the anterograde AV nodal limb of the circuit (**Fig. 1**).[19,20] In patients with dual AV nodal physiology, adenosine's depressant effect is most potent on the anterograde fast pathway followed by the anterograde slow pathway.[21] Retrograde AV nodal conduction is most resistant to adenosine and up to 40% of patients may not demonstrate ventriculoatrial block in response to adenosine.[22–24]

In patients with an AT, adenosine may result in transient AV block, helping determine the diagnosis. Occasionally, adenosine may terminate an AT, especially if the arrhythmia is caused by a triggered or automatic mechanism and can be used to differentiate the tachycardia between a focal and reentrant mechanism.[25] Adenosine is particularly effective on beta-adrenergic–dependent atrial tachycardias,[26] and transient suppression may be seen when given to patients with an automatic atrial tachycardia, whereas there is no effect on intra-arterial reentrant tachyarrhythmias.[27] Adenosine's ultra-short duration of action makes it a preferred agent before resorting to emergent direct current cardioversion in patients with a tenuous hemodynamic state. Caution has to be exercised when using adenosine because of a potential proarrhythmic effect stemming from a transient increase in atrial vulnerability to atrial fibrillation (AF).[28–30]

Adenosine's antiarrhythmic effects are mediated by activation of the adenosine A1 receptor, which activates the inwardly rectifying K+ current I[KACh,Ado],[31] resulting in the negative chronotropic and dromotropic effects. Expected adverse effects such as high-grade AV block and sinus pauses are the result of activation of the A1 receptor. Other adenosine receptors, A2A, A2B, and A3, cause coronary dilatation, inhibition of platelet aggregation, and neuronal stimulation.[32] Side effects such as facial flushing, shortness of breath, and chest discomfort are attributable to adenosine's nonselective activation of these other receptors. Selective adenosine A1 receptor agonists, such as tecadenoson, are currently

Table 1
Pharmacologic agents commonly used in the acute treatment of paroxysmal SVT

Therapeutic Agent	Intravenous Dosage	Oral Dosage	Predominant Site of Action
Adenosine Receptor Agonists			
Adenosine	6–12 mg bolus	–	AVN, focal AT
Beta-Adrenergic Blockers			
Esmolol	0.5 g/kg load, then 0.05–0.2 mg/kg/min	–	AVN
Metoprolol	5 mg q 5 min (up to 15 mg)	25 – 50 mg	AVN
Propranolol	0.25–0.5 mg q 5 min (up to 0.2 mg/kg)	20 – 80 mg	AVN
Calcium Channel Antagonists			
Diltiazem	20–25 mg over 1–2 min, then 10–15 mg/h	120 – 240 mg	AVN
Verapamil	5–10 mg over 1–2 min, then 10–15 mg/h	120 – 240 mg	AVN
Antiarrhythmic Agents			
Amiodarone	150 mg over 10 min	–	AVN, AP
Flecainide	–	200 – 300 mg	AP, retrograde AVN, AT
Ibutilide	1 mg over 10 min, repeat after 10 min	–	AP, preexcited AF
Procainamide	25–50 mg/min (up to 1000 mg)	500 – 1000 mg	AP, reentrant AT, preexcited AF
Propafenone	–	300 – 600 mg	AP, AVN, AT

Abbreviations: AP, accessory pathway; AT, atrial tachycardia; AVN, atrioventricular node.

under development and have been shown in early trials to be effective with fewer side effects.[33,34]

Overall, the side effects of adenosine are usually very transient because of the drug's short half-life.[18] Because the density of K^+ACh,Ado channels is much less in ventricular than atrial myocytes, serious ventricular proarrhythmias are not common. Transient ventricular ectopy and nonsustained ventricular tachycardia, however, can be seen in up to 50% or more of patients and can be either monomorphic or polymorphic in appearance.[35,36] Although rare, sustained ventricular arrhythmias have been reported.[37,38] When given to patients with preexcited atrial fibrillation or ventricular tachycardia, degeneration of the arrhythmia to ventricular fibrillation has also been reported.[39–42]

Calcium Channel Antagonists and Beta-Blockers

The nondihydropyridine calcium channel blockers, diltiazem and verapamil, are also effective at depressing conduction in the AV node and potentially terminating SVT. Intravenous verapamil and diltiazem have a later onset of action than adenosine, but also have a longer effect. Like adenosine, calcium channel blockers can occasionally terminate AT but the most common outcome is slowing down the ventricular response rate, making the tachycardia more hemodynamically stable without terminating it.[43,44] Intravenous beta-blockers have also been used for the acute termination of SVT, and although effective in decreasing the heart rate during SVT, acute termination with restoration to sinus rhythm is less commonly seen.[45–47]

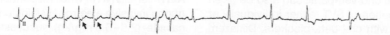

Fig. 1. Termination of SVT with adenosine. The rhythm strip (Lead II) shows an atrioventricular reentrant tachycardia terminating after the intravenous administration of 6 mg of adenosine. The arrow marks retrograde activation of the atrium during SVT. The tachycardia terminates in the anterograde AV nodal limb of the circuit and a slight increase in the PR interval occurs before AV nodal block.

Verapamil is administered in 5 mg intravenous (IV) boluses, up to 20 mg, and compared with adenosine, verapamil is slightly less effective in terminating SVT. In a study by Sethi and colleagues,[20] the overall efficacy of verapamil was 61% compared with 89% for adenosine. Other studies have shown more comparable effectiveness between the drugs.[15,48] Termination of the arrhythmia by verapamil usually occurs in the anterograde slow pathway during AVNRT and in the anterograde AV nodal pathway during AVRT.[20] Retrograde conduction via the fast AV nodal pathway is less likely to be affected by verapamil.[49] Verapamil tends to be better tolerated than adenosine with fewer noncardiac side effects,[50] but is more likely to cause hypotension.[51] The hypotensive effects of verapamil can be avoided by pretreatment with calcium chloride[52] and limited by using a slow infusion.[53] Verapamil should therefore not be used in patients with profound hypotension or with severely depressed ventricular systolic function[4] and should also be avoided in patients with preexcited atrial fibrillation because of its potential to accelerate the ventricular response rate.[54,55]

Diltiazem is another calcium channel blocker commonly used for supraventricular tachycardia. Given as a bolus of 0.25 to 0.45 mg/kg IV, termination of SVT can occur in up to 90% of patients.[56,57] In a trial comparing a slow infusion of diltiazem (2.5 mg/min up to 50 mg) or verapamil (1 mg/min up to 20 mg) with adenosine (6-mg bolus followed by a 12-mg bolus), the conversion rate for SVT was 98% in the calcium channel blocker group and 86.5% in the adenosine group.[53] Although well tolerated, hypotension can occur in about 10% of patients,[57] but is usually mild with a reduction in systolic pressure of less than 20 mm Hg.[58,59]

IV beta-blockers, such as esmolol and metoprolol, are less effective in the acute treatment of SVT. In a trial comparing IV diltiazem and esmolol, termination of SVT occurred in only 25% of the beta-blocker group, whereas all patients given IV diltiazem were successfully converted, including the esmolol failures.[60] Side effects with IV beta-blockers are mostly limited to hypotension, and are usually asymptomatic. In critically ill patients, however, esmolol's short half-life and duration of action make it a safer option for rate control of SVT.[47,61]

Both diltiazem and verapamil can also be given orally for termination of SVT, either individually or in combination with oral beta-blockers. Diltiazem has been given as a single oral dose of 120 mg along with 160 mg of propranolol and resulted in termination of SVT in 14 of 15 patients in an average of 27 ± 15 minutes.[62] A more recent trial also demonstrated similar effectiveness with this combination, terminating SVT in 94% of patients within 32 ± 22 minutes.[63] Monotherapy with verapamil appears to be less effective, terminating SVT in only 10% of patients when given as a single oral dose of up to 240 mg.[64] However, when combined with a beta-blocker such as pindolol (20 mg with 120 mg of verapamil), the efficacy increases to 75%.[65]

Sodium Channel Blockers

IV procainamide is a class IA agent that depresses conduction and prolongs refractoriness in atrial and ventricular myocardium, accessory pathways, and the His-Purkinje system.[66,67] Its effect on the AV node includes a lengthening of the retrograde AV nodal refractory period but has no discernable effect on anterograde AV nodal refractoriness.[6] Procainamide is most effective in terminating reentrant atrial tachycardia and AVRT and is less effective in terminating AVNRT. In a recent review of children presenting with SVT, intravenous procainamide was effective in terminating the arrhythmia in 50% of the patients and resulting in clinical improvement in an additional 21%. Other studies have also demonstrated similar effectiveness in patients with AVRT,[68] but procainamide has limited efficacy in patients with ectopic automatic atrial arrhythmias.[69] In patients presenting with a wide QRS complex tachycardia of unknown etiology, procainamide is considered one of the safest and most effective drugs to administer.[70] Its electrophysiologic effects may result in the termination of both ventricular tachycardias as well as antidromic AVRT.

Flecainide is a class 1C sodium channel blocker that also can be used in the acute treatment of SVT. Its predominant effect is the slowing of conduction in atrial, His-Purkinje, and ventricular conduction with a lesser effect on prolonging the refractory periods in these tissues. Flecainide has marked effects on accessory atrioventricular pathways and retrograde AV nodal conduction,[71,72] but minimal effect on anterograde AV nodal conduction.[73] In patients with SVT, intravenous flecainide terminated both AVNRT and AVRT by inducing retrograde block in either the fast AV nodal pathway or the accessory pathway, respectively.[74] In a study of 22 patients with recurrent AVRT or AVNRT who responded to flecainide during invasive electrophysiologic testing, oral flecainide (2.5–3.3 mg/kg) successfully terminated 127 of 134 spontaneous episodes over 2 years.[75] Flecainide can also cause prolongation of the sinus node recovery time in patients with preexisting sinus node disease[71] and should be avoided in patients with underlying His-Purkinje disease and sinus node dysfunction.[76]

Propafenone is a class 1C sodium channel blocker that also has beta adrenergic-blocking effects.[77] Propafenone has a significant inhibitory effect on accessory pathway conduction, and in a study by Sethi and colleagues[78] using dosages of 300 mg 3 times daily, complete suppression of anterograde conduction was seen in 4 of 5 subjects and retrograde conduction in 6 of 9 subjects. In addition, electrophysiologic testing revealed significant increase in the effect refractory periods of the atrium, AV node, and ventricle and markedly prolonged the AV nodal Wenckebach cycle length from 288 ± 51 msec to 389 ± 51 msec. Its beta-blocking effects, however, are relatively weak,[79,80] but enhanced in patients who are genetically deficient in the hydroxylation of the agent.[81] The acute administration of propafenone has been successful in terminating SVT in approximately 84% of patients, but mostly using the intravenous formulation.[82]

Other Antiarrhythmic Agents

Ibutilide is a Class III antiarrhythmic agent that prolongs cardiac repolarization by enhancing the slow, inward sodium current. It has been approved for the acute termination of atrial fibrillation and flutter, but has been shown to have modest efficacy in the treatment of atrial tachycardia.[83] Its

effects on accessory pathway conduction include prolongation of both the anterograde and retrograde refractory periods and can also increase the shortest RR interval during preexcited atrial fibrillation.[84] These properties have made ibutilide useful in the acute management of patients with preexcited atrial fibrillation (**Fig. 2**).[2]

Amiodarone is predominantly a class III antiarrhythmic agent but has electrophysiologic properties that span all 4 Vaughan Williams classes and is the most commonly used antiarrhythmic agent for the treatment of atrial fibrillation.[85] Administered intravenously, amiodarone causes significant prolongation of AV nodal conduction and the AV nodal refractory period and can also be used in the acute termination of paroxysmal SVT,[86,87] although it is less effective than procainamide.[88] In contrast to the Class I agents, amiodarone is more likely to terminate AVRT in the AV nodal limb of the circuit rather than the accessory pathway.[89] Intravenous amiodarone should be avoided in the acute treatment of preexcited atrial fibrillation because of its potential for proarrhythmia.[90,91]

CHRONIC PHARMACOTHERAPY IN THE TREATMENT OF SVT

The goals of long-term maintenance therapy for SVT are to suppress future episodes and to control the rate of the ventricular response if episodes do

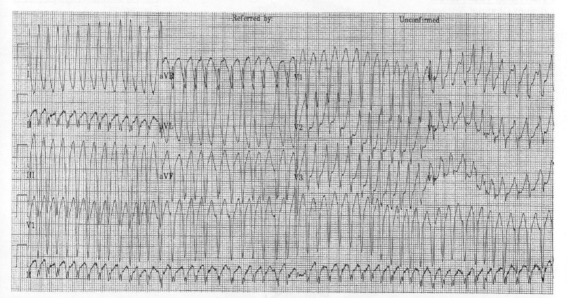

Fig. 2. Preexcited atrial fibrillation. Twelve-lead electrocardiogram (ECG) showing rapidly conducting atrial fibrillation in a patient with Wolff-Parkinson-White syndrome and a posteroseptal accessory pathway. Acute treatment with AV nodal blocking agents, such as verapamil and adenosine, should be avoided, as they may enhance anterograde conduction though the accessory pathway and potentially lead to hemodynamic instability or ventricular fibrillation. In patients who are clinically stable, intravenous procainamide or ibutilide is recommended.

recur. The selection of a pharmacologic agent is based on the unique electrophysiologic properties of the arrhythmia and patient characteristics such as existing comorbidities, cardiac function, severity of symptoms during SVT, and drug sensitivities. Pharmacologic agents that are well tolerated with low organ toxicity are preferred (**Fig. 3**). Commonly used pharmacologic agents along with their mechanism of action are listed in **Table 2**.

AV Nodal and Atrioventricular Reentry

Agents with AV nodal–specific activity, such as beta-blockers, calcium channel blockers, and, to a lesser extent, digoxin, are most commonly used as first-line therapy for AV nodal dependent arrhythmias. Overall, these agents may improve symptoms in up to 60% to 80% of patients,[4] but are sometimes inadequate as monotherapy because of their inability to directly slow conduction and alter the refractoriness of an accessory pathway or to significantly reduce the frequency of arrhythmia-triggering ectopy.[92–94]

Suppression of SVT using AV nodal blocking agents has been evaluated by testing the ability to induce the arrhythmia during electrophysiologic testing. Verapamil has been shown to be more effective in preventing the induction of AV nodal reentrant tachycardia than orthodromic AV reentry,[95,96] and its overall efficacy can be improved with the addition of a beta-blocker.[97] In patients with successful prevention of SVT induction, chronic therapy was generally effective in preventing clinical recurrences.[95,97] Similar efficacy has been shown in response to diltiazem, with two-thirds of subjects who responded to acute testing having no recurrences and one-third having less frequent and better tolerated events.[53]

Digitalis is more effective in the treatment of AV nodal reentry than AV reentry with its effect predominantly on anterograde AV nodal conduction, resulting in an increase in refractoriness and conduction time of the AV node, a narrowing of the zone of induction of atrial premature beats, and a decrease in the tachycardia rate.[98] In children, digoxin may be considered as a first line of therapy for the chronic treatment of SVT,[99–101] and its effectiveness can be increased in combination with beta-blockers.[102] Digoxin is less effective in children and infants with Wolff-Parkinson-White syndrome,[103] and its use as monotherapy in this group is not recommended.[104]

Less commonly used in the chronic treatment of paroxysmal SVT are the class 1C antiarrhythmic agents. Flecainide's affect on accessory pathway and retrograde AV nodal conduction, however,

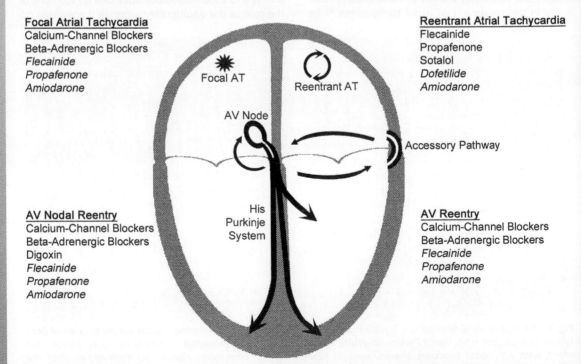

Focal Atrial Tachycardia
Calcium-Channel Blockers
Beta-Adrenergic Blockers
Flecainide
Propafenone
Amiodarone

Reentrant Atrial Tachycardia
Flecainide
Propafenone
Sotalol
Dofetilide
Amiodarone

AV Nodal Reentry
Calcium-Channel Blockers
Beta-Adrenergic Blockers
Digoxin
Flecainide
Propafenone
Amiodarone

AV Reentry
Calcium-Channel Blockers
Beta-Adrenergic Blockers
Flecainide
Propafenone
Amiodarone

Focal AT
Reentrant AT
AV Node
Accessory Pathway
His Purkinje System

Fig. 3. Mechanisms of SVT and their pharmacologic treatment. Different mechanisms of SVT are shown with commonly used pharmacologic agents for their treatment. Drugs shown in italics are generally considered second-line agents because of their increased potential for side effects.

Table 2
Common pharmacologic agents used for suppression of paroxysmal SVT

Therapeutic Agent	Dosage	Predominant Mechanism of Action
AV Nodal Blocking Agents		
Atenolol	50 – 200 mg daily	Beta-adrenergic blocker
Digoxin	0.125 – 0.25 mg daily	Na+/K+ ATPase pump inhibitor and enhances vagal activity
Diltiazem	120 – 360 mg daily	Ca^{++} channel blocker
Metoprolol	25 – 100 mg BID	Beta-adrenergic blocker
Verapamil	120 – 240 mg daily	Ca^{++} channel blocker
Membrane-Active Antiarrhythmic Agents		
Amiodarone	100 – 200 mg daily	Na+ and K+-channel blocker, with beta-adrenergic and Ca^{++} channel blocking activity
Dofetilide	0.125 – 0.5 mg BID	K$^+$ channel blocker, I[Kr]
Flecainide	50 – 150 mg BID	Class 1C Na$^+$ channel blocker
Procainamide	500 – 1000 mg	Class 1A Na$^+$ channel blocker
Propafenone	150 – 300 mg TID	Class 1C Na$^+$ channel blocker and modest beta-adrenergic blocker
Sotalol	120 – 160 mg BID	K$^+$ channel blocker, I[Kr] and Beta-adrenergic blocker

Abbreviations: BID, twice daily; TIC, 3 times daily.

makes it a useful agent in the suppression of AVRT and AVNRT.[73,105–108] In a series of 102 patients with frequent episodes of recurrent SVT, approximately two-thirds of whom had AVNRT or AVRT, 89% remained symptom free on oral flecainide over a mean follow-up period of 3.9 years.[109] The Flecainide Supraventricular Tachycardia Study included 67 patients with paroxysmal SVT, 87% of whom had symptomatic improvement on flecainide.[110] In a comparison study, both oral flecainide (200 mg/d) and oral verapamil (240 mg/d) were found to markedly decrease the frequency of arrhythmias with 11% of the flecainide group and 19% of the verapamil group discontinuing the drugs by 1 year because of lack of effectiveness.[111]

Propafenone is a class 1C agent that has similar electrophysiologic effects to flecainide, but also causes an increase in the anterograde AV nodal conduction time and anterograde AV nodal effective refractory period. Chronic therapy with propafenone has showed it to be effective in both AV nodal reentry and AV reentry.[112] A large placebo-controlled trial of 2 dosing regimens in patients with both paroxysmal SVT and atrial fibrillation found propafenone to be effective at a dosage of 300 mg twice a day for patients with SVT and had fewer side effects than at the higher dosage of 300 mg 3 times a day.[113] An important contraindication to the use of Class 1C agents is the presence of known coronary disease or structural heart disease, as the risk of proarrhythmic effects in those settings is increased.[114]

Other antiarrhythmic agents that are effective in the treatment of paroxysmal SVT include sotalol,[115,116] dofetilide,[117,118] and amiodarone.[119–121] The chronic use of amiodarone results in different electrophysiologic effects than those that occur with the acute administration. Although IV amiodarone causes significant prolongation in AV nodal conduction, a greater effect on the atrial, ventricular, and accessory pathway effective refractory periods is seen with chronic use,[122] along with a decrease in the ventricular response rate of induced atrial fibrillation.[123] These other antiarrhythmic agents are best considered as second-line agents, however, because of their side-effect profiles and increased risk of proarrhythmia.

Atrial Tachycardia

Although atrial tachycardia is less common than AVNRT and AVRT, chronic therapy for suppression of these arrhythmias is sometimes necessary and the choice of agent depends on the underlying mechanism. Focal atrial tachycardias can be of either an automatic or triggered mechanism and may respond to adenosine, calcium channel antagonists, beta-blockers, or amiodarone acutely.[43,69,124,125] Chronic therapy with calcium channel antagonists or beta-blockers is recommended as initial therapy because of their low toxicity and side effects, with Class 1C agents and amiodarone for resistant arrhythmias.[2,126] In children, focal atrial tachycardias can be difficult to control and amiodarone has been shown to be the most effective agent, followed by the Class 1C antiarrhythmics.[127]

In patients with reentrant atrial arrhythmias, the role of AV nodal blocking agents is limited to controlling the ventricular response rate, as these agents have little effect in suppressing the primary arrhythmia. Instead, Class 1A, Class 1C, and Class III agents are typically required for adequate control of the arrhythmia.[126] As most patients with this type of atrial tachycardia are older and have structural heart disease, class 1C agents should be used only after coronary artery disease is excluded.[2] In a small series of 19 patients with intra-atrial reentrant tachycardia, only 6 patients could be successfully treated long-term with a Class 1A agent, whereas amiodarone was effective in 11 patients.[128]

Multifocal atrial tachycardia (MAT) is an irregular rhythm with at least 3 different P-wave morphologies at different rates and is most commonly associated with underlying pulmonary disease. This arrhythmia can be quite difficult to treat and antiarrhythmic agents are generally ineffective, although some success with amiodarone has been reported.[129] The agents most commonly used for this arrhythmia are beta-blockers and calcium channel antagonists. In one series of critically ill patients, verapamil was effective in either controlling the ventricular rate or suppressing the arrhythmia, but also had a tendency to aggravate preexisting hypoxemia.[130] Salerno and colleagues[131] reported on 16 consecutive patients with MAT in whom verapamil (total 6–30 mg at a rate of 1 mg/min) was successful in decreasing the heart rate by 21% and restoring sinus rhythm in 8 of 16 patients with no effect on arterial blood gases. Beta-blocking agents, however, may be more effective in the treatment of this arrhythmia. Despite concerns for the use of beta-blockers in patients with significant pulmonary disease,

Arsura and colleagues[132] reported on a series of 11 patients with serious underlying respiratory disease and MAT, who were given metoprolol in a dose of 25 to 50 mg orally with no adverse pulmonary effects, while successfully restoring sinus rhythm in all patients. In a randomized trial comparing metoprolol and verapamil with placebo, metoprolol was most effective with an 89% response rate (defined as restoration of sinus rhythm or ventricular rate <100 bpm), compared with 44% in the verapamil group and 20% in the placebo group.[133]

SUMMARY

Paroxysmal SVTs are a diverse group of arrhythmias with most being attributable to either AV nodal reentry or atrioventricular reentry. Pharmacologic therapy with adenosine and calcium channel blockers is most commonly used in the acute treatment of these arrhythmias, although other antiarrhythmic agents may also be effective. For long-term treatment, the efficacy of catheter ablation therapy has made it the treatment of choice in paroxysmal SVT, but pharmacotherapy is still used in patients who are either not candidates for or have failed a catheter-based approach. In these patients, careful consideration needs to be given to the mechanism of the arrhythmia and the patient's comorbidities for choosing the most effective and safest agent.

REFERENCES

1. Orejarena LA, Vidaillet HJ, DeStefano F, et al. Paroxysmal supraventricular tachycardia in the general population. J Am Coll Cardiol 1998;31: 150–7.
2. Blomstrom-Lundqvist C, Scheinman MM, Aliot EM, et al. ACC/AHA/ESC guidelines for the management of patients with supraventricular arrhythmias—executive summary: a report of the American College of Cardiology/American Heart Association Task Force on Practice Guidelines and the European Society of Cardiology Committee for Practice Guidelines (writing committee to develop guidelines for the management of patients with supraventricular arrhythmias). Circulation 2003;108:1871–909.
3. Ganz LI, Friedman PL. Supraventricular tachycardia. N Engl J Med 1995;332:162–73.
4. Ferguson JD, DiMarco JP. Contemporary management of paroxysmal supraventricular tachycardia. Circulation 2003;107:1096–9.
5. Shah D, Jais P, Haissaguerre M. Electrophysiological evaluation and ablation of atypical right atrial flutter. Card Electrophysiol Rev 2002;6:365–70.

6. Akhtar M, Jazayeri MR, Sra J, et al. Atrioventricular nodal reentry. Clinical, electrophysiological, and therapeutic considerations. Circulation 1993;88: 282–95.

7. Cranefield PF. Action potentials, afterpotentials, and arrhythmias. Circ Res 1977;41:415–23.

8. Wit AL, Rosen MR. Pathophysiologic mechanisms of cardiac arrhythmias. Am Heart J 1983;106: 798–811.

9. Akhtar M, Tchou PJ, Jazayeri M. Mechanisms of clinical tachycardias. Am J Cardiol 1988;61: 9A–19A.

10. Marchlinski FE, Miller JM. Atrial arrhythmias exacerbated by theophylline. Response to verapamil and evidence for triggered activity in man. Chest 1985;88:931–4.

11. O'Hara GE, Philippon F, Champagne J, et al. Catheter ablation for cardiac arrhythmias: a 14-year experience with 5330 consecutive patients at the Quebec Heart Institute, Laval Hospital. Can J Cardiol 2007;23(Suppl B):67B–70B.

12. Scheinman MM, Huang S. The 1998 NASPE prospective catheter ablation registry. Pacing Clin Electrophysiol 2000;23:1020–8.

13. Parker RB, McCollam PL. Adenosine in the episodic treatment of paroxysmal supraventricular tachycardia. Clin Pharm 1990;9:261–71.

14. McIntosh-Yellin NL, Drew BJ, Scheinman MM. Safety and efficacy of central intravenous bolus administration of adenosine for termination of supraventricular tachycardia. J Am Coll Cardiol. 1993;22:741–5.

15. DiMarco JP, Miles W, Akhtar M, et al. Adenosine for paroxysmal supraventricular tachycardia: dose ranging and comparison with verapamil. Assessment in placebo-controlled, multicenter trials. The Adenosine for PSVT Study Group. Ann Intern Med 1990;113:104–10.

16. Rankin AC, Brooks R, Ruskin JN, et al. Adenosine and the treatment of supraventricular tachycardia. Am J Med 1992;92:655–64.

17. Biaggioni I, Paul S, Puckett A, et al. Caffeine and theophylline as adenosine receptor antagonists in humans. J Pharmacol Exp Ther 1991;258: 588–93.

18. Lerman BB, Belardinelli L. Cardiac electrophysiology of adenosine. Basic and clinical concepts. Circulation 1991;83:1499–509.

19. Donahue JK, Orias D, Berger RD, et al. Comparison of adenosine effects on atrioventricular node reentry and atrioventricular reciprocating tachycardias. Clin Cardiol 1998;21:743–5.

20. Sethi KK, Singh B, Kalra GS, et al. Comparative clinical and electrophysiologic effects of adenosine and verapamil on termination of paroxysmal supraventricular tachycardia. Indian Heart J 1994;46: 141–4.

21. Lai WT, Lee KT, Wu JC, et al. Differential effects of adenosine on antegrade fast pathway, antegrade slow pathway, and retrograde fast pathway in atrioventricular nodal reentry. Cardiology 2002;97: 147–54.

22. Souza JJ, Zivin A, Flemming M, et al. Differential effect of adenosine on anterograde and retrograde fast pathway conduction in patients with atrioventricular nodal reentrant tachycardia. J Cardiovasc Electrophysiol 1998;9:820–4.

23. Miyata A, Kobayashi Y, Jinbo Y, et al. Effects of adenosine triphosphate on ventriculoatrial conduction—usefulness and problems in assessment of catheter ablation of accessory pathways. Jpn Circ J 1997;61:323–30.

24. Mewis C, Kuhlkamp V, Mermi J, et al. High variability of retrograde fast pathway sensitivity to adenosine. Clin Cardiol 2000;23:576–8.

25. Iwai S, Markowitz SM, Stein KM, et al. Response to adenosine differentiates focal from macroreentrant atrial tachycardia: validation using three-dimensional electroanatomic mapping. Circulation 2002;106:2793–9.

26. Kall JG, Kopp D, Olshansky B, et al. Adenosine-sensitive atrial tachycardia. Pacing Clin Electrophysiol 1995;18:300–6.

27. Engelstein ED, Lippman N, Stein KM, et al. Mechanism-specific effects of adenosine on atrial tachycardia. Circulation 1994;89:2645–54.

28. Pelleg A, Pennock RS, Kutalek SP. Proarrhythmic effects of adenosine: one decade of clinical data. Am J Ther 2002;9:141–7.

29. Kaltman JR, Tanel RE, Shah MJ, et al. Induction of atrial fibrillation after the routine use of adenosine. Pediatr Emerg Care 2006;22:113–5.

30. Strickberger SA, Man KC, Daoud EG, et al. Adenosine-induced atrial arrhythmia: a prospective analysis. Ann Intern Med 1997;127:417–22.

31. Belardinelli L, Shryock JC, Song Y, et al. Ionic basis of the electrophysiological actions of adenosine on cardiomyocytes. FASEB J 1995;9:359–65.

32. Cheung JW, Lerman BB. CVT-510: a selective A1 adenosine receptor agonist. Cardiovasc Drug Rev 2003;21:277–92.

33. Ellenbogen KA, O'Neill G, Prystowsky EN, et al. Trial to evaluate the management of paroxysmal supraventricular tachycardia during an electrophysiology study with tecadenoson. Circulation 2005;111:3202–8.

34. Prystowsky EN, Niazi I, Curtis AB, et al. Termination of paroxysmal supraventricular tachycardia by tecadenoson (CVT-510), a novel A1-adenosine receptor agonist. J Am Coll Cardiol 2003;42: 1098–102.

35. Tan HL, Spekhorst HH, Peters RJ, et al. Adenosine induced ventricular arrhythmias in the emergency room. Pacing Clin Electrophysiol 2001;24:450–5.

36. Ertan C, Atar I, Gulmez O, et al. Adenosine-induced ventricular arrhythmias in patients with supraventricular tachycardias. Ann Noninvasive Electrocardiol 2008;13:386–90.

37. Huemer M, Boldt LH, Rolf S, et al. Sustained monomorphic ventricular tachycardia after adenosine infusion. Int J Cardiol 2009;131:e97–100.

38. Ben-Sorek ES, Wiesel J. Ventricular fibrillation following adenosine administration. A case report. Arch Intern Med 1993;153:2701–2.

39. Gupta AK, Shah CP, Maheshwari A, et al. Adenosine induced ventricular fibrillation in Wolff-Parkinson-White syndrome. Pacing Clin Electrophysiol 2002;25:477–80.

40. Shah CP, Gupta AK, Thakur RK, et al. Adenosine-induced ventricular fibrillation. Indian Heart J 2001;53:208–10.

41. Parham WA, Mehdirad AA, Biermann KM, et al. Case report: adenosine induced ventricular fibrillation in a patient with stable ventricular tachycardia. J Interv Card Electrophysiol 2001;5:71–4.

42. Walsh RC, Felice KL, Meehan TJ, et al. Adenosine-induced cardiopulmonary arrest in a patient with paroxysmal supraventricular tachycardia. Am J Emerg Med 2009;27:901.e1–2.

43. Markowitz SM, Stein KM, Mittal S, et al. Differential effects of adenosine on focal and macroreentrant atrial tachycardia. J Cardiovasc Electrophysiol 1999;10:489–502.

44. Gonzalez R, Scheinman MM. Treatment of supraventricular arrhythmias with intravenous and oral verapamil. Chest 1981;80:465–70.

45. Olukotun AY, Klein GJ. Efficacy and safety of intravenous nadolol for supraventricular tachycardia. Am J Cardiol 1987;60:59D–62D.

46. Intravenous esmolol for the treatment of supraventricular tachyarrhythmia: results of a multicenter, baseline-controlled safety and efficacy study in 160 patients. The Esmolol Research Group. Am Heart J 1986;112:498–505.

47. Abrams J, Allen J, Allin D, et al. Efficacy and safety of esmolol vs propranolol in the treatment of supraventricular tachyarrhythmias: a multicenter double-blind clinical trial. Am Heart J 1985;110:913–22.

48. Madsen CD, Pointer JE, Lynch TG. A comparison of adenosine and verapamil for the treatment of supraventricular tachycardia in the prehospital setting. Ann Emerg Med 1995;25:649–55.

49. Klein GJ, Gulamhusein S, Prystowsky EN, et al. Comparison of the electrophysiologic effects of intravenous and oral verapamil in patients with paroxysmal supraventricular tachycardia. Am J Cardiol 1982;49:117–24.

50. Belhassen B, Glick A, Laniado S. Comparative clinical and electrophysiologic effects of adenosine triphosphate and verapamil on paroxysmal reciprocating junctional tachycardia. Circulation 1988;77:795–805.

51. Brady WJJ, DeBehnke DJ, Wickman LL, et al. Treatment of out-of-hospital supraventricular tachycardia: adenosine vs verapamil. Acad Emerg Med 1996;3:574–85.

52. Haft JI, Habbab MA. Treatment of atrial arrhythmias. Effectiveness of verapamil when preceded by calcium infusion. Arch Intern Med 1986;146:1085–9.

53. Lim SH, Anantharaman V, Teo WS, et al. Slow infusion of calcium channel blockers compared with intravenous adenosine in the emergency treatment of supraventricular tachycardia. Resuscitation 2009;80:523–8.

54. Gulamhusein S, Ko P, Carruthers SG, et al. Acceleration of the ventricular response during atrial fibrillation in the Wolff-Parkinson-White syndrome after verapamil. Circulation 1982;65:348–54.

55. Jacob AS, Nielsen DH, Gianelly RE. Fatal ventricular fibrillation following verapamil in Wolff-Parkinson-White syndrome with atrial fibrillation. Ann Emerg Med 1985;14:159–60.

56. Huycke EC, Sung RJ, Dias VC, et al. Intravenous diltiazem for termination of reentrant supraventricular tachycardia: a placebo-controlled, randomized, double-blind, multicenter study. J Am Coll Cardiol 1989;13:538–44.

57. Dougherty AH, Jackman WM, Naccarelli GV, et al. Acute conversion of paroxysmal supraventricular tachycardia with intravenous diltiazem. IV Diltiazem study group. Am J Cardiol 1992;70:587–92.

58. Boudonas G, Lefkos N, Efthymiadis AP, et al. Intravenous administration of diltiazem in the treatment of supraventricular tachyarrhythmias. Acta Cardiol 1995;50:125–34.

59. Sternbach GL, Schroeder JS, Eliastam M, et al. Intravenous diltiazem for the treatment of supraventricular tachycardia. Clin Cardiol 1986;9:145–9.

60. Gupta A, Naik A, Vora A, et al. Comparison of efficacy of intravenous diltiazem and esmolol in terminating supraventricular tachycardia. J Assoc Physicians India 1999;47:969–72.

61. Angaran DM, Schultz NJ, Tschida VH. Esmolol hydrochloride: an ultrashort-acting, beta-adrenergic blocking agent. Clin Pharm 1986;5:288–303.

62. Yeh SJ, Lin FC, Chou YY, et al. Termination of paroxysmal supraventricular tachycardia with a single oral dose of diltiazem and propranolol. Circulation 1985;71:104–9.

63. Alboni P, Tomasi C, Menozzi C, et al. Efficacy and safety of out-of-hospital self-administered single-dose oral drug treatment in the management of infrequent, well-tolerated paroxysmal supraventricular tachycardia. J Am Coll Cardiol 2001;37:548–53.

64. Hamer AW, Tanasescu DE, Marks JW, et al. Failure of episodic high-dose oral verapamil therapy to

convert supraventricular tachycardia: a study of plasma verapamil levels and gastric motility. Am Heart J 1987;114:334–42.

65. Rose JS, Bhandari A, Rahimtoola SH, et al. Effective termination of reentrant supraventricular tachycardia by single dose oral combination therapy with pindolol and verapamil. Am Heart J 1986;112:759–65.

66. Wellens HJ, Durrer D. Effect of procaine amide, quinidine, and ajmaline in the Wolff-Parkinson-White syndrome. Circulation 1974;50:114–20.

67. Windle J, Prystowsky EN, Miles WM, et al. Pharmacokinetic and electrophysiologic interactions of amiodarone and procainamide. Clin Pharmacol Ther 1987;41:603–10.

68. Hiejima K, Suzuki F, Takahashi M, et al. Electrophysiologic evaluation of antiarrhythmic drugs on supraventricular tachyarrhythmias. Jpn Circ J 1983;47:98–104.

69. Mehta AV, Sanchez GR, Sacks EJ, et al. Ectopic automatic atrial tachycardia in children: clinical characteristics, management and follow-up. J Am Coll Cardiol 1988;11:379–85.

70. Saoudi N, Cosio F, Waldo A, et al. Classification of atrial flutter and regular atrial tachycardia according to electrophysiologic mechanism and anatomic bases: a statement from a joint expert group from the working group of Arrhythmias of the European Society of Cardiology and the North American Society of Pacing and Electrophysiology. J Cardiovasc Electrophysiol 2001;12:852–66.

71. NA 3rd Estes, Garan H, Ruskin JN. Electrophysiologic properties of flecainide acetate. Am J Cardiol 1984;53:26B–9B.

72. Hellestrand KJ, Nathan AW, Bexton RS, et al. Cardiac electrophysiologic effects of flecainide acetate for paroxysmal reentrant junctional tachycardias. Am J Cardiol 1983;51:770–6.

73. Musto B, D'Onofrio A, Cavallaro C, et al. Electrophysiologic effects and clinical efficacy of flecainide in children with recurrent paroxysmal supraventricular tachycardia. Am J Cardiol 1988;62:229–33.

74. Gambhir DS, Bhargava M, Arora R, et al. Electrophysiologic effects and therapeutic efficacy of intravenous flecainide for termination of paroxysmal supraventricular tachycardia. Indian Heart J 1995;47:237–43.

75. Musto B, Cavallaro C, Musto A, et al. Flecainide single oral dose for management of paroxysmal supraventricular tachycardia in children and young adults. Am Heart J 1992;124:110–5.

76. Vik-Mo H, Ohm OJ, Lund-Johansen P. Electrophysiologic effects of flecainide acetate in patients with sinus nodal dysfunction. Am J Cardiol 1982;50:1090–4.

77. Dukes ID, Vaughan Williams EM. The multiple modes of action of propafenone. Eur Heart J 1984;5:115–25.

78. Sethi KK, Prasad GS, Mohan JC, et al. Electrophysiologic effects of oral propafenone in Wolff-Parkinson-White syndrome studied by programmed electrical stimulation. Indian Heart J 1991;43:5–10.

79. Siddoway LA, Roden DM, Woosley RL. Clinical pharmacology of propafenone: pharmacokinetics, metabolism and concentration-response relations. Am J Cardiol 1984;54:9D–12D.

80. Cheriex EC, Krijne R, Brugada P, et al. Lack of clinically significant beta-blocking effect of propafenone. Eur Heart J 1987;8:53–6.

81. Lee JT, Kroemer HK, Silberstein DJ, et al. The role of genetically determined polymorphic drug metabolism in the beta-blockade produced by propafenone. N Engl J Med 1990;322:1764–8.

82. Reimold SC, Maisel WH, Antman EM. Propafenone for the treatment of supraventricular tachycardia and atrial fibrillation: a meta-analysis. Am J Cardiol 1998;82:66N–71N.

83. Eidher U, Freihoff F, Kaltenbrunner W, et al. Efficacy and safety of ibutilide for the conversion of monomorphic atrial tachycardia. Pacing Clin Electrophysiol 2006;29:358–62.

84. Glatter KA, Dorostkar PC, Yang Y, et al. Electrophysiological effects of ibutilide in patients with accessory pathways. Circulation 2001;104:1933–9.

85. Andrade JG, Connolly SJ, Dorian P, et al. Antiarrhythmic use from 1991 to 2007: insights from the Canadian Registry of Atrial Fibrillation (CARAF I and II). Heart Rhythm 2010.

86. Waleffe A, Nzayinambaho K, Rodriguez LM, et al. Mechanisms of termination of supraventricular tachycardias by intravenous class III antiarrhythmic agents. A comparison of amiodarone and sotalol. Eur Heart J 1989;10:1084–9.

87. Gomes JA, Kang PS, Hariman RJ, et al. Electrophysiologic effects and mechanisms of termination of supraventricular tachycardia by intravenous amiodarone. Am Heart J 1984;107:214–21.

88. Chang PM, Silka MJ, Moromisato DY, et al. Amiodarone versus procainamide for the acute treatment of recurrent supraventricular tachycardia in pediatric patients. Circ Arrhythm Electrophysiol 2010;3:134–40.

89. Kuga K, Yamaguchi I, Sugishita Y. Effect of intravenous amiodarone on electrophysiologic variables and on the modes of termination of atrioventricular reciprocating tachycardia in Wolff-Parkinson-White syndrome. Jpn Circ J 1999;63:189–95.

90. Tijunelis MA, Herbert ME. Myth: intravenous amiodarone is safe in patients with atrial fibrillation and Wolff-Parkinson-White syndrome in the emergency department. CJEM 2005;7:262–5.

91. Simonian SM, Lotfipour S, Wall C, et al. Challenging the superiority of amiodarone for rate control in

Wolff-Parkinson-White and atrial fibrillation. Intern Emerg Med 2010.

92. Akhtar M, Tchou P, Jazayeri M. Use of calcium channel entry blockers in the treatment of cardiac arrhythmias. Circulation 1989;80:IV31–9.

93. Gmeiner R, Ng CK. Metoprolol in the treatment and prophylaxis of paroxysmal reentrant supraventricular tachycardia. J Cardiovasc Pharmacol 1982;4: 5–13.

94. Lindsay BD, Saksena S, Rothbart ST, et al. Long-term efficacy and safety of beta-adrenergic receptor antagonists for supraventricular tachycardia. Am J Cardiol 1987;60:63D–7D.

95. Sakurai M, Yasuda H, Kato N, et al. Acute and chronic effects of verapamil in patients with paroxysmal supraventricular tachycardia. Am Heart J 1983;105:619–28.

96. Hamer A, Peter T, Platt M, et al. Effects of verapamil on supraventricular tachycardia in patients with overt and concealed Wolff-Parkinson-White syndrome. Am Heart J 1981;101:600–12.

97. Yee R, Gulamhusein SS, Klein GJ. Combined verapamil and propranolol for supraventricular tachycardia. Am J Cardiol 1984;53:757–63.

98. Wellens HJ, Duren DR, Liem DL, et al. Effect of digitalis in patients with paroxysmal atrioventricular nodal tachycardia. Circulation 1975;52:779–88.

99. Bouhouch R, El Houari T, Fellat I, et al. Pharmacological therapy in children with nodal reentry tachycardia: when, how and how long to treat the affected patients. Curr Pharm Des 2008;14:766–9.

100. Pfammatter JP, Stocker FP. Results of a restrictive use of antiarrhythmic drugs in the chronic treatment of atrioventricular reentrant tachycardias in infancy and childhood. Am J Cardiol 1998;82: 72–5.

101. Strasburger JF. Cardiac arrhythmias in childhood. Diagnostic considerations and treatment. Drugs 1991;42:974–83.

102. Hung JS, Kou HC, Wu D. Digoxin, propranolol, and atrioventricular reentrant tachycardia in the Wolff-Parkinson-White syndrome. Ann Intern Med 1982; 97:175–82.

103. Tortoriello TA, Snyder CS, Smith EO, et al. Frequency of recurrence among infants with supraventricular tachycardia and comparison of recurrence rates among those with and without preexcitation and among those with and without response to digoxin and/or propranolol therapy. Am J Cardiol 2003;92:1045–9.

104. Luedtke SA, Kuhn RJ, McCaffrey FM. Pharmacologic management of supraventricular tachycardias in children. Part 1: Wolff-Parkinson-White and atrioventricular nodal reentry. Ann Pharmacother 1997;31:1227–43.

105. Ward DE, Jones S, Shinebourne EA. Use of flecainide acetate for refractory junctional tachycardias

in children with the Wolff-Parkinson-White syndrome. Am J Cardiol 1986;57:787–90.

106. Kim SS, Lal R, Ruffy R. Treatment of paroxysmal reentrant supraventricular tachycardia with flecainide acetate. Am J Cardiol 1986;58:80–5.

107. Cockrell JL, Scheinman MM, Titus C, et al. Safety and efficacy of oral flecainide therapy in patients with atrioventricular re-entrant tachycardia. Ann Intern Med 1991;114:189–94.

108. Zee-Cheng CS, Kim SS, Ruffy R. Flecainide acetate for treatment of bypass tract mediated reentrant tachycardia. Am J Cardiol 1988;62: 23D–8D.

109. Hellestrand KJ. Efficacy and safety of long-term oral flecainide acetate in patients with responsive supraventricular tachycardia. Am J Cardiol 1996; 77:83A–8A.

110. Hopson JR, Buxton AE, Rinkenberger RL, et al. Safety and utility of flecainide acetate in the routine care of patients with supraventricular tachyarrhythmias: results of a multicenter trial. The Flecainide Supraventricular Tachycardia Study Group. Am J Cardiol 1996;77:72A–82A.

111. Dorian P, Naccarelli GV, Coumel P, et al. A randomized comparison of flecainide versus verapamil in paroxysmal supraventricular tachycardia. The Flecainide Multicenter Investigators Group. Am J Cardiol 1996;77:89A–95A.

112. Musto B, D'Onofrio A, Cavallaro C, et al. Electrophysiological effects and clinical efficacy of propafenone in children with recurrent paroxysmal supraventricular tachycardia. Circulation 1988;78: 863–9.

113. A randomized, placebo-controlled trial of propafenone in the prophylaxis of paroxysmal supraventricular tachycardia and paroxysmal atrial fibrillation. UK Propafenone PSVT Study Group. Circulation 1995;92:2550–7.

114. Echt DS, Liebson PR, Mitchell LB, et al. Mortality and morbidity in patients receiving encainide, flecainide, or placebo. The Cardiac Arrhythmia Suppression Trial. N Engl J Med 1991;324: 781–8.

115. Mitchell LB, Wyse DG, Duff HJ. Electropharmacology of sotalol in patients with Wolff-Parkinson-White syndrome. Circulation 1987;76:810–8.

116. Kunze KP, Schluter M, Kuck KH. Sotalol in patients with Wolff-Parkinson-White syndrome. Circulation 1987;75:1050–7.

117. Tendera M, Wnuk-Wojnar AM, Kulakowski P, et al. Efficacy and safety of dofetilide in the prevention of symptomatic episodes of paroxysmal supraventricular tachycardia: a 6-month double-blind comparison with propafenone and placebo. Am Heart J 2001;142:93–8.

118. Kobayashi Y, Atarashi H, Ino T, et al. Clinical and electrophysiologic effects of dofetilide in

patients with supraventricular tachyarrhythmias. J Cardiovasc Pharmacol 1997;30:367—73.

119. Rosenbaum MB, Chiale PA, Ryba D, et al. Control of tachyarrhythmias associated with Wolff-Parkinson-White syndrome by amiodarone hydrochloride. Am J Cardiol 1974;34:215—23.

120. Wellens HJ, Lie KI, Bar FW, et al. Effect of amiodarone in the Wolff-Parkinson-White syndrome. Am J Cardiol 1976;38:189—94.

121. Feld GK, Nademanee K, Weiss J, et al. Electrophysiologic basis for the suppression by amiodarone of orthodromic supraventricular tachycardias complicating pre-excitation syndromes. J Am Coll Cardiol 1984;3:1298—307.

122. Wellens HJ, Brugada P, Abdollah H, et al. A comparison of the electrophysiologic effects of intravenous and oral amiodarone in the same patient. Circulation 1984;69:120—4.

123. Feld GK, Nademanee K, Stevenson W, et al. Clinical and electrophysiologic effects of amiodarone in patients with atrial fibrillation complicating the Wolff-Parkinson-White syndrome. Am Heart J 1988;115:102—7.

124. Barbarash RA, Bauman JL, Lukazewski AA, et al. Verapamil infusions in the treatment of atrial tachyarrhythmias. Crit Care Med 1986;14:886—8.

125. Khongphatthanayothin A, Chotivitayatarakorn P, Lertsupcharoen P, et al. Atrial tachycardia from enhanced automaticity in children: diagnosis and initial management. J Med Assoc Thai 2001;84: 1321—8.

126. Steinbeck G, Hoffmann E. 'True' atrial tachycardia. Eur Heart J 1998;19(Suppl E):E10—2, E48—49.

127. von Bernuth G, Engelhardt W, Kramer HH, et al. Atrial automatic tachycardia in infancy and childhood. Eur Heart J 1992;13:1410—5.

128. Haines DE, DiMarco JP. Sustained intraatrial reentrant tachycardia: clinical, electrocardiographic and electrophysiologic characteristics and long-term follow-up. J Am Coll Cardiol 1990;15: 1345—54.

129. Kouvaras G, Cokkinos DV, Halal G, et al. The effective treatment of multifocal atrial tachycardia with amiodarone. Jpn Heart J 1989;30:301—12.

130. Hazard PB, Burnett CR. Verapamil in multifocal atrial tachycardia. Hemodynamic and respiratory changes. Chest 1987;91:68—70.

131. Salerno DM, Anderson B, Sharkey PJ, et al. Intravenous verapamil for treatment of multifocal atrial tachycardia with and without calcium pretreatment. Ann Intern Med 1987;107:623—8.

132. Arsura EL, Solar M, Lefkin AS, et al. Metoprolol in the treatment of multifocal atrial tachycardia. Crit Care Med 1987;15:591—4.

133. Arsura E, Lefkin AS, Scher DL, et al. A randomized, double-blind, placebo-controlled study of verapamil and metoprolol in treatment of multifocal atrial tachycardia. Am J Med 1988;85:519—24.

Pharmacologic Conversion of Atrial Fibrillation and Atrial Flutter

Alessandro Marinelli, MD*, Alessandro Capucci, MD

KEYWORDS

• Atrial fibrillation • Atrial flutter
• Pharmacologic cardioversion • Antiarrhythmic drugs

Atrial fibrillation (AF) and atrial flutter (AFl) are the most common sustained tachyarrhythmias occurring in the clinical setting.[1] The management of these arrhythmias includes two different approaches, a rate-control and a rhythm-control strategy. A rhythm control strategy is preferable for achieving a quality-of-life goal; nevertheless, no differences in long-term survival were found between the two strategies in several clinical trials.[2–6] In addition, medical therapy with currently available antiarrhythmic drugs (AADs) is moderately effective, with a high rate of recurrences (approximately 50% at 12 months) and is associated with risks of adverse effects (AEs) and multiorgan toxicity.[7] Direct current cardioversion (CV) is more effective than pharmacologic CV in the long-lasting forms.[1]

AADs have a high rate of efficacy to restore normal sinus rhythm (SR) in patients with arrhythmias lasting less than 48 hours' duration. Agents currently approved for this indication are dofetilide, ibutilide, flecainide, and propafenone. New drugs with different mechanisms and time to efficacy are under investigation.

TIME FROM ONSET OF ARRHYTHMIA IN THE CHOICE OF AADS AND IN EVALUATING THEIR REAL EFFICACY

Time from onset and duration influence strongly the effectiveness of the attempts to restore SR, especially if pharmacologic CV is performed.[1]

Pharmacologic CV is most effective when initiated within 7 days after onset of AF and is markedly reduced in AF of longer duration.[1]

The relevance of time is underlined in the definition of AF present in the international guidelines on AF treatment: AF is defined as paroxysmal when it terminates spontaneously (generally lasting <7 days but most lasting <24 hours), as persistent when it does not self-terminate and is sustained beyond 7 days until effective pharmacologic or electrical CV is performed, and as permanent if CV has failed or has not been attempted and in cases of long-lasting AF (ie, lasting more than 1 year).[1]

Another important consideration is related to the high rate of spontaneous conversion to SR occurring in patients with recent-onset AF (lasting <48 hours): spontaneous conversions rates have been reported s high as 73% within the first 24 hours[8] and even higher (76%–83%) in the first 48 hours.[9]

This high rate of spontaneous conversion underlines the need for performing placebo-controlled trials and evaluating the time to efficacy of every drug, considering its pharmacokinetics properties and its expected peak of action. The evaluation of the real efficacy of AADs may be difficult in some cases, especially in recent-onset arrhythmias, and some investigators suggest the clinical usefulness of a watchful waiting period, allowing spontaneous SR conversion to occur before active treatment is adopted.[10]

Clinica di Cardiologia, Azienda Ospedaliero Universitaria Ospedali Riuniti, Università Politecnica delle Marche, Via Conca 71, Località Torrette, Ancona 60126, Italy
* Corresponding author.
E-mail address: marinelli.doc@gmail.com

Card Electrophysiol Clin 2 (2010) 393–407
doi:10.1016/j.ccep.2010.06.002
1877-9182/10/$ — see front matter © 2010 Elsevier Inc. All rights reserved.

Evidence on effectiveness of pharmacologic CV of AF and AFl is limited by lack of standard criteria of inclusion and variable drug dosages and intervals from drug administration to assessment of outcome.[1] The majority of patients included is represented by recent-onset AF (<48 hours), and little is known about the role of pharmacologic conversion in long-lasting AF or AFl.

AGENTS AVAILABLE FOR PHARMACOLOGIC CV OF AF OR AFL

Several drugs are available and commonly used for converting AF and AFl to normal SR. Nevertheless, only some of these agents are formally approved by the United States Food and Drug Administration (FDA) for this specific indication. Currently approved drugs for intravenous administration are flecainide, propafenone, and ibutilide, whereas quinidine and dofetilide are approved as oral agents.

Class IA Drugs

Quinidine
Quinidine is an antiarrhythmic agent with class IA activity: depressing the rapid inward depolarizing sodium current, it slows conduction velocity and prolongs the effective refractory period. It can interrupt and prevent re-entrant arrhythmias and arrhythmias due to increased automaticity, including AF, AFl, and paroxysmal supraventricular tachycardia (PSVT).

Quinidine is currently approved for acute conversion of symptomatic AF and AFl. The preparation commonly used for oral administration is quinidine sulfate, and recommended dose is 750 to 1500 mg in divided doses over 6 to 12 hours.[1] It is usually administered after digoxin or verapamil has been given to control the ventricular response rate, because its anticholinergic activity can facilitate rapid conduction through atrioventricular node.

In the studies performed on recent-onset AF,[11,12] quinidine was administered orally in repeated doses of 200 to 275 mg every 2 hours, up to 1100 mg. Other regimens adopted were 300 to 400 mg three times daily or 300 to 600 mg oral loading dose.[13] Reported rate of conversion to SR is variable (ranging between 59% and 86% within the first 24 hours); nevertheless, it seems moderately effective compared with placebo. There was a delayed time to conversion compared with class IC agents.[11,12]

Few studies have been performed to analyze the efficacy of quinidine for conversion of long-lasting AF to SR with different results. In a group of 49 patients with persistent AF lasting more than 48 hours but less than 6 months, the rate of conversion was 79.6%.[14] In another small study of 40 patients with chronic AF (lasting more than 4 weeks up to 2 years), SR was achieved only in 25% of patients.[15] A rate of conversion of 47% was reported by Kerin and colleagues[16] in another small group of chronic AF patients.

In conclusion, inconsistent data exist to support the employment of quinidine in the setting of long-term AF, but the drug is effective in pharmacologic conversion of recent-onset AF at a mean longer time to conversion. Nevertheless, its use in clinical practice is limited, due to its side effects, most often affecting the gastrointestinal tract, and concern about its safety. The most dangerous AE after quinidine administration is torsades de pointes, reported in 1% to 8% of patients treated.[17] In addition, meta-analyses performed on quinidine use for prevention of AF recurrences showed an increased all-cause mortality trend compared with control,[18,19] contributing to its dramatic decrease in use. No meta-analysis is available for the CV setting.

Procainamide
Procainamide hydrochloride is another group IA cardiac AAD, currently approved for the treatment of documented ventricular life-threatening arrhythmias.

Intravenous procainamide has been used extensively for conversion of recent-onset AF and AFl, and several studies suggest that it may be superior to placebo.[20,21] Commonly used dosages are an initial loading dose of 5 to 15 mg/kg (maximum dose 1000 mg) delivered over 15 to 30 minutes, followed by continuous infusion of 2 to 6 mg per minute.

A recent study conducted on 362 patients who had AF less than 48 hours' duration, evaluated the effectiveness in SR conversion and the safety of intravenously administered procainamide, propafenone, and amiodarone within the first 24 hours. The rate of success of procainamide was 68.5%, superior to placebo (61.1%) but inferior to amiodarone and propafenone (rate of success of 89.1 and 80.2, respectively).[22] Ibutilide resulted superior to procainamide for SR conversion in patients with both recent-onset AF or AFl in another multicenter study.[23] Previous studies reported variable results,[24,25] but in conclusion it seems that procainamide has a limited efficacy compared with other currently available agents.

Procainamide has not been tested adequately in patients with long-lasting AF and its efficacy in this setting is unknown. The most common AE during intravenous administration is hypotension with depressed cardiac function. Procainamide is also associated with an increased risk of torsades de pointes due to QT prolongation.[26]

Disopyramide

Disopyramide, another class IA agent used for ventricular arrhythmias, has not been tested adequately for pharmacologic CV of AF and it is not currently recommended for this indication.

It may be effective when administered intravenously,[27] but data regarding its efficacy are mainly limited to prevention of AF recurrences after direct current CV.[28]

In any case, its use is limited by poor tolerability due to anticholinergic AEs, such as constipation, urinary retention, dry mouth, and depression of left ventricle contractility.

Class IC Drugs

Flecainide

Flecainide is a class IC antiarrhythmic drug that acts (1) depressing the rate of depolarization of action potential blocking the rapid sodium channel with marked use-dependent effects. It has a substantial effect on conduction velocity with modest effect on refractoriness.[29] It is approved by the FDA for the prevention of PSVT and for the treatment of symptomatic paroxysmal AF and AFI in patients without structural heart disease.

Flecainide has been highly effective in CV of recent-onset AF (**Table 1**). Its effectiveness in this setting was proved orally[30,31] and intravenously,[32–35] with a rate of conversion ranging from 51% at 3 hours to 72% at 8 hours for the oral administration and from 57% to 82% at 1 hour for the intravenous administration.

In comparison with oral flecainide, intravenous flecainide is no more effective for pharmacologic CV of recent-onset AF (conversion rate of 72 vs 75% at 8 hours), although it has a more rapid onset of action (mean time to CV 55 minutes vs 110 minutes).[36]

Conversion rates of oral flecainide were similar to rates obtained with oral propafenone.[31] Flecainide had similar efficacy to ibutilide[37] and greater efficacy than procainamide[20] and sotalol.[38]

Currently used dosages are a bolus of 1.5 to 3.0 mg/kg over 10 to 20 minutes, followed by 0.007 mg/kg/min continuous infusion for the intravenous administration, or single oral loading dose of 200 to 300 mg for the oral assumption.[1]

As with the other class IC AADs, AFI with rapid ventricular rate and bradycardia after conversion may occur, despite their relatively rare complications. Concomitant use of atrioventricular node blocking agents might be practical, because flecainide lacks the β-adrenergic blocking effects inherent in propafenone.

Flecainide should be avoided in patients with underlying organic heart disease involving abnormal ventricular function[1] because of its negative inotropic effect and because its use in these patients resulted in increased mortality.[39]

Flecainide seems to have a limited efficacy in the CV of AFI, despite that solid data are currently lacking, because patients with AFI are only a small number of patients included in AADs studies. Flecainide is much less effective in CV of long-lasting AF and, therefore, is not an advisable therapeutic option in this setting. Reported conversion rates range from 0 to 46% in heterogeneous groups of patients.[9]

Propafenone

Propafenone is another class IC agent, that acts blocking the fast inward sodium current in Purkinje fibers and to a lesser degree in ventricular muscle, in a use-dependent manner. In addition, it has a weak β-adrenoceptor blocking activity. It is currently approved to prolong time to recurrence of symptomatic paroxysmal AF, AFI, and PSVT in patients without structural heart disease.

The efficacy of propafenone in converting recent-onset AF has been evaluated in several trials, with both intravenous and oral administration (**Table 2**).

Intravenous propafenone had a conversion rate ranging from 50% to 80% within the first 2 to 3 hours in AF lasting less than 48 hours, significantly higher than placebo.[40–43] It was equally effective as intravenous amiodarone in restoring SR within the first 24 hours and with a more rapid effect.[22]

Oral administration of propafenone as a single oral loading dose also was more effective than placebo, with conversion rates of 45% to 55% at 3 hours and 69% to 78% at 8 hours.[44] The success rate of oral propafenone in previous studies available in literature ranges from 58% to 83%, depending on the duration of AF and follow-up after administration of the drug.[31,45–49]

There was comparable efficacy between intravenous and oral administration in a population of 123 patients with recent-onset AF. Intravenous propafenone was superior in the first hour of observation (rate of conversion 48% vs 15% of oral propafenone), whereas the overall efficacy of oral administered propafenone was superior at 8 hours (78% vs 53% of intravenous propafenone).[48] Oral propafenone was as efficacious as oral flecainide[31] and superior both to oral amiodarone[50] and quinidine plus digoxin within the first 4 hours,[51] although this superiority was lost after a longer periods of observation (>6 hours).

Currently used dosages for intravenous administration are 1.5 to 2.0 mg/kg over 10 to 20 minutes, followed by 0.007 mg/kg/min infusion. The oral administration route is started with a single

Table 1
Summary of randomized comparative trials on efficacy of flecainide in pharmacologic cardioversion of atrial fibrillation and atrial flutter

Authors	Year Published	No. of Patients	Route of Administration	AF Duration	Control (s)	Assessment of Efficacy	Efficacy		P
							Flecainide	Control	
Suttorp et al[32]	1989	40	IV	NA	Verapamil	1 Hour	82%	6%	NA
Suttorp et al[33]	1990	50	IV	NA	Propafenone	1 Hour	90%	55%	<0.002
Donovan et al[34]	1991	102	IV	<72 Hours	Placebo	1 Hour / 6 Hours	57% / 67%	14% / 35%	0.0001 / <0.03
Donovan et al[35]	1995	98	IV	<72 Hours	Placebo	2 Hours / 8 Hours	59% / 68%	22% / 59%	<0.005 / NS
Reisinger et al[38]	1998	71	IV	<24 Hours	Sotalol	2 Hours	69%	31%	<0.004
Reisinger et al[37]	2004	207	IV	<48 Hours	Ibutilide	1.5 Hours	56%	50%	NS
Kochiadakis et al[22]	2007	182	IV	<48 Hours	Placebo	24 Hours	89%	61%	<0.05
Madrid et al[20]	1993	80	IV	<24 Hours	Procainamide	1 Hour	92%	65%	0
Capucci et al[30]	1992	62	PO	<7 Days	Placebo / Amiodarone	8 Hours	91%	48% / 37%	<0.01 / <0.001
Capucci et al[31]	1994	181	PO	<7 Days	Placebo / Propafenone	8 Hours	78%	39% / 72%	<0.001 / NS

Abbreviations: IV, intravenous administration; NA, data not available; NS, nonsignificant; PO, oral administration.

Table 2
Summary of randomized comparative trials on efficacy of propafenone in pharmacologic cardioversion of atrial fibrillation and atrial flutter

Authors	Year Published	No. of Patients	Route of Administration	AF Duration	Control (s)	Assessment of Efficacy	Efficacy Propafenone	Efficacy Control	P
Kochiadakis et al[22]	2007	273	IV	<48 Hours	Placebo Amiodarone	24 Hours	80%	61% 89%	<0.05 NS
Kochiadakis et al[43]	1999	100	IV	<48 Hours	Placebo Amiodarone	24 hours	78%	55% 83%	<0.02 NS
Fresco et al[41]	1996	75	IV	<72 Hours	Placebo	3 Hours	59%	29%	<0.01
Bianconi and Mennuni[40]	1998	83	IV	<72 Hours	Placebo Digoxin	1 Hour	49%	14% 32%	<0.01 NS
Ganau and Lenzi[42]	1998	156	IV	<72 Hours	Placebo	2 Hours	70%	17%	<0.001
Botto et al[47]	1997	105	PO	<72 Hours	Placebo	2 Hours 8 Hours 24 Hours	43% 69% 80%	11% 34% 69%	<0.004 <0.001 NS
Botto et al[48]	1998	123	PO	<72 Hours	Placebo	4 Hours 8 Hours	71% 78%	33% 48%	<0.001 <0.01
Capucci et al[31]	1994	181	PO	<7 Days	Placebo	3 Hours 8 Hours	51% 72%	18% 39%	<0.001 <0.001
Boriani et al[46]	1997	240	PO	<7 Days	Placebo	3 Hours 8 Hours	45% 76%	18% 37%	<0.001 <0.001
Azpitarte et al[49]	1997	55	PO	<7 Days	Placebo	2 Hours 6 Hours 12 Hours 24 Hours	41% 65% 69% 79%	8% 31% 42% 73%	<0.005 <0.001 0.06 NS

Abbreviations: IV, intravenous administration; NS, nonsignificant; PO, oral administration.

oral loading dose of 600 mg in patients with body weight greater than or equal to 70 kg, followed by maintenance dosage of 450 to 900 mg/d.

Limited data suggest reduced efficacy in patients with persistent AF and AFI. The rate of conversion at 6 to 8 hours for persistent AF with a duration of less than 7 days ranges from 65% [1] to 72%, resulting more effective than placebo (rate of conversion from 17% to 39%).[31,49,51,52] Propafenone added to ibutilide showed an increase in the rate of SR conversion compared with ibutilide alone in patients with persistent AF lasting more than 1 month but less than 1 year.[53] Propafenone was used to terminate chronic AF and compared with amiodarone in a prospective, randomized, placebo-controlled study involving 101 patients with AF lasting from more than 3 weeks. Conversion rate within 4 weeks was 41% in propafenone group and 47% in amiodarone group, with no conversions in the control subjects.[54] Nevertheless, lower rate of conversion are reported in previous studies.[55]

The same recommendations given for flecainide are valid for the use of propafenone, and administration of propafenone should be limited to patients without organic heart disease and heart failure. AEs are uncommon and include rapid conduction atrial flutter, ventricular tachycardia, intraventricular conduction disturbance, hypotension, and bradycardia at conversion. Milder adverse side effects include gastrointestinal symptoms, such as nausea.

Class III Drugs

Amiodarone

Amiodarone is classified into the group of class III antiarrhythmic agent, because its main action is to block the rapid component of delayed rectifier potassium current. Nevertheless, it has additional class I, II, and IV properties, also blocking sodium and calcium channels and inhibiting α- and β-receptors, without clinically relevant negative inotropic effect.[56] It increases the action potential duration and the cardiac refractory period in all cardiac tissues, without influencing resting membrane potential, except in automatic cells where the slope of the prepotential is reduced, generally reducing automaticity.

Because of its side effects, amiodarone is currently approved only for the treatment of the life-threatening recurrent ventricular arrhythmias, when these have not responded to documented adequate doses of other available antiarrhythmics or when alternative agents could not be tolerated, but not for the management of AF. Nevertheless, intravenous administration of amiodarone is the most widely used strategy to treat AF in every patient with contraindications to class IC agents.

Evidence regarding the efficacy of intravenous amiodarone in the conversion of recent-onset AF is confusing, with reported efficacy ranging from 25% to 89% within the first 12 hours,[9] with some studies reporting no efficacy compared with placebo (**Table 3**).[22,43,57–61]

Data from meta-analyses are also inconclusive, with some studies reporting no differences between intravenous amiodarone and placebo,[62–64] and others finding amiodarone more effective than placebo after a longer observation period (6–24 hours).[65,66]

Regarding oral loading dose of amiodarone for the conversion of recent-onset AF, few and small studies are available. Superiority to placebo within the first 24 hours was reported in one study[67] and there was comparable efficacy to oral propafenone, despite a longer mean time to conversion (rate of conversion 47% and mean time to conversion 6.9 hours for amiodarone vs 56% and 2.4 hours for propafenone).[50]

Higher rate of conversion was reported in a recent study performed on 223 patients with AF lasting less than 48 hours, evaluating the safety and efficacy of oral versus intravenous amiodarone. After an observation of 24 hours, conversion to SR occurred in 85% in the group who received 600 mg oral amiodarone and 82% in the group receiving intravenous amiodarone, with a longer mean time to conversion in the oral administration group (20 vs 12 hours).[68] This similarity in efficacy between oral and intravenous amiodarone was reported in another previous small study.[69]

Comparative trials between amiodarone and other AADs conventionally used for the pharmacologic CV of recent-onset AF, such as flecainide and propafenone, showed that amiodarone is not superior in efficacy,[63,64] but it is the only drug that is safe in the setting of patients with structural heart disease, including those with depressed left ventricle, for whom administration of class IC drugs is contraindicated.

Currently recommended dosages are 5 to 7 mg/kg over 30 to 60 minutes, followed by 1.2 to 1.8 g over 24 hours intravenously. The oral route of administration is started with an initial dose of 600 to 800 mg/d in divided doses until 10 g total, followed by maintenance dosage of 200 to 400 mg/d.

Amiodarone seems to play a role also in the CV of long-lasting AF, with oral or intravenous initial loading dose followed by maintenance oral administration.[16] In the Sotalol Amiodarone Atrial Fibrillation Efficacy Trial (SAFE-T), a study involving 665 patients with persistent (lasting more than 72

Table 3
Summary of randomized comparative trials on efficacy of amiodarne in pharmacologic cardioversion of atrial fibrillation and atrial flutter

Authors	Year Published	No of Patients	Route of Administration	AF Duration	Control (s)	Assessment of Efficacy	Efficacy Amiodarone	Control	P
Kochiadakis et al[43]	1998	97	IV	<48 Hours	Placebo	24 Hours	83%	55%	<0.002
Cotter et al[57]	1999	100	IV	<48 Hours	Placebo	8 Hours 24 Hours	62% 92%	58% 64%	NS <0.001
Vardas[58]	2000	106	IV	<48 Hours	Placebo	1 Hour 24 Hours	61% 96%	45% 63%	NS <0.05
Joseph and Ward[59]	2001	120	IV	<24 Hours	Digoxin	4 Hours 24 Hours	31% 69%	25% 50%	NS NS
Cybulski et al[60]	2003	160	IV	<24 Hours	Placebo	8 Hours 20 Hours	50% 83%	26% 44%	<0.05 <0.001
Thomas et al[61]	2004	140	IV	<48 Hours	Digoxin Sotalol	12 Hours	51%	50% 44%	NS NS
Kochiadakis et al[22]	2007	182	IV	<48 Hours	Placebo	24 Hours	89%	61%	<0.05
Peuhkurinen et al[67]	2000	62	PO	<48 Hours	Placebo	8 Hours 24 Hours	50% 87%	20% 35%	NA NA
Galve et al[63]	1996	100	IV	<7 Days	Placebo	12 Hours 24 Hours	56% 78%	50% 60%	NS NS
Boriani et al[64]	1998	172	IV	<7 Days	Placebo	8 Hours	57%	37%	NS
Blanc et al[50]	1999	86	PO	<2 Weeks	Propafenone	24 Hours	47%	56%	NS
Singh et al[70]	2005	665	PO	>72 Hours (including >1 year)	Placebo Sotalol	1 Month	27%	1% 24%	<0.001 NS
Kerin et al[16]	1996	32	IV bolus followed by oral maintenance	>3 Weeks	Quinidine	24 Hours 9 Months	44% 67%	47% /	NS /
Kochiadakis et al[54]	1999	101	IV bolus followed by oral maintenance	>3 Weeks	Placebo Propafenone	4 Weeks	47%	40% 0%	<0.001 <0.001
Zehender et al[15]	1994	40	IV bolus followed by oral maintenance	>4 Weeks; <2 Years	Verapamil/ Quinidine	3 Months	60%	55%	NS

Abbreviations: IV, intravenous administration; NA, data not available; NS, nonsignificant; PO, oral administration.

hours) and chronic AF, the rate of CV with oral amiodarone was 27% after 28 days of treatment, compared with 24% with sotalol and 0.8% with placebo.[70] In a comparative study, intravenous amiodarone and propafenone followed by oral regimen were associated with similar rates (40% after 2 weeks) of converting persistent AF averaging 5 months in duration,[54] and Zehender and colleagues[15] confirmed the same rate of CV (40%) with oral amiodarone in patients with AF lasting at least 1 month evaluated after 2 weeks.

Taken together, available studies on amiodarone in CV of long-lasting AF suggest that approximately 30% to 40% of patients are likely to convert within 2 to 4 weeks of oral amiodarone administration.[9]

Limited information is available about the specific role of amiodarone in AFI, but a similar efficacy was demonstrated in the available studies involving AF and AFI together.

The use of amiodarone is limited by immediate AEs, such us bradycardia and hypotension, and by long-term extracardiac and toxic adverse effects, such as thyroid abnormalities, visual disturbances, and hepatotoxicity.

Dofetilide

Dofetilide is an antiarrhythmic drug with class III properties, blocking the cardiac ion channels carrying the rapid component of the delayed rectifier potassium current, without effects on sodium channels, α-adrenergic receptors, or β-adrenergic receptors. It is currently approved for the conversion of persistent AF and AFI to SR and for the prevention of recurrences in patients with AF or AFI lasting more than 1 week who have been successfully converted to normal SR. It does not posses negative inotropic effects and there was no evidence of increase in heart failure or mortality in patients with significant left ventricular dysfunction (ejection fraction <35%) or recent myocardial infarction (<7 days).[71,72] Thus, like amiodarone, it is considered safe to use in these patients.

A situation in which dofetilide might be particularly useful would be the treatment of persistent AF or AFI in patients with reduced left ventricular ejection fraction as an alternative to amiodarone, avoiding the multiple noncardiac side effects of amiodarone.

Dofetilide is the only oral drug that have a clear indication for converting both recent-onset and long-lasting persistent AF and AFI.

Dofetilide can be administered intravenously or orally, but only the oral formulation is currently approved for clinical use. Currently used oral dosages are 500 µg twice a day in patients with normal renal function, 250 µg twice a day in patients with creatinine clearance between 40 and 60 mL/min, and 125 µg twice a day if creatinine clearance is between 20 and 40 mL/min. The use of dofetilide is not recommended in patients with severe renal failure (creatinine clearance <20 mL/min).[1]

The major prospective studies conducted on oral dofetilide were performed in patients with persistent or chronic AF and AFI,[73] including patients with structural heart disease and depressed left ventricular function,[71] and their results showed dofetilide more effective than placebo in the CV of AF lasting more than 1 week. Subgroup analyses showed the superior efficacy of dofetilide in AFI.[74]

Oral dofetilide was more efficacious than sotalol in converting AF to SR in 535 patients with persistent AF or AFI (rate of conversion 29% with dofetilide vs 6% with sotalol) in the European and Australian Multicenter Evaluative Research on Atrial Fibrillation Dofetilide (EMERALD) trial.[75] Intravenous dofetilide was significantly more effective than intravenous amiodarone or placebo in restoring SR in patients with AF or AFI lasting less than 6 months (35% for dofetilide vs 4% for amiodarone).[76] It was associated, however, with a significant incidence of torsades de pointes (8%).

For recent-onset AF, few data are available, because studies performed on dofetilide included long-lasting and recent-onset forms together. Studies on intravenous dofetilide have shown an overall efficacy ranging between 14% and 53%.[9] Its efficacy seemed considerably higher in AFI than in AF (rate of conversion of approximately 70% in AFI vs 30% in AF).[76,77]

Dofetilide is generally well tolerated; however, torsades de pointes is the AE of primary concern,[78] with an incidence ranging from 0.3% to 4.7% in dofetilide clinical trials.[1] The kidneys play an important role in elimination of dofetilide; therefore, dosage reduction is required for patients with renal impairment. Additionally, initiation of therapy should be performed on an inpatient basis to minimize the risk of proarrhythmia.

Ibutilide

Ibutilide is an AAD with predominantly class III properties, prolonging action potential duration as its primary mechanism of action. It acts by activating a slow, inward current (predominantly sodium), in addition to the block of the outward potassium currents, which is the mechanism by which most other class III antiarrhythmics act.[79] It is currently approved for the rapid conversion of AF or AFI of recent-onset to SR. Atrial arrhythmias of longer duration are less likely to respond to ibutilide, and its effectiveness has not been determined in patients with arrhythmias of more than 90 days in duration.

Ibutilide is available only for intravenous administration, due to a high first-pass clearance by the liver. The recommended dose for acute CV of AF and AFI is 1 mg over 10 minutes (0.01 mg/kg in patients weighing <60 kg). A second 10-minute infusion of equal strength may be administered 10 minutes after completion of the first infusion, if the arrhythmia does not terminate within 10 minutes after the end of the initial infusion.[1]

Intravenous ibutilide has been evaluated for conversion of both AF and AFI of duration ranging from 3 hours to 45 or 90 days in two placebo-controlled trials,[80,81] and the overall success rate of patients with AFI (38%–60%) tended to be higher than for those with AF (29%–31%).

Ibutilide was more effective than intravenous amiodarone in converting recent-onset AFI to SR, whereas both drugs were equally effective in converting recent-onset AF.[82] There were no differences between the rate of conversion in 207 patients with recent-onset AF (<48 hours duration) treated with intravenous flecainide (56%) or ibutilide (50%) within the first 90 minutes of observation.[37] Ibutilide may be used in patients who fail to convert after treatment with propafenone or in those in whom the arrhythmia recurs during treatment with propafenone or flecainide.[83,84]

Available data are insufficient to establish the efficacy of intravenous ibutilide in conversion of AF or AFI lasting more than 90 days.

Major AEs related to ibutilide use are polymorphic ventricular arrhythmias, including torsades de pointes (risk of approximately 2%–4%), with women more susceptible than men to this complication (5.6% vs 3%).[85] Ibutilide should be avoided in patients with very low ejection fractions or heart failure because of the higher risk of ventricular proarrhythmia.[86]

Sotalol
Sotalol is a drug with combined class II (β-adrenoceptor blocking) and class III (cardiac action potential duration prolongation) antiarrhythmic properties. Sotalol is currently approved for the treatment of life-threatening ventricular arrhythmias and for maintenance of normal SR in patients with symptomatic AF and AFI. It is not approved for the CV of AF or AFI and its use in this setting is not recommended by current guidelines.[1]

Available data show that intravenous sotalol for conversion of acute AF is inferior to quinidine[11] or flecainide[38] and only slightly superior to placebo.[87]

Data about efficacy of oral sotalol in converting long-lasting forms of AF came from the SAFE-T trial.[70] Patients included had AF lasting more than 72 hours and also long-lasting forms (>1 year). The rate of conversion was 24% in 244 patients treated with oral sotalol, similar to the rate obtained in the group assuming oral amiodarone (27.1%) and significantly higher than spontaneous conversions (0.8% in placebo-group) after 28 days' follow-up.

Additional studies about oral sotalol for CV of AF or AFI, however, are needed to confirm these results, and at the moment its use remains limited to prevention of recurrences.

New AADs

The limited efficacy, the AEs, and the increased risk of proarrhythmia related to current available therapeutic options for pharmacologic CV of AF and AFI have made new drug development crucial. New antiarrhythmic agents with improved efficacy, safety, and tolerability could lead clinicians to re-examine the debate about the rate- versus rhythm-control strategy.

Innovative drugs are under development and clinical efficacy has already been demonstrated in others. Among these, it is possible to find the selective atrial ion channels blockers, vernakalant and ranolazine, and the nonselective amiodarone-derived multiple ion channels blockers, dronedarone.

Vernakalant
Vernakalant is a mixed sodium and potassium channel blocker currently under review for approval by the FDA for acute conversion of AF. Human electrophysiology studies showed an atrial selectivity in the action of the drug, with greater atrial than ventricular refractoriness prolongation.[88]

Most studies were performed on patients with recent-onset AF (lasting <3 or 7 days) and conversion rate ranged from 45% to 61% within the first 10 to 15 minutes after intravenous administration with the most commonly used regimen (2 mg/kg bolus followed by 3 mg/kg 30 minutes later if AF continued).[89–91]

Rate of rapid conversion in short-duration AF was much greater than with placebo yet much lower (6% to 9%) in studies that included patients with onset of AF within 8 to 45 days.[90,92]

Vernakalant may be also useful for prevention of recurrence of AF, and preliminary results showed that high-dose oral vernakalant prevented recurrence of AF without proarrhythmia; however, no phase 3 trial data are available. Vernakalant was not effective in converting AFI to SR.

Commonly reported AEs during vernakalant treatment include dysgeusia, sneezing, and paresthesia. Proarrhythmia with the use of vernakalant has not been reported to date and will be important in weighing the risks versus the benefits of this agent.

Ranolazine

Ranolazine has antianginal properties of unknown mechanism and is currently approved for use in chronic angina. Ranolazine has atrial-selective sodium channel blocking properties.

The efficacy of ranolazine as antianginal in acute coronary syndrome was investigated in the Metabolic Efficiency with Ranolazine for Less Ischemia in Non–STElevation Acute Coronary Syndromes 36 trial in 6500 patients,[93] and occasionally less frequent AF was reported in the ranolazine group (1.7% vs 2.4%) than in the placebo group.

Subsequent findings of two small nonrandomized studies showed that oral ranolazine safely converts new-onset or paroxysmal AF[94] and promotes SR maintenance.[95] Prospective studies of oral ranolazine in suppression of AF are in progress.[96]

Dronedarone

Dronedarone is a recently FDA-approved antiarrhythmic agent with electrophysiologic effects that are similar to those of amiodarone.[97] The chemical structure of dronedarone differs from that of amiodarone in its lack of iodine, which could minimize the impact of dronedarone on thyroid function. The lack of iodine also makes dronedarone less lipophilic and limits its distribution and potential for extracardiac toxicities.[97]

It is currently indicated to reduce the risk of recurrences and cardiovascular hospitalization in patients with paroxysmal or persistent AF or AFI, with a recent episode of AF or AFL and without signs of moderate or severe heart failure, with left ventricle ejection fraction greater than 35%, who are in SR, or who will be cardioverted.[98]

Several trials conducted on dronedarone assessed the effectiveness of the drug in maintaining SR after successful CV, including a large variety of patients.[99–101] It was more effective than placebo in prolonging time to recurrence in patients with paroxysmal or persistent AF and AFI and reduced the incidence of cardiovascular hospitalization.[102]

Nevertheless, its role and efficacy in pharmacologic conversion of recent-onset or long-lasting AF remains unknown and its use for this purpose is not recommended. Data from one study reported conversion to SR superior to placebo and associated with a significant dose-effect relationship,[99] but additional studies are needed.

THE PILL-IN-THE-POCKET APPROACH

A frequent issue related to pharmacologic CV of AF is whether or not to initiate AADs therapy in hospital or on an outpatient basis. Certain patients with recurrent episodes of symptomatic AF may be candidates for outpatient self-administration of single oral loading dose of the AAD to improve quality of life, decrease hospital admissions, and reduce costs.[103]

The efficacy and safety of this approach were demonstrated in 210 patients with mild or no heart disease who came to the emergency room with recent-onset AF that was hemodynamically well tolerated. If flecainide or propafenone was successful in converting patients from AF in the emergency room, they were eligible for inclusion in the study.[104] Treatment was successful in 94% of the episodes occurred during the 15 months' follow-up period, with conversion occurring over a mean of 2 hours. The numbers of monthly visits to emergency rooms and hospitalizations were significantly lower during follow-up than during the year before the target episode.

The major concern of this approach is the potential for serious AEs after oral assumption of the drug, including ventricular tachyarrhythmias. The incidence of major AEs during in-hospital treatment with a loading oral dose of flecainide or propafenone was 5%, and only one patient among the selected for enrolment (0.7%) experienced a major AE (AFI at a rapid ventricular rate) during out-of-hospital treatment.

Current guidelines recommend that this approach may be used with class IC drugs in patients with lone AF or in other selected patients only if they have had a safe response to single-dose therapy as an inpatients.[1]

Oral flecainide and propafenone, however, are rarely used for the conversion of AF in emergency departments, because intravenous administration is generally preferred due to a more rapid action. Consequently, the pill-in-the-pocket treatment is largely underused, because of lack of in-hospital initial screening treatment. In addition, in a recent study, intravenous administration of flecainide or propafenone did not seem to predict AEs during out-of-hospital self-administration of these drugs,[105] and then it was not able to select patients eligible for this approach.

The concomitant use of a β-blocker or nondihydropyridine calcium channel antagonist is generally recommended to prevent rapid atrioventricular conduction in the event of AFI, and this requires an accurate selection of the patients. The exclusion of sick sinus syndrome is important because it could became symptomatic when a class IC and and an atrioventricular node slowing agent are used together and marked bradycardia can occur early after the termination of the arrhythmia.

PHARMACOLOGIC TREATMENT IN THE ENHANCEMENT OF EFFICACY AND PREVENTION OF RECURRENCES AFTER SUCCESSFUL DIRECT CURRENT CV

The role of the pharmacologic treatment in AF and AFl conversion is more established in recent-onset (<48 hours) forms, because the efficacy of this strategy decreases as the duration of the arrhythmias increases.

Conversion to normal SR of episodes of longer duration might be best done with electrical CV, which is the current gold standard for the conversion of these forms.[106] Electrical CV is also the therapy of choice when pharmacologic conversion is ineffective.

After the widespread use of biphasic waveform shocks that increased success rate from 79% to 94%,[107] drugs may play only a minor role in enhancing the success of the procedure. Nevertheless, prophylactic administration of some AADs can be useful and effective in preventing early and late recurrences after a successful direct current CV is achieved. Among these agents are amiodarone, flecainide, propafenone, ibutilide, and sotalol.

Oral amiodarone, administered 6 weeks before and after CV, was shown to increased the conversion rate, to prolong fibrillatory cycle length and atrial effective refractory period, and to preserve SR maintenance after CV in persistent AF patients by suppressing the atrial ectopics that may involved in the initiation of AF.[108] In another study performed in 92 patients with persistent AF, pretreatment with amiodarone improved CV success rate and reduced the defibrillation threshold and AF recurrences in the first 2 months after CV compared with oral diltiazem or glucose-insulin-potassium treatments.[109] Both amiodarone and sotalol facilitated successful electro-CV in the SAFE-T trial compared with placebo.[110] Oral propafenone started 2 days before direct current CV decreased early recurrences of AF after shock, despite influencing neither the rate of success nor the defibrillation threshold.[55] Intravenous flecainide did not show to improve efficacy of electrical CV in a group of 54 patients with persistent AF.[111] Intravenous ibutilide not only enhanced the efficacy of transthoracic CV of AF to SR compared with placebo but also converted those patients in whom CV initially failed when the procedure was repeated after treatment with ibutilide.[86]

SUMMARY

Pharmacologic conversion remains a simple and widely used approach. Many drugs are currently available and commonly used for this purpose, with a good efficacy rate.

Promising results due to a very short time to efficacy came from the studies performed with vernakalant, a new agent that is shown safe and effective in converting AF to SR. This could be a useful alternative to electrical CV when a prompt restoration of SR is needed.

In addition, the employment of IC AADs by oral route, such as in the pill-in-the-pocket approach, could be a new strategy allowing patients to self-terminate the arrhythmia after the onset, thus not recurring hospitalization. This may be an important way to improve quality of life, particularly in patients with symptomatic recurrent persistent AF episodes.

REFERENCES

1. Fuster V, Rydén LE, Cannom DS, et al. ACC/AHA/ESC 2006 guidelines for the management of patients with atrial fibrillation: a report of the American College of Cardiology/American Heart Association Task Force on practice guidelines and the European Society of Cardiology Committee for Practice Guidelines (Writing Committee to Revise the 2001 guidelines for the management of patients with atrial fibrillation) developed in collaboration with the European Heart Rhythm Association and the Heart Rhythm Society. J Am Coll Cardiol 2006;48(4):854–906.

2. Van Gelder IC, Hagens VE, Bosker HA, et al. A comparison of rate control and rhythm control in patients with recurrent persistent atrial fibrillation. N Engl J Med 2002;347:1834–40.

3. Hohnloser SH, Kuck KH, Lilienthal J. Rhythm or rate control in atrial fibrillation. Parmacological Intervention in Atrial Fibrillation (PIAF): a randomised trial. Lancet 2000;356:1789–94.

4. Carlsson J, Miketic S, Windeler J, et al. Randomized trial of rate-control versus rhythm-control in persistent atrial fibrillation: the Strategies of Treatment of Atrial Fibrillation (STAF) study. J Am Coll Cardiol 2003;41:1690–6.

5. Opolski G, Torbicki A, Kosior DA, et al. Rate control vs. rhythm control in patients with nonvalvular persistent atrial fibrillation: the results of the Polish How to Treat Chronic Atrial Fibrillation (HOT CAFE) Study. Chest 2004;126:476–86.

6. Roy D, Talajic M, Nattel S, et al. Rhythm control versus rate control for atrial fibrillation and heart failure. N Engl J Med 2008;358(25):2667–77.

7. Naccarelli GV, Deborah LW, Mazhar K, et al. Old and new antiarrhythmic drugs for converting and maintaining sinus rhythm in atrial fibrillation: comparative efficacy and results of trials. Am J Cardiol 2003;91(Suppl):15D–26D.

8. Klein AL, Grimm RA, Murray RD, et al. Use of trans-esophageal echocardiography to guide cardioversion in patients with atrial fibrillation. N Engl J Med 2001;344:1411–20.

9. Boriani G, Diemberger I, Biffi M, et al. Pharmacological cardioversion of atrial fibrillation: current management and treatment options. Drugs 2004; 64(24):2741–62.

10. Hiatt WR, Lincoff AM, Harrington RA. Acute pharmacological conversion of atrial fibrillation to sinus rhythm. Is short symptomatic therapy worth it? A report from the December 2007 Meeting of the Cardiovascular and Renal Drugs Advisory Committee of the Food and Drug Administration. Circulation 2008;117:2956–7.

11. Halinen MO, Hattunen M, Paakinen S, et al. Comparison of sotalol with digoxin-quinidine for conversion of acute atrial fibrillation to sinus rhythm (the sotalol-digoxin-quinidine trial). Am J Cardiol 1995;76:495–8.

12. Capucci A, Villani GQ, Aschieri D, et al. Safety of oral propafenone in the conversion of recent onset atrial fibrillation to sinus rhythm: a prospective parallel placebo-controlled multicentre study. Int J Cardiol 1999;68:187–96.

13. Kowey PR, Marinchack RA, Rials SJ, et al. Acute treatment of atrial fibrillation. Am J Cardiol 1998; 81(Suppl 5A):16C–22C.

14. Kirpizidis C, Stavrati A, Geleris P, et al. Safety and effectiveness of oral quinidine in cardioversion of persistent atrial fibrillation. J Cardiol 2001;38(6): 351–4.

15. Zehender M, Hohnloser S, Müller B, et al. Effects of amiodarone versus quinidine and verapamil in patients with chronic atrial fibrillation: results of a comparative study and a 2-year follow-up. J Am Coll Cardiol 1992;19(5):1054–9.

16. Kerin NZ, Faitel K, Naini M. The efficacy of intravenous amiodarone for the conversion of chronic atrial fibrillation: amiodarone vs quinidine for conversion of atrial fibrillation. Arch Intern Med 1996;156(1):49–53.

17. Falk RH. Proarrhythmia in patients treated for atrial fibrillation or flutter. Ann Intern Med 1992;117(2):141–50.

18. Coplen SE, Antman EM, Berlin JA, et al. Efficacy and safety of quinidine therapy for maintenance of sinus rhythm after cardioversion: a meta-analysis of randomized control trials. Circulation 1990;82(4):1106–16.

19. Lafuente-Lafuente C, Mouly S, Longas-Tejero MA, et al. Antiarrhythmics for maintaining sinus rhythm after cardioversion of atrial fibrillation. Cochrane Database Syst Rev 2007;(4):CD005049.

20. Madrid AH, Moro C, Marin-Huerta E, et al. Comparison of flecainide and procainamide in cardioversion of atrial fibrillation. Eur Heart J 1993;14: 1127–31.

21. Kochiadakis GE, Igoumenidis NE, Solomou MC, et al. Conversion of atrial fibrillation to sinus rhythm using acute intravenous procainamide infusion. Cardiovasc Drugs Ther 1998;12:75–81.

22. Kochiadakis GE, Igoumenidis NE, Hamilos ME, et al. A comparative study of the efficacy and safety of procainamide versus propafenone versus amiodarone for the conversion of recent-onset atrial fibrillation. Am J Cardiol 2007;99:1721–5.

23. Volgman AS, Carberry PA, Stambler B, et al. Conversion efficacy and safety of intravenous ibutilide compared with intravenous procainamide in patients with atrial flutter or fibrillation. J Am Coll Cardiol 1998;31:1414–9.

24. Stiell IG, Clement CM, Symington C, et al. Emergency department use of intravenous procainamide for patients with acute atrial fibrillation or flutter. Acad Emerg Med 2007;14:1158–64.

25. Fenster PE, Comess KA, Marsh R, et al. Conversion of atrial fibrillation to sinus rhythm by acute intravenous procainamide infusion. Am Heart J 1983;106: 501–4.

26. Drew BJ, Ackerman MJ, Funk M, et al. Prevention of Torsade de Pointes in hospital settings: a scientific statement from the American Heart Association and the American College of Cardiology Foundation. Circulation 2010;121:1047–60.

27. Nakazawa H, Lythall DA, Noh J, et al. Is there a place for the late cardioversion of atrial fibrillation? A long-term follow-up study of patients with post-thyrotoxic atrial fibrillation. Eur Heart J 2000; 21:327–33.

28. Karlson BW, Torstensson I, Abjornj C, et al. Disopyramide in the maintenance of sinus rhythm after electroconversion of atrial fibrillation. A placebo-controlled one-year follow-up study. Eur Heart J 1988;9:284–90.

29. Mehta D, Camm AJ, Ward DE. Clinical electrophysiologic effects of flecainide acetate. Cardiovasc Drugs Ther 1988;1(6):599–603.

30. Capucci A, Lenzi T, Boriani G, et al. Effectiveness of loading oral flecainide for converting recent-onset atrial fibrillation to sinus rhythm in patients without organic heart disease or with only systemic hypertension. Am J Cardiol 1992;70:69–72.

31. Capucci A, Boriani G, Rubino I, et al. Conversion of recent onset atrial fibrillation by a single oral loading dose of propafenone or flecainide. Am J Cardiol 1994;74:503–5.

32. Suttorp MJ, Kingma JH, Lie-A-Huen L, et al. Intravenous flecainide versus verapamil for acute conversion of paroxysmal atrial fibrillation or flutter to sinus rhythm. Am J Cardiol 1989;63 (11):693–6.

33. Suttorp MJ, Kingma JH, Jessurun ER, et al. The value of class IC antiarrhythmic drugs for acute conversion of paroxysmal atrial fibrillation or flutter

to sinus rhythm. J Am Coll Cardiol 1990;16(7): 1722–7.

34. Donovan KD, Dobb GJ, Coombs LJ, et al. Reversion of recent-onset atrial fibrillation to sinus rhythm by intravenous flecainide. Am J Cardiol 1991;67(2): 137–41.

35. Donovan KD, Power BM, Hockings BE, et al. Intravenous flecainide versus amiodarone for recent-onset atrial fibrillation. Am J Cardiol 1995;75(10): 693–7.

36. Alp NJ, Bell JA, Shahi M. Randomised double blind trial of oral versus intravenous flecainide for the cardioversion of acute atrial fibrillation. Heart 2000;84:37–40.

37. Reisinger J, Gatterer E, Lang W, et al. Flecainide versus ibutilide for immediate cardioversion of atrial fibrillation of recent onset. Eur Heart J 2004; 25:1318–24.

38. Reisinger J, Gatterer E, Heinze G, et al. Prospective comparison of flecainide versus sotalol for immediate cardioversion of atrial fibrillation. Am J Cardiol 1998;81:1450–4.

39. Echt DS, Liebson PR, Mitchell LB, et al. Mortality and morbidity in patients receiving encainide, flecainide, or placebo. The Cardiac Arrhythmia Suppression Trial. N Engl J Med 1991;324(12):781–8.

40. Bianconi L, Mennuni M. Comparison between propafenone and digoxin administered intravenously to patients with acute atrial fibrillation. PAFIT-3 Investigators. The Propafenone in Atrial Fibrillation Italian Trial. Am J Cardiol 1998;82(5): 584–8.

41. Fresco C, Proclemer A, Pavan A, et al. Intravenous propafenone in paroxysmal atrial fibrillation: a randomized, placebo-controlled, double-blind, multicenter clinical trial. Paroxysmal Atrial Fibrillation Italian Trial (PAFIT)-2 Investigators. Clin Cardiol 1996;19(5):409–12.

42. Ganau G, Lenzi T. Intravenous propafenone for converting recent onset atrial fibrillation in emergency departments: a randomized placebo-controlled multicenter trial. FAPS Investigators Study Group. J Emerg Med 1998;16(3):383–7.

43. Kochiadakis GE, Igoumenidis NE, Simantirakis EN, et al. Intravenous propafenone versus intravenous amiodarone in the management of atrial fibrillation of recent onset: a placebo-controlled study. Pacing Clin Electrophysiol 1998;21(11 Pt 2):2475–9.

44. Boriani G, Martignani C, Biffi M, et al. Oral loading with propafenone for conversion of recent-onset atrial fibrillation: a comparison review on in-hospital treatment. Drugs 2002;62(3):415–23.

45. Khan IA. Single oral loading dose of propafenone for pharmacological cardioversion of recent-onset atrial fibrillation. J Am Coll Cardiol 2001;37:542–7.

46. Boriani G, Biffi M, Capucci A, et al. Oral propafenone to convert recent-onset atrial fibrillation in patients with and without underlying heart disease: a randomized, controlled trial. Ann Intern Med 1997;126:621–5.

47. Botto GL, Capucci A, Bonini W, et al. Conversion of recent onset atrial fibrillation to sinus rhythm using a single loading oral dose of propafenone: comparison of two regimens. Int J Cardiol 1997;58:55–61.

48. Botto GL, Bonini W, Broffoni T, et al. Randomized, crossover, controlled comparison of oral loading versus intravenous infusion of propafenone in recent-onset atrial fibrillation. Pacing Clin Electrophysiol 1998;21(11 Pt 2):2480–4.

49. Azpitarte J, Alvarez M, Baun O, et al. Value of single oral loading dose of propafenone in converting recent onset atrial fibrillation: results of a randomized, double-blind, controlled study. Eur Heart J 1997;18:1649–54.

50. Blanc JJ, Voinov C, Maarek M. Comparison of oral loading dose of propafenone and amiodarone for converting recent-onset atrial fibrillation. PARSIFAL Study Group. Am J Cardiol 1999;84:1029–32.

51. Capucci A, Boriani G, Rubino I, et al. A controlled study on oral propafenone versus digoxin plus quinidine in converting recent onset atrial fibrillation to sinus rhythm. Int J Cardiol 1994;43:305–13.

52. Boriani G, Capucci A, Lenzi T, et al. Propafenone for conversion of recent-onset atrial fibrillation. A controlled comparison between oral loading dose and intravenous administration. Chest 1995;108: 355–8.

53. Korantzopoulos P, Kolettis TM, Papathanasiou A, et al. Propafenone added to ibutilide increases conversion rates of persistent atrial fibrillation. Heart 2006;92(5):631–4.

54. Kochiadakis GE, Igoumenidis NE, Parthenakis FI, et al. Amiodarone versus propafenone for conversion of chronic atrial fibrillation: results of a randomized, controlled study. J Am Coll Cardiol 1999;33(4):966–71.

55. Bianconi L, Mennuni M, Lukic V, et al. Effects of oral propafenone administration before electrical cardioversion of chronic atrial fibrillation: a placebo-controlled study. J Am Coll Cardiol 1996;28(3): 700–6.

56. Roden DM. Antiarrhythmic drugs: from mechanisms to clinical practice. Heart 2000;84:339–46.

57. Cotter G, Blatt A, Kaluski E, et al. Conversion of recent onset paroxysmal atrial fibrillation to normal sinus rhythm: the effect of no treatment and high-dose amiodarone. A randomized, placebo-controlled study. Eur Heart J 1999;20(24): 1833–42.

58. Vardas PE, Kochiadakis GE, Igoumenidis, et al. Amiodarone as a first-choice drug for restoring sinus rhythm in patients with atrial fibrillation: a randomized, controlled study. Chest 2000; 117(6):1538–45.

59. Joseph AP, Ward MR. A prospective, randomized controlled trial comparing the efficacy and safety of sotalol, amiodarone, and digoxin for the reversion of new-onset atrial fibrillation. Ann Emerg Med 2000;36(1):1–9.

60. Cybulski J, Kułakowski P, Budaj A, et al. Intravenous amiodarone for cardioversion of recent-onset atrial fibrillation. Clin Cardiol 2003;26(7):329–35.

61. Thomas SP, Guy D, Wallace E, et al. Rapid loading of sotalol or amiodarone for management of recent onset symptomatic atrial fibrillation: a randomized, digoxin-controlled trial. Am Heart J 2004;147(1):E3.

62. Khan IA, Mehta NJ, Gowda RM. Amiodarone for pharmacological cardioversion of recent-onset atrial fibrillation. Int J Cardiol 2003;89:239–48.

63. Galve E, Rius T, Ballester R, et al. Intravenous amiodarone in treatment of recent-onset atrial fibrillation: results of a randomized, controlled study. J Am Coll Cardiol 1996;27(5):1079–82.

64. Boriani G, Biffi M, Capucci A, et al. Conversion of recent-onset atrial fibrillation to sinus rhythm: effects of different drug protocols. Pacing Clin Electrophysiol 1998;21(11 Pt 2):2470–4.

65. Chevalier P, Durand-Dubief A, Burri H, et al. Amiodarone versus placebo and class IC drugs for cardioversion of recent-onset atrial fibrillation: a meta-analysis. J Am Coll Cardiol 2003;41:255–62.

66. Hilleman DE, Spinler SA. Conversion of recent-onset atrial fibrillation with intravenous amiodarone: a meta-analysis of randomized controlled trials. Pharmacotherapy 2002;22:66–74.

67. Peuhkurinen K, Niemelä M, Ylitalo A, et al. Effectiveness of amiodarone as a single oral dose for recent-onset atrial fibrillation. Am J Cardiol 2000;85(4):462–5.

68. Xanthos T, Bassiakou E, Vlachos IS, et al. Intravenous and oral administration of amiodarone for the treatment of recent onset atrial fibrillation after digoxin administration. Int J Cardiol 2007;121(3):291–5.

69. Andrivet P, Boubakri E, Dove PJ, et al. A clinical study of amiodarone as a single oral dose in patients with recent-onset atrial tachyarrhythmia. Eur Heart J 1994;15(10):1396–402.

70. Singh BN, Singh SN, Reda DJ, et al. Amiodarone versus sotalol for atrial fibrillation. N Engl J Med 2005;352:1861–72.

71. Torp-Pedersen C, Møller M, Block-Thomsen PE, et al. Dofetilide in patients with congestive heart failure and left ventricular dysfunction. Danish Investigations of Arrhythmia and Mortality on Dofetilide Study Group. N Engl J Med 1999;341(12):857–65.

72. DIAMOND Study Group. Dofetilide in patients with left ventricular dysfunction and either heart failure or acute myocardial infarction: rationale, design, and patient characteristics of the DIAMOND studies: Danish Investigations of Arrhythmia and Mortality ON Dofetilide. Clin Cardiol 1997;20:704–10.

73. Singh S, Zoble RG, Yellen L, et al. Efficacy and safety of oral dofetilide in converting to and maintaining sinus rhythm in patients with chronic atrial fibrillation or atrial flutter: the symptomatic atrial fibrillation investigative research on dofetilide (SAFIRE-D) study. Circulation 2000;102:2385–90.

74. Pedersen OD, Bagger H, Keller N, et al. Efficacy of dofetilide in the treatment of atrial fibrillation-flutter in patients with reduced left ventricular function: a Danish Investigations of Arrhythmia and Mortality ON Dofetilide (DIAMOND) sub-study. Circulation 2001;104(3):292–6.

75. Tikosyn (dofetilide) package insert. New York: Pfizer Inc.; 2000.

76. Bianconi L, Castro A, Dinelli M, et al. Comparison of intravenously administered dofetilide versus amiodarone in the acute termination of atrial fibrillation and flutter. a multicentre, randomized, double-blind, placebo-controlled study. Eur Heart J 2000;21(15):1265–73.

77. Falk RH, Pollak A, Singh SN, et al. Intravenous dofetilide, a class III antiarrhythmic agent, for the termination of sustained atrial fibrillation or flutter. Intravenous Dofetilide Investigators. J Am Coll Cardiol 1997;29(2):385–90.

78. Kalus JS, Mauro VF. Dofetilide: a class III-specific antiarrhythmic agent. Ann Pharmacother 2000;34(1):44–6.

79. Murray KT. Ibutilide. Circulation 1998;97(5):493–7.

80. Ellenbogen KA, Stambler BS, Wood MA, et al. Efficacy of intravenous ibutilide for rapid termination of atrial fibrillation and atrial flutter: a dose-response study. J Am Coll Cardiol 1996;28:130–6.

81. Stambler BS, Wood MA, Ellenbogen KA, et al. Efficacy and safety of repeated intravenous doses of ibutilide for rapid conversion of atrial flutter or fibrillation. Circulation 1996;94:1613–21.

82. Kafkas NV, Patsilinakos SP, Mertzanos GA, et al. Conversion efficacy of intravenous ibutilide compared with intravenous amiodarone in patients with recent-onset atrial fibrillation and atrial flutter. Int J Cardiol 2007;118(3):321–5.

83. Chiladakis JA, Kalogeropoulos A, Patsouras N, et al. Ibutilide added to propafenone for the conversion of atrial fibrillation and atrial flutter. J Am Coll Cardiol 2004;44:859–63.

84. Hongo RH, Themistoclakis S, Raviele A, et al. Use of ibutilide in cardioversion of patients with atrial fibrillation or atrial flutter treated with class IC agents. J Am Coll Cardiol 2004;44:864–8.

85. Gowda RM, Khan IA, Punukollu G, et al. Female preponderance in ibutilide-induced torsade de pointes. Int J Cardiol 2004;95:219–22.

86. Oral H, Souza JJ, Michaud GF, et al. Facilitating transthoracic cardioversion of atrial fibrillation with ibutilide pretreatment. N Engl J Med 1999;340:1849–54.

87. Sung RJ, Tan HL, Karagounis L, et al. Intravenous sotalol for the termination of supraventricular tachycardia and atrial fibrillation and flutter: a multicenter, randomized, double-blind, placebo-controlled study. Sotalol Multicenter Study Group. Am Heart J 1995;129(4):739–48.

88. Dorian P, Pinter A, Mangat I, et al. The effect of vernakalant (RSD1235), an investigational antiarrhythmic agent, on atrial electrophysiology in humans. J Cardiovasc Pharmacol 2007;50:35–40.

89. Roy D, Rowe BH, Stiell IG, et al. A randomized, controlled trial of RSD1235, a novel antiarrhythmic agent, in the treatment of recent onset atrial fibrillation. J Am Coll Cardiol 2004;44: 2355–61.

90. Roy D, Pratt CM, Torp-Pedersen C, et al. Vernakalant hydrochloride for rapid conversion of atrial fibrillation: a phase 3, randomized, placebo-controlled trial. Circulation 2008;117:1518–25.

91. Kowey PR, Mitchell LB, Pratt CM, et al. Vernakalant hydrocholoride for the rapid conversion of atrial fibrillation after cardiac surgery: a randomized, double-blind, placebo-controlled trial. Circ Arrhythm Electrophysiol 2009;2:652–9.

92. Cheng JW. Vernakalant in the management of atrial fibrillation. Ann Pharmacother 2008;42(4):533–42.

93. Scirica BM, Morrow DA, Hod H, et al. Effect of ranolazine, an antianginal agent with novel electrophysiological properties, on the incidence of arrhythmias in patients with non ST-segment elevation acute coronary syndrome: results from the Metabolic Efficiency With Ranolazine for Less Ischemia in Non ST-Elevation Acute Coronary Syndrome Thrombolysis in Myocardial Infarction 36 (MERLIN-TIMI 36) randomized controlled trial. Circulation 2007;116:1647–52.

94. Murdock DK, Kersten M, Kaliebe J, et al. The use of oral ranolazine to convert new or paroxysmal atrial fibrillation: a review of experience with implications for possible "pill in the pocket" approach to atrial fibrillation. Indian Pacing Electrophysiol J 2009;9:260–7.

95. Murdock DK, Overton N, Kersten M, et al. The effect of ranolazine on maintaining sinus rhythm in patients with resistant atrial fibrillation. Indian Pacing Electrophysiol J 2008;8:175–81.

96. Burashnikov A, Antzelevitch C. Atrial-selective sodium channel blockers: do they exist? J Cardiovasc Pharmacol 2008;52:121–8.

97. Laughlin JC, Kowey PR. Dronedarone: a new treatment for atrial fibrillation. J Cardiovasc Electrophysiol 2008;19(11):1220–6.

98. Sanofi-Aventis website. Available at: http://products.sanofi-aventis.us/multaq/multaq.html. Accessed May 12, 2010.

99. Touboul P, Brugada J, Capucci A, et al. Dronedarone for prevention of atrial fibrillation: a dose-ranging study. Eur Heart J 2003;24:1481–7.

100. Singh BN, Connolly SJ, Crijns HJ, et al. for the EURIDIS and ADONIS Investigators Dronedarone for maintenance of sinus rhythm in atrial fibrillation or flutter. N Engl J Med 2007;357:987–99.

101. Davy JM, Herold M, Hoglund C, et al. for the ERATO Study Investigators Dronedarone for the control of ventricular rate in permanent atrial fibrillation: the Efficacy and safety of dRonedArone for The cOntrol of ventricular rate during atrial fibrillation (ERATO) study. Am Heart J 2008;156 (527):e1–9.

102. Hohnloser SH, Crijns HJ, van Eickels M, et al. for the ATHENA Investigators. Effect of dronedarone on cardiovascular events in atrial fibrillation. N Engl J Med 2009;360:668–78.

103. Capucci A, Villani GQ, Piepoli MF, et al. The role of oral 1C antiarrhythmic drugs in terminating atrial fibrillation. Curr Opin Cardiol 1999;14:4–8.

104. Alboni P, Botto GL, Baldi N, et al. Outpatient treatment of recent-onset atrial fibrillation with the "pill-in-the-pocket" approach. N Engl J Med 2004;351: 2384–91.

105. Alboni P, Botto GL, Boriani G, et al. Intravenous administration of flecainide or propafenone in patients with recent-onset atrial fibrillation does not predict adverse effects during 'pill-in-the-pocket' treatment. Heart. 2010;96(7): 546–9.

106. Lip GY, Tse HF. Management of atrial fibrillation. Lancet 2007;370(9587):604–18.

107. Page RL, Kerber RE, Russell JK, et al. Biphasic versus monophasic shock waveform for conversion of atrial fibrillation: the results of an international randomized, double-blind multicenter trial. J Am Coll Cardiol 2002;39:1956–63.

108. Manios EG, Mavrakis HE, Kanoupakis EM, et al. Effects of amiodarone and diltiazem on persistent atrial fibrillation conversion and recurrence rates: a randomized controlled study. Cardiovasc Drugs Ther 2003;17:31–9.

109. Capucci A, Villani GQ, Aschieri D, et al. Oral amiodarone increases the efficacy of direct-current cardioversion in restoration of sinus rhythm in patients with chronic atrial fibrillation. Eur Heart J 2000; 21(1):66–73.

110. Singh SN, Tang XC, Reda D, et al. Systematic electrocardioversion for atrial fibrillation and role of antiarrhythmic drugs: a substudy of the SAFE-T trial. Heart Rhythm 2009;6:152–5.

111. Climent VE, Marin F, Mainar L, et al. Effects of pretreatment with intravenous flecainide on efficacy of external cardioversion of persistent atrial fibrillation. Pacing Clin Electrophysiol. 2004;27(3): 368–72.

Chronic Maintenance of Sinus Rhythm in Patients with Atrial Fibrillation Using Antiarrhythmic Drugs: Update 2010

John P. Morrow, MD[a],*, James A. Reiffel, MD[a,b]

KEYWORDS

- Atrial fibrillation • Ion channels • Antiarrhythmic drugs
- Ranolazine • Dronedarone

Atrial fibrillation (AF) is a growing public health concern. It has a prevalence of almost 1% in the adult United States population. As the population ages, it will become even more frequent.[1] In most patients the treatment of AF involves antiarrhythmic drugs (AADs). In the AFFECTS Registry, for example, a rhythm control strategy was selected for 65% of patients.[2] Despite the widespread use of AADs for the conversion of AF and maintenance of normal sinus rhythm (NSR), their use is limited by modest efficacy, frequent intolerance, and the potential for organ toxicity and serious ventricular proarrhythmia. Ablation techniques for AF have gained acceptance, but there are significant safety risks and concerns about long-term efficacy, and the logistical impossibility of ablation for all AF patients given the current and near-term laboratory capacity and the anticipated growth of the incidence of AF. Better drugs are needed and many are under active investigation. This article focuses on medications for maintaining NSR after AF.

THE SCOPE OF THE PROBLEM

The morbidity and mortality associated with AF are significant. AF causes considerable suffering and frequent outpatient visits and hospitalizations by causing dyspnea, palpitations, strokes, and precipitating (or worsening) heart failure (HF). Contemporary drug therapy for maintaining NSR is often inadequate. Most patients with AF, in the absence of a transient cause, have a recurrence of AF even with treatment. Furthermore, many trials of different AADs have shown increased mortality in the presence of structural heart disease (SHD), for example the Cardiac Arrhythmia Suppression Trial[3] and Survival With Oral d-Sotalol trial.[4] SHD is common in patients with AF, particularly older patients. The role for AAD therapy for AF has been questioned.

RATIONALE FOR AAD TREATMENT

There are two reasons to do anything in health care: to help people live longer or to help them feel better. AF is associated with higher mortality, at least with older patients, but it is difficult to say how much of this is caused by comorbidities rather than the AF itself. Certainly, developing a tachycardia-induced cardiomyopathy or having a large stroke can lead to death. Regardless of mortality, reducing the morbidity of AF is clearly necessary and can involve any or all of the

[a] Division of Cardiology, Department of Medicine, Columbia University Medical Center, New York, NY 10032, USA
[b] 161 Fort Washington Avenue, Columbia University Medical Center, New York, NY 10032, USA
* Corresponding author. PH 10-203, 622 West 168th Street, New York, NY 10032.
E-mail address: jpm46@columbia.edu

Card Electrophysiol Clin 2 (2010) 409–418
doi:10.1016/j.ccep.2010.06.003
1877-9182/10/$ – see front matter © 2010 Elsevier Inc. All rights reserved.

following: reducing symptoms, hospitalizations, long-term consequences of the disease, adverse effects of therapy, and the economic impact of the disease and its therapy (**Fig. 1**).

Management of AF usually involves a decision between rate control and rhythm control. The choice of one over the other is dependent on the duration and pattern of AF, the severity of symptoms, the presence of cardiovascular disease, intrinsic atrioventricular node function, and the safety profiles of the rhythm control treatments under consideration. Prevention of thromboembolism must be considered regardless of treatment strategy. The indication for anticoagulation therapy is based on the overall risk of stroke, not on the restoration or maintenance of sinus rhythm. In most circumstances, rate control is also incorporated into a rhythm control strategy.

The need for pharmacotherapy to restore and maintain NSR has been questioned, given the results of recent trials, such as the Atrial Fibrillation Follow-up Investigation of Rhythm Management (AFFIRM),[5] Rate Control versus Electrical Cardioversion for Persistent Atrial Fibrillation,[6] Pharmacologic Intervention in Atrial Fibrillation,[7] and others that do not show a mortality benefit with a strategy to attempt to restore NSR. Despite the lack of outcome data supporting rhythm control, many physicians do not believe that rate-controlled AF is equivalent to NSR.

It is possible that NSR is better but the toxicities and proarrhythmic risks of current AADs cancel out the benefits. For example, on-treatment analysis in AFFIRM suggests that NSR was associated with improved survival compared with AF, and AADs were associated with an increase in mortality when rhythm was taken into effect in a regression model.[8] That is, NSR was associated with a mortality reduction similar to the increased mortality risk seen in patients taking AADs (often amiodarone). Furthermore, now that dronedarone has been shown to decrease hospitalizations and cardiovascular deaths in some patient populations, there is evidence that safer AADs may result in better survival than rate control.[9]

Rhythm control often improves symptoms more than rate control. A substantial number of patients with AF have significantly impaired quality of life with rate control. In such patients, restoring sinus rhythm is necessary to allow them to live their lives satisfactorily. Even for patients who undergo ablation procedures or surgery to cure AF, AADs are sometimes needed afterward. For example, in the trial of AF ablation by Pappone and colleagues,[10] AADs were needed in 14% of patients in the ablation group after the initial procedure. If one considers AADs for ablation or surgery failures, and AADs as hybrid therapy in some of the published efficacy data for ablation, it seems likely that many of the patients who have AF ablations or surgery are likely to take an AAD after the procedure.

NOT ALL AF PATIENTS BENEFIT FROM CHRONIC AADS: INTERMITTENT THERAPY AS AN ALTERNATIVE

It should also be noted that the rhythm control strategy does not always require chronic AADs. Some patients have infrequent episodes of

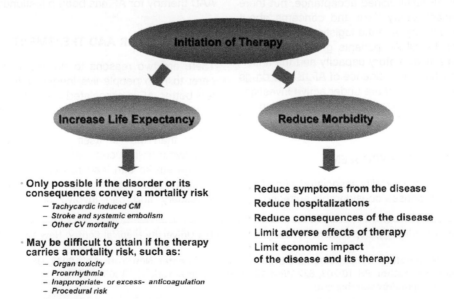

Fig. 1. Therapy goals in AF.

paroxysmal AF and may only need periodic cardi-oversion, either electric or pharmacologic (including the "pill-in-the-pocket" approach). This approach to maintaining NSR for patients with infrequent, tolerable episodes was recently re-viewed; for more detail we refer the interested reader to a prior publication.[11] For example, the patient with only one or a few AF episodes per year may be better treated with intermittent cardi-oversion than with a daily antiarrhythmic drug or an ablative approach, especially if this can be done rapidly, reproducibly, without risk, and at home pharmacologically (see later). Also, some patients with paroxysmal AF (perhaps 15%) are asymp-tomatic and may need only rate control and prophylaxis for thromboemoblic events.

CURRENT PRACTICE

Because AF should not be a lethal arrhythmia (if the patient has effective rate-control and anticoa-gulation), and because AADs are similar in efficacy for AF, the current guidelines for AAD selection for AF focus primarily on safety as the prime selection factor (**Fig. 2**).[12] For most patients, AADs are not given after the first episode. Infrequent, well-tolerated events can be treated with intermittent cardioversion. For most, however, with more frequent symptomatic events, chronic antiar-rhythmic therapy is required. The American Heart Association (AHA)/American College of Cardiology (ACC)/European Society of Cardiology (ESC)

guidelines for therapy to maintain sinus rhythm are based on the premise that limiting the risk of organ toxicity and ventricular proarrhythmia and minimizing adverse drug interactions should be considered before absolute efficacy rates when selecting an agent for AF. For example, these guidelines list sotalol, propafenone, and flecainide as the first-line agents for patients without SHD rather than amiodarone or ablation.

CLASS 1C

Both flecainide and propafenone can be effective at maintaining sinus rhythm, with recurrences rates of 31% to 37% in most series and as high as 70% in the RAFT trial with sustained release propafenone.[13] The most common adverse-event profiles of these agents (tremor, blurred vision, headache, ataxia, and HF with flecainide; constipation, dizziness, headache, metallic taste, and asthma exacerbation with propafenone) are not trivial, but fewer than 15% of patients discon-tinue treatment with class IC agents because of adverse effects. Both flecainide and propafenone have been used in pill-in-the-pocket protocols for rapid conversion of recent-onset AF. For this purpose, a single dose of immediate-release prop-afenone (600 mg) or of flecainide (300 mg) is given. A rate control agent (eg, 80 mg of verapamil) is also given unless the patient is on such a drug chroni-cally. Conversion rates of 70% to 80% have typi-cally been reported[11] with excellent tolerance

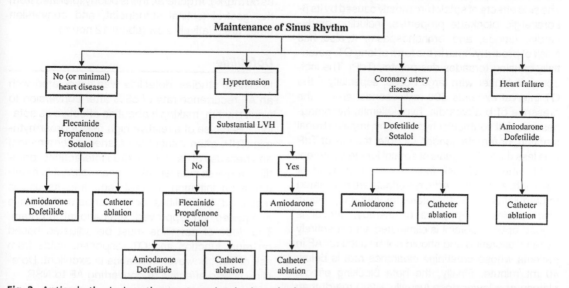

Fig. 2. Antiarrhythmic drug therapy to maintain sinus rhythm in patients with recurrent paroxysmal or persistent atrial fibrillation. *From* Fuster V, Ryden LE, Cannom DS, et al. ACC/AHA/ESC 2006 guidelines for the management of patients with atrial fibrillation–executive summary: a report of the American College of Cardiology/American Heart Association Task Force on Practice Guidelines and the European Society of Cardiology Committee for Prac-tice Guidelines [Writing Committee to Revise the 2001 Guidelines for the Management of Patients With Atrial Fibrillation]. J Am Coll Cardiol 2006;48(4):854–906; with permission.

and mean conversion times of just under 4 hours. If a patient is taking propafenone or flecainide chronically as maintenance therapy and a breakthrough AF event occurs, the pill-in-the-pocket approach can still be used, but with smaller doses such that the total daily dose of the drug for that day does not exceed the maximal allowable total daily dose chronically (eg, 400 mg of flecainide in 24 hours or 900 mg of immediate-release propafenone or its sustained-release equivalent in 24 hours). Flecainide and propafenone can be initiated in the outpatient setting, so long as sinus node function and atrioventricular conduction are normal. When used for atrial arrhythmias, the class IC agents should only be given to patients without SHD, including those with hypertension but without ischemia or marked left ventricular hypertrophy, somewhat limiting their use in elderly patients.

CLASS 3
Sotalol

Sotalol is similarly effective in the prevention of recurrences of AF, with recurrence rates being approximately 50% to 60% depending on the time frame.[14] Comparing absolute efficacy rates from one study to another is difficult, however, because the populations are not the same. In trials in which sotalol and class IC drugs have been studied in the same patients, their efficacy rates have been similar. The side effects of sotalol are mostly caused by its β-adrenergic blockade properties, including bradycardia, fatigue, and bronchospasm. It also has a risk of proarrhythmia in the form of long QT, potentially causing torsades des pointes (TdP). The incidence is higher with large doses, especially if the QT interval exceeds 500 milliseconds, and in the presence of bradycardia, hypokalemia, hypomagnesemia, left ventricular hypertrophy, impaired renal function, or female gender. Of note, the risk of TdP was less than 1% in trials of sotalol for the treatment of AF when such risk factors were minimized or taken into account.[15] Adverse effects are not related to cumulative dose; therefore, for younger patients who require many years of therapy, sotalol is a good option. Sotalol is eliminated almost entirely by renal excretion and should not be used for AF in patients whose creatinine clearance rate is below 40 mL/minute. Finally, the beta blocking effects plateau at a lower dose (usually ≤240 mg/d) than does its class III antiarrhythmic actions. Sotalol is not effective for pharmacologic cardioversion of AF, likely related to its degree of reverse use dependence and, hence, is not useful as pill-in-the-pocket therapy.

Amiodarone

Amiodarone and dofetilide are second line for patients without heart disease, but are first line for patients with HF. Amiodarone is only approved for treating ventricular tachycardia but it is probably the most effective drug for the prevention of AF, with recurrence rates about 30%. The frequent and sometimes severe adverse reactions make it a less attractive option when other agents are not contraindicated. Amiodarone is associated with adverse effects involving nearly every organ system except the kidney. Adverse reactions include gastrointestinal disorders (eg, nausea and anorexia); hepatotoxicity; neuropathy; corneal opacification; optic neuritis and blindness; chronic interstitial pneumonitis; acute pulmonary reactions; hypothyroidism and hyperthyroidism; skin photosensitivity; and skin discoloration.

Given that the risk of organ toxicity increases with lifetime cumulative dose, maintenance doses for AF no higher than 200 mg/day should be used after an initial loading regimen. Regular monitoring for adverse reactions is necessary for all patients. Even with 200 mg/day dosing thyroid abnormalities have been noted in up to 15% of patients and pulmonary toxicity has been seen in up to 2% annually. The prescriber should consider at least twice yearly assessment of pulmonary, hepatic, eye, and thyroid function during amiodarone therapy. Oral amiodarone has been used in very limited reports as pill-in-the-pocket therapy, administered as 50 mg/kg. In general, this is poorly tolerated from the gastrointestinal standpoint, and conversion times are relatively slow (about 12 hours).

Dofetilide

In clinical studies, dofetilide was associated with an AF recurrence rate of 58% after conversion to sinus rhythm, making it about as effective as sotalol.[14] Because of a relative high risk of proarrhythmia (TdP, often without spontaneous termination) and because of its multiple drug interactions, dofetilide requires inpatient electrocardiographic monitoring on initiation of treatment, and its use is restricted to facilities or prescribers that have completed an approved educational program. The dose of dofetilide must be adjusted based on renal function and QT response. Aside from risk of TdP, however, tolerance is excellent. Dofetilide is also effective at converting AF to NSR.

Older Drugs

Several members of the 1A class (disopyramide, procainamide, and quinidine) have been considered third-line agents for AF in patients without heart disease; these drugs are now rarely used. Because class IA agents have significant potassium channel blocking activity in addition to their sodium channel blocking activity, they can prolong QT and induce TdP. They should be avoided in the presence of ventricular hypertrophy, bradycardia, hypokalemia, hypomagnesemia, or other situations that can lead to long QT. It is recommended to initiate class IA agents in the in-patient setting with heart rhythm monitoring. Of this group, quinidine is likely the most proarrhythmic and can have significant adverse gastrointestinal effects, whereas disopyramide is the most vagolytic, which can contribute both to its side effect profile and its use in patients in whom vagal activation contributes to the production of their AF.

ION-CHANNEL ACTIVE AGENTS

In addition to the established antiarrhythmic agents, a number of new agents are now available. It is likely that these new agents will in large part replace many of the current medications. These are reviewed in detail elsewhere in this issue, and are not discussed in detail here. We do include, however, some additional considerations beyond those in the other article.

Ranolazine

Ranolazine, developed as an antianginal medication, blocks sodium channels in the inactive state, and also I_{Kr}. Because of differences in the inactivation characteristics of atrial sodium channels compared with ventricular sodium channels, ranolazine is relatively atrial specific and has been shown to decrease AF in canine atrial tissue preparations.[16] A clinical trial of ranolazine for patients with acute coronary syndromes showed a significant decrease in both ventricular and supraventricular tachycardias.[17] Although ranolazine can increase the QT interval modestly, it has not produced TdP in clinical trials and has blocked induction of TdP by other agents in some experimental models. Ranolazine is also known to have anti-ischemic properties without affecting heart rate and blood pressure. In January 2006, the Food and Drug Administration approved its use for the treatment of chronic angina pectoris based on its efficacy and favorable side-effect profile. The mechanism of action of its antianginal effects has not yet been determined, but may involve the fact that it is a partial fatty oxidation inhibitor.[18] This causes a shift in ATP production away from fatty acid oxidation toward carbohydrate oxidation. Myocardial oxygen demand is then reduced without any substantial decrease in cardiac work, alleviating angina.

I_{NaL} AND THE PATHOPHYSIOLOGY OF HF AND AF

The late sodium current is increased in ventricular myocytes in both animal models of HF and in patients with HF, and this may have a role in the pathophysiology of both HF and AF.[19] Elevated intracellular sodium levels can lead to calcium overload, because sodium is not only regulated through the sodium channel, but also through the Na-Ca exchanger. Increased I_{NaL} increases the intracellular concentration of Na^+, resulting in Na^+-Ca^{2+} exchange though Na-Ca exchanger, and increased Ca^{2+} entry into myocytes. Prolonged late sodium current may contribute to arrhythmias by two mechanisms: by preventing timely repolarization and causing early afterdepolarizations; and by triggering delayed afterdepolarizations attributable to calcium oscillations in calcium overload. Decreasing the late sodium current could be useful in treating AF. Although all class I AADs inhibit sodium current, ranolazine has been shown to be a more specific and potent blocker of the late sodium current.[20]

PRECLINICAL STUDIES OF RANOLAZINE AND AF

Ranolazine can decrease early afterdepolarizations and delayed afterdepolarizations–mediated triggered activity in canine pulmonary vein sleeve preparations.[21] These findings were demonstrated in vivo by Kumar and colleagues,[22] in which episodes of AF were induced by intrapericardial acetylcholine injections in pigs. Ranolazine decreased both the duration of AF and the dominant frequency.

CLINICAL STUDIES OF RANOLAZINE AND AF

The largest clinical trial with ranolazine to date was MERLIN-TIMI 36. In this trial 6560 patients hospitalized with a non–ST-elevation acute coronary syndrome were randomized to ranolazine or placebo.[23] In this trial ranolazine had a beneficial effect on supraventricular tachycardias in. Using a cut-off of 4 beats or more, supraventricular tachycardia was less common in the group treated with ranolazine (44.7% vs 55%; significant). AF was infrequent in this trial but was also reduced with ranolazine (1.7% vs 2.4%; significant). Interestingly, pauses of 3 seconds or more were also less frequent with ranolazine (3.1% vs 4.3%; significant), so it does not seem to have negative chronotropic effects or block the atrioventricular node. Clinical trials of ranolazine in patients with AF are being planned and in progress to assess its effectiveness in this patient population. In one, presented at the Annual Scientific Sessions of the ACC in March 2010 by Murdock and Reiffel and co-workers,[22] ranolazine was shown to have efficacy as pill-in-the-pocket therapy for AF. Using 2 g, conversion rates around 70% by 6 hours were seen in patients with new-onset or recurrent recent-onset AF. Importantly, these patients had SHD and hence did not have the exclusions necessary for pill-in-the-pocket therapy with a class IC agent. A larger scale trial seems warranted. In another ongoing series in our own patients (not yet published), ranolazine has demonstrated efficacy in AF reduction in some patients who broke through previously effective class IC agents or sotalol.

ATRIAL-SPECIFIC AGENTS

Because different ion channels are found in atrial tissue compared with the ventricles, AADs that have specific activity for ion channels found predominantly in the atria might provide effective treatment for AF without promoting ventricular arrhythmias. Furthermore, early in the course of AF electrical remodeling occurs and the relative contribution of ion channels changes (**Fig. 3**). This is manifest by shortening of the action potential duration, with a relatively greater contribution from the ultrarapid potassium current I_{Kur}, the transient outward potassium current I_{to}, and the muscarinic acetylcholine potassium current I_{KACh}, and a decreased influence of the delayed rectifying potassium current (which has two components: rapid- I_{Kr} and slow- I_{Ks}) and the calcium current. I_{Kur} and I_{KACh} in particular seem to be important for atrial myocytes but not ventricular myocytes.

Currently available AADs that target potassium channels tend to block the late-phase 3 repolarizing currents, I_{Kr} and I_{Ks}, which may make them less effective during AF because this phase is shortened in the atria as a part of electrical remodeling, as illustrated in **Fig. 3**. They also target the same channels in the ventricle, which can prolong the QT interval, resulting in TdP. Drugs with selectivity for the atrial channels that are most active subsequent to the electrical remodeling of AF (early phase 3 repolarizing channels) could provide effective rhythm control with minimal ventricular proarrhythmia.

AZD7009 is an agent that is relatively atrial-specific. It blocks the sodium current I_{Na}, the atrial potassium current I_{Kur}, and the potassium current I_{Kr} to some extent. AZD7009 has shown only a small effect on the ventricular effective refractory period and QT interval.[24] Small clinical trials support AZD7009 as safe and effective for cardioversion with conversion rates of about 80% for AF of short duration.[25,26] However, the presence of mild prolongation of the QT interval, probably mediated by ventricular I_{Kr} current, suggests that some risk of TdP may exist, and one patient did have a short, asymptomatic run of polymorphic ventricular tachycardia. It has not been tested for chronic administration.

Vernakalant (previously called RSD1235) is another relatively atrial-specific AAD. It has mild frequency-dependent sodium channel block and I_{Kur} and I_{to} block.[27] It is the most thoroughly studied atrial-specific agent currently and is adequately discussed elsewhere in this issue. It is being developed for both conversion (intravenous administration) and prevention (oral administration) of AF. The intravenous studies seem to demonstrate superiority over placebo in the conversion of AF, but no significant efficacy for atrial flutter. This may at least in part be reflective of the observations seen to date with several of the "atrial-specific" agents that their actions on

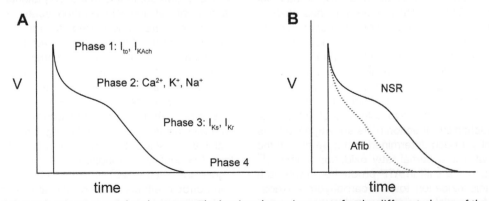

Fig. 3. (*A*) Atrial action potential and currents. The key ion channel currents for the different phases of the action potential are shown. (*B*) Atrial action potential in normal sinus rhythm (NSR) and atrial fibrillation (Afib). As the action potential shortens, the relative contribution of the ion channel currents is altered.

refractoriness can be significantly greater on left atrial than right atrial tissue, which is opposite to that of ibutilide and dofetilide, both of which are more effective in the conversion of atrial flutter than fibrillation.

Dronedarone

Dronedarone is a derivative of amiodarone with similar mechanisms of action, blocking calcium, potassium, and sodium channels in addition to having antiadrenergic effects. Dronedarone does not contain iodine, and has shown no thyroid or pulmonary toxicity in its clinical trials to date. It has fewer drug interactions than amiodarone. Dronedarone blocks multiple ion channels in the heart. Dronedarone's relevant pharmacology and the clinical trials that led to its marketing for AF and flutter in 2009 are well detailed elsewhere in this issue and in a prior review.[29] Dronedarone's striking results in ATHENA, in which an antiarrhythmic drug shown to be effective for AF reduction was now also shown effective in decreasing cardiovascular mortality and hospitalization, are unique for AADs. Dronedarone was approved by the Food and Drug Administration in July 2009 and by the European regulators later in the same year. Dronedarone's indication in the United State is to reduce the risk of cardiovascular hospitalization in patients with paroxysmal or persistent AF or atrial flutter, who are in sinus rhythm or who will be

cardioverted, and who have a recent episode of AF or atrial flutter and one or more associated cardiovascular risk factors: age greater than 70 years, hypertension, diabetes, prior cerebrovascular accident, or left atrial diameter greater than or equal to 50 mm or left ventricular ejection fraction less than 40%.

These criteria derive strongly from the ATHENA trial. Similarly, based on the ANDROMEDA trial (discussed elsewhere in this issue), dronedarone is contraindicated in patients with New York Heart Association Class IV HF or Class II to III HF with a recent decompensation requiring hospitalization or referral to a specialized HF clinic.

Dronedarone's release has come subsequent to the most recent (2006) ACC/AHA/ESC guidelines for AF management, and as such it is not discussed in their recommended algorithm approach for the maintenance of sinus rhythm. Based on that algorithm schematic and the indication and contraindication status noted, previously, however, the suggested pattern for dronedarone use in this context is described in **Fig. 4**.

REMODELING

It is said that AF begets AF, and animal models have demonstrated that rapid atrial pacing promotes AF.[28] AF changes the electrical and anatomic properties of the atria, a process termed "remodeling." Electrical remodeling includes

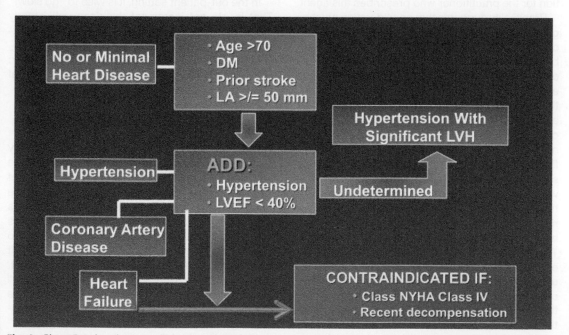

Fig. 4. Given Food and Drug Administration approval for dronedarone to reduce cardiovascular hospitalizations, for patients meeting certain criteria, this flow chart illustrates how dronedarone could be used for rhythm management of AF.

shortening of the effective refractory period. Structural remodeling can be demonstrated by histology, with increased inflammation, fibrosis, and myocyte apoptosis. Remodeling may be the mechanism by which AF begets AF. The concept of "upstream therapy" aims to reverse or prevent the substrate for AF. Upstream therapy has also been detailed elsewhere in this issue and in a prior review.[29] The large scale (approximately 600 patients), double-blind, prospective, multicenter trial of prescription-grade purified omega-3 fish oil versus placebo was completed (last patient, last visit) in January 2010 and its results are expected later in 2010.

SWITCHING MEDICATION FOR AF

When one is treating AF pharmacologically, it is not unusual for reasons of tolerance, suboptimal efficacy, or safety to need to change from one antiarrhythmic drug to another. Unfortunately, for the most part, formal guidelines based on clinical trials for this exercise are generally lacking, and available information data sets can be confusing. For example, with dronedarone, in EURIDIS/ADONIS investigators could discontinue amiodarone the day before initiating dronedarone, whereas in ATHENA investigators could not initiate dronedarone until 4 weeks after amiodarone's discontinuation. These data are in the package insert for dronedarone without any specific recommendation for the practitioner who prescribes this agent.

Practicality suggests that consideration must be given to the half-life of the drug that is being discontinued, so that the patient does not have bradycardia or proarrhythmic risk from the effects of two drugs at once, and the time to steady state expected for the agent being started. Generally, three or four half-lives are sufficient to allow almost all drug to be out of the system, but active metabolites can be an issue for propafenone and procainamide. For most patients with paroxysmal atrial fibrillation, going without drugs for a few days should not be difficult. Discontinuing amiodarone, with its long half-life, is a problem regarding the timing of starting a new AAD. In the authors' experience, it may be guided by serum concentrations, heart rate, and electrocardiogram (ECG) intervals. That is, when an agent is discontinued, its ECG effects, such as those on sinus rate, atrioventricular conduction, or the QRS or QT interval should dissipate as it is cleared from the body. When these effects reach a level at which the effects of the drug to be added would not seem to pose an additive risk, the new agent can be started. In this regard, the use of daily transtelephonic ECGs from home, for those occasions when the drug is initiated as an out-patient, can be quite useful for the patient and the physician.

SITE OF INITIATION

Some antiarrhythmic medications can be initiated in the out-patient setting, whereas others require in-patient initiation (or dose escalation). Those that require in-patient initiation do so because of proarrhythmic or bradycardic or hemodynamic concerns. These include the class IA agents (eg, quinidine) regardless of the arrhythmia being treated, dofetilide, and sotalol in most circumstances. According to the ACC/AHA/ESC guidelines, however, sotalol may be initiated in the out-patient setting for AF if the patient is both in sinus rhythm and does not have high risk markers for TdP (eg, bradycardia, a long QT, concomitant QT prolonging drugs, hypokalemia, hypomagnesemia, female gender) as was the case in its pivotal trials for AF. Out-patient initiation is allowed for AF when class IC agents are used (ie, in the absence of SHD or significant sinus node or conduction system disease), and for dronedarone. The pivotal clinical trials for these agents support this position. Amiodarone is customarily started in the out-patient setting for AF, not because it is free of risk of bradycardia or proarrhythmia (although the latter is rare) but largely because its long time to steady state makes in-patient initiation impractical and not cost effective.

In the out-patient setting, it is wise to "go slow." That is, do not increment the dose until steady state is reached, and use the longest $T_{1/2}$ expected for the drug, rather than its average $T_{1/2}$ to calculate this time period. Transtelephonic ECG monitoring can be extremely useful in lieu of more cumbersome and expensive daily ECGs.

ANTIARRHYTHMIC DRUGS AFTER ABLATION

Because ablation is often not effective in totally curing AF, antiarrhythmic drugs may still be required to provide the patient adequate relief from recurrent episodes. This therapy may be considered in three broad settings. The first is during the first 3 months postablation until lesions are fully matured, the period frequently referred to as the "blanking period" when AF may recur but without a later recurrent pattern. In this context, an AAD may be used with expectation that it will be discontinued after the first 3 months and the outcome observed. The second is for the suppression of recurrent events after the "blanking period" until such time that the patient undergoes a repeat ablation attempt. The third is for the suppression of recurrent events after the "blanking period" for chronic administration in lieu of a repeat ablation attempt.

In the postablation setting, antiarrhythmic drugs have the same indications and contraindications that they have in the absence of ablation and all have been tried. Not infrequently, an antiarrhythmic drug may be effective after ablation when it was less so before ablation. Recognize that the atrial substrate is altered by the procedure and this may affect the actions of the drug. Unfortunately, to date, there have been no large-scale prospective comparative trials across the antiarrhythmic drug spectrum to assess whether or not any particular drug or drug class has enhanced or reduced efficacy in this setting, so the drug choice, when one is made, remains for now empiric.

REFERENCES

1. Go AS, Hylek EM, Phillips KA, et al. Prevalence of diagnosed atrial fibrillation in adults: national implications for rhythm management and stroke prevention: the AnTicoagulation and risk factors in Atrial Fibrillation (ATRIA) Study. JAMA 2001;285(18):2370–5.

2. Reiffel J. The AFFECTS Registry Steering Committee and Investigators. The selection of a rate versus rhythm control strategy for atrial fibrillation management following AFFIRM and RACE [abstract 2029]. 2007;116:II_439.

3. Ruskin JN. The cardiac arrhythmia suppression trial (CAST). N Engl J Med 1989;321(6):386–8.

4. Waldo AL, Camm AJ, deRuyter H, et al. Effect of d-sotalol on mortality in patients with left ventricular dysfunction after recent and remote myocardial infarction. The SWORD Investigators. Survival With Oral d-Sotalol. Lancet 1996;348(9019):7–12.

5. Wyse DG, Waldo AL, DiMarco JP, et al. A comparison of rate control and rhythm control in patients with atrial fibrillation. N Engl J Med 2002; 347(23):1825–33.

6. Van Gelder IC, Hagens VE, Bosker HA, et al. A comparison of rate control and rhythm control in patients with recurrent persistent atrial fibrillation. N Engl J Med 2002;347(23):1834–40.

7. Hohnloser SH, Kuck KH, Lilienthal J. Rhythm or rate control in atrial fibrillation–Pharmacological Intervention in Atrial Fibrillation (PIAF): a randomised trial. Lancet 2000;356(9244):1789–94.

8. Corley SD, Epstein AE, DiMarco JP, et al. Relationships between sinus rhythm, treatment, and survival in the Atrial Fibrillation Follow-Up Investigation of Rhythm Management (AFFIRM) study. Circulation 2004;109(12):1509–13.

9. Hohnloser SH, Crijns HJ, van Eickels M, et al. Effect of dronedarone on cardiovascular events in atrial fibrillation. N Engl J Med 2009;360(7):668–78.

10. Pappone C, Augello G, Sala S, et al. A randomized trial of circumferential pulmonary vein ablation versus antiarrhythmic drug therapy in paroxysmal atrial fibrillation: the APAF Study. J Am Coll Cardiol 2006;48(11):2340–7.

11. Reiffel JA. Cardioversion for atrial fibrillation: treatment options and advances. Pacing Clin Electrophysiol 2009;32(8):1073–84.

12. Fuster V, Ryden LE, Cannom DS, et al. ACC/AHA/ESC 2006 guidelines for the management of patients with atrial fibrillation–executive summary: a report of the American College of Cardiology/American Heart Association Task Force on Practice Guidelines and the European Society of Cardiology Committee for Practice Guidelines (Writing Committee to Revise the 2001 Guidelines for the Management of Patients With Atrial Fibrillation). J Am Coll Cardiol 2006;48(4):854–906.

13. Pritchett ELC, Page RL, Carlson M, et al. For the Rythmol Atrial Fibrillation Trial (RAFT) Investigators. Efficacy and safety of sustained-release propafenone (propafenone SR) for patients with atrial fibrillation. Am J Cardiol 2003;92:941–6.

14. Lafuente-Lafuente C, Mouly S, Longas-Tejero MA, et al. Antiarrhythmic drugs for maintaining sinus rhythm after cardioversion of atrial fibrillation: a systematic review of randomized controlled trials. Arch Intern Med 2006;166(7):719–28.

15. Singh BN, Singh SN, Reda DJ, et al. Amiodarone versus sotalol for atrial fibrillation. N Engl J Med 2005;352(18):1861–72.

16. Burashnikov A, Di Diego JM, Zygmunt AC, et al. Atrium-selective sodium channel block as a strategy for suppression of atrial fibrillation: differences in sodium channel inactivation between atria and ventricles and the role of ranolazine. Circulation 2007;116(13):1449–57.

17. Scirica BM, Morrow DA, Hod H, et al. Effect of ranolazine, an antianginal agent with novel electrophysiological properties, on the incidence of arrhythmias in patients with non ST-segment elevation acute coronary syndrome: results from the Metabolic Efficiency With Ranolazine for Less Ischemia in Non ST-Elevation Acute Coronary Syndrome Thrombolysis in Myocardial Infarction 36 (MERLIN-TIMI 36) randomized controlled trial. Circulation 2007; 116(15):1647–52.

18. Conti CR. Partial fatty acid oxidation (pFOX) inhibition: a new therapy for chronic stable angina. Clin Cardiol 2003;26(4):161–2.

19. Valdivia CR, Chu WW, Pu J, et al. Increased late sodium current in myocytes from a canine heart failure model and from failing human heart. J Mol Cell Cardiol 2005;38(3):475–83.

20. Belardinelli L, Shryock JC, Fraser H. Inhibition of the late sodium current as a potential cardioprotective principle: effects of the late sodium

current inhibitor ranolazine. Heart 2006;92(Suppl 4):iv6–14.

21. Sicouri S, Glass A, Belardinelli L, et al. Antiarrhythmic effects of ranolazine in canine pulmonary vein sleeve preparations. Heart Rhythm 2008;5(7):1019–26.

22. Kumar K, Nearing BD, Carvas M, et al. Ranolazine exerts potent effects on atrial electrical properties and abbreviates atrial fibrillation duration in the intact porcine heart. J Cardiovasc Electrophysiol 2009;20(7):796–802.

23. Morrow DA, Scirica BM, Karwatowska-Prokopczuk E, et al. Effects of ranolazine on recurrent cardiovascular events in patients with non-ST-elevation acute coronary syndromes: the MERLIN-TIMI 36 randomized trial. JAMA 2007;297(16):1775–83.

24. Persson F, Andersson B, Duker G, et al. Functional effects of the late sodium current inhibition by AZD7009 and lidocaine in rabbit isolated atrial and ventricular tissue and Purkinje fibre. Eur J Pharmacol 2007;558(1–3):133–43.

25. Crijns HJ, Van Gelder IC, Walfridsson H, et al. Safe and effective conversion of persistent atrial fibrillation to sinus rhythm by intravenous AZD7009. Heart Rhythm 2006;3(11):1321–31.

26. Geller JC, Egstrup K, Kulakowski P, et al. Rapid conversion of persistent atrial fibrillation to sinus rhythm by intravenous AZD7009. J Clin Pharmacol 2009;49(3):312–22.

27. Fedida D, Orth PM, Chen JY, et al. The mechanism of atrial antiarrhythmic action of RSD1235. J Cardiovasc Electrophysiol 2005; 16(11):1227–38.

28. Wijffels MC, Kirchhof CJ, Dorland R, et al. Atrial fibrillation begets atrial fibrillation. A study in awake chronically instrumented goats. Circulation 1995;92(7): 1954–68.

29. Morrow JP, Reiffel JA. Drug therapy for atrial fibrillation: what will its role be in the era of increasing use of catheter ablation? Pacing Clin Electrophysiol 2009;32(1):108–18.

Rate Control in Atrial Fibrillation

Isabelle C. Van Gelder, MD, FESC[a,b],*,
Hessel F. Groenveld, MD[a]

KEYWORDS

- Atrial fibrillation • Rate control
- Negative dromotropic drugs

Atrial fibrillation (AF) is not a benign condition[1] and may cause symptoms, and is associated with stroke and heart failure. The first step in treating patients with AF is searching for and treating the associated disease, which is often hypertension or heart failure. Thereafter, AF itself should be treated. Therapy is aimed at reducing symptoms, improving quality of life, and preventing cardiovascular morbidity and mortality. There are 2 treatment strategies: rhythm control and rate control. The goal of rhythm control is achieving and maintaining sinus rhythm by serial cardioversions and antiarrhythmic drugs or by nonpharmacologic approaches, such as atrial catheter ablation. However, the problem of pharmacologic rhythm control therapy is that recurrences of AF occur frequently. In the Atrial Fibrillation Follow-up Investigation of Rhythm Management (AFFIRM) and the RAte Control versus Electrical cardioversion for persistent atrial fibrillation (RACE) studies, rhythm control treatment was effective in maintaining sinus rhythm in only 39% to 63% of patients after a mean of 2.3 to 3.5 years.[2,3] Efficacy of catheter ablation of AF is increasing and evolving rapidly, but AFFIRM and RACE made clear that most patients with AF can be treated with rate control. These studies showed that rate control therapy is not inferior to rhythm control treatment with regard to cardiovascular morbidity and mortality. Since then, acceptance of the arrhythmia with therapy aimed at achieving adequate ventricular rate control to prevent heart failure and symptoms is

an appropriate strategy in many patients with AF.[2,3] This article discusses for whom rate control is indicated and how it may be instituted.

INDICATIONS FOR RATE CONTROL: RATE CONTROL FOR WHOM AND WHEN

The wide heterogeneity in the presentation and underlying causes of AF calls for an individual approach to therapy, for either rate control or rhythm control. Such an approach requires selection of patients depending on the nature, intensity, and frequency of symptoms, patient preferences, comorbid conditions, and the risk on recurrent AF and complications associated with pharmacologic and nonpharmacologic therapies, and should be openly discussed with the patient.[4] In AFFIRM and RACE, predominantly elderly patients with underlying heart diseases were included. Most patients had at least one previous electrical cardioversion, and only a small number of patients with paroxysmal AF were included. Patients with (severely) symptomatic AF and advanced heart failure were excluded. Additional analyses of prespecified subgroups of patients in the AFFIRM study showed that patients who are 65 years or older and patients without a history of chronic heart failure had significantly better outcome (lower all-cause mortality) with rate control therapy (P<.01).[5] Subanalyses of the RACE trial showed enhanced cardiovascular morbidity and mortality in patients

The authors have nothing to disclose.
[a] Department of Cardiology, University Medical Center Groningen, University of Groningen, PO Box 30.001, 9700 RB Groningen, Groningen, The Netherlands
[b] Interuniversity Cardiology Institute Netherlands, Utrecht, Groningen, The Netherlands
* Corresponding author. Department of Cardiology, University Medical Center Groningen, University of Groningen, PO Box 30.001, 9700 RB Groningen, Groninger, The Netherlands.
E-mail address: I.C.van.Gelder@thorax.umcg.nl

Card Electrophysiol Clin 2 (2010) 419–427
doi:10.1016/j.ccep.2010.07.004
1877-9182/10/$ – see front matter © 2010 Published by Elsevier Inc.

cardiacEP.theclinics.com

with a history of hypertension or with hypertension, and in women treated with rhythm control.[6,7] Thus, depending on the severity of symptoms, which can easily be assessed by either the European Heart Rhythm Association symptom score or the Canadian Cardiovascular Society score,[8,9] rate control may be a reasonable therapy in the elderly, even more so in women, with persistent AF who have hypertension or other underlying heart diseases (**Box 1**). This condition also holds for patients with heart failure. The Atrial Fibrillation and Congestive Heart Failure Trial recently showed no difference in cardiovascular mortality between patients randomized to rate and rhythm control therapy in patients with AF, chronic heart failure, and a left ventricular ejection fraction less than or equal to 35%.[10] Limited efficacy of maintaining sinus rhythm and the potential harmful effects of current antiarrhythmic therapy in these patients may explain the earlier-mentioned results. A post hoc analysis of the AFFIRM trial suggested that deleterious effects of antiarrhythmic drugs (mortality increase of 49%) may have offset the benefits of sinus rhythm (which was associated with a 53% reduction in mortality),[11] whereas an analysis of the RACE data suggested that underlying heart disease impacts prognosis more than AF itself.[12] In favor of rhythm control is that subanalyses from several studies suggest that maintenance of sinus rhythm improves quality of life.[13,14]

Box 1
Criteria for choice of pharmacologic treatment strategy in persistent AF

Rhythm control

First episode of AF

(Severely) symptomatic AF

Young age

Poor control of ventricular rate during AF

Reversible tachycardiomyopathy

Possible discontinuation of anticoagulation

Rate control

No or minor complaints of AF (also lone AF)

Older age (>75 years)

High-risk recurrence of AF (severe AF)

Indication for anticoagulation irrespective of the rhythm

Certain subgroups (women, hypertensives)

OPTIMAL HEART RATE TARGET

Goal of rate control therapy is to reduce symptoms, improve quality of life, and minimize the development of heart failure. Guidelines, though empiric and not evidence based, have always recommended strict rate control, which is a resting heart rate between 60 and 80 beats per minute and a heart rate between 90 and 115 beats per minute during moderate exercise.[1] Strict rate control, on the other hand, could cause drug-related adverse effects, including bradycardia, syncope, and pacemaker implantation. Recently, the RAte Control Efficacy in permanent AF: a comparison between lenient versus strict rate control (RACE II) study was conducted to investigate the optimal level of heart-rate control during permanent AF.[15,16] The hypothesis of RACE II was that lenient rate control is not inferior to strict rate control in patients with permanent AF in terms of cardiovascular mortality and morbidity, quality of life, and costs. Therapy for strict rate control was defined as a mean resting heart rate (12-lead resting electrocardiogram) of less than 80 beats per minute and a heart rate of less than 110 beats per minute during moderate exercise (heart rate present at 25% of the maximal achieved exercise time during bicycle exercise test). Lenient heart rate control was defined as a heart rate of less than 110 beats per minute on a 12-lead resting electrocardiogram. A total of 614 patients were randomized to lenient or strict rate control. These patients were typical AF, the mean age was 68 ± 8 years, 66% were men patients, and hypertension was the associated disease in more than 60% of patients. The primary outcome was a composite of cardiovascular mortality and morbidity, and was reached in 81 patients (38 in the lenient and 43 in the strict group). The cumulative incidence of the primary outcome at 3 years of follow-up was 12.9% in the lenient and 14.9% in the strict group. This 2% difference in the primary outcome between both groups indicated noninferiority for lenient rate control as compared with strict rate control. More patients in the lenient group met the heart rate target (304 [98%] vs 203 [67%] in the strict group, P<.001) with fewer visits (mean 0.2 ± 0.6 vs 2.3 ± 1.4, P<.001) and with use of fewer rate control drugs. Symptoms, quality of life, and adverse events were also comparable between both groups. From RACE II, together with previous observations in nonrandomized studies and a post hoc analysis comparing data of AFFIRM (strict rate control) and RACE (lenient rate control),[17–19] it may be concluded that lenient rate control is as effective as strict rate control and easier to achieve. Rate control therapy, therefore, should be instituted with the aim to reduce symptoms rather than to "treat the electrocardiogram." In a lenient rate control approach there is only one heart-rate target, a resting heart rate less than 110 beats per minute. Dosages of rate control drugs can be increased and drugs can be combined until this target has been achieved. If patients remain symptomatic, with either an excessive rate or irregularity during exercise, or develop symptomatic heart failure, a stricter rate control target should be attempted. The heart rate may be reduced until the patient is asymptomatic or symptoms are tolerable, or when it is recognized that symptoms are caused by the underlying disease rather than the rhythm or the rate. When a strict rate control policy is adopted, an exercise test may be performed for assessing heart rate during moderate exercise. Eventually, a 24-hour Holter monitoring should be performed to check for pauses and bradycardia.

DRUGS USED TO ACHIEVE ADEQUATE RATE CONTROL

The main determinants of the ventricular rate during AF are the conduction characteristics and refractoriness of the atrioventricular node, and the sympathetic and parasympathetic tone. Negative dromotropic drugs are commonly used to lower the ventricular rate. These drugs include β-blockers, nondihydropyridine calcium channel antagonists, and digitalis; they can be instituted alone or in combination and at various doses. Dronedarone may also effectively reduce heart rate at the moment of recurrent AF and during permanent AF, but this drug is not approved for permanent AF.[20,21]

Which rate control drug or combination is the most effective is at present uncertain. Comparative evaluation of rate control drugs is difficult. There is a wide heterogeneity between trials in terms of objectives, patient selection, agents and doses used, duration of therapy, outcome measures (both quantitative and qualitative), and trial size (**Table 1**).[20,22–37] During chronic treatment, β-blockers are effective and safe as compared with placebo and digoxin in reducing heart rate. The data available also indicate that an improvement in exercise tolerance occurs. Farshi and colleagues[25] compared the effects of 5 standard drug regimens consisting of digoxin, diltiazem, atenolol, the combination digoxin/diltiazem, and the combination digoxin/atenolol on the mean 24-hour heart rates, circadian patterns of ventricular responses, and programmed exercise in patients with persistent AF. Least effective

were the use of digoxin and diltiazem alone. The combination of digoxin and atenolol produced the most effective rate control, reflecting a synergistic effect on the atrioventricular node. For the long term, the combination of a β-blocker and digitalis may be beneficial in patients with heart failure. Khand and colleagues[26] randomized patients with heart failure (left ventricular ejection fraction averaging 24%) and AF to carvedilol plus digoxin or to digoxin alone. These investigators observed that in patients with an impaired left ventricular function and AF, after a follow-up of 4 months heart rate was significantly lower in the patients treated with the combination of drugs than in those treated with digoxin alone (65 ± 15 beats per minute vs 75 ± 11 beats per minute, $P<.0001$). Compared with placebo, the addition of carvedilol to digoxin significantly improved left ventricular ejection fraction (24% ± 7% to 31% ± 10%, $P<.05$). However, uncertainty about the role of β-blockers under these circumstances remains because the Cardiac Insufficiency Bisoprolol Studies did not show a survival benefit with β-blockade in the subgroup of patients with heart failure who also had AF.[38] However, in the AFFIRM study the most effective rate control drug to achieve their (strict) rate control target were β-blockers.[39] Sotalol, being a β-blocker with additional class III antiarrhythmic activity, is strongly discouraged for rate control only because this relatively complex drug may induce life-threatening ventricular arrhythmias (torsades de pointes). Nondihydropyridine calcium channel antagonists (verapamil and diltiazem) should be avoided in patients with systolic heart failure because of their negative inotropic effect. Digoxin should be recommended with care because data suggest that digoxin increases mortality in patients with AF.[2,11,17,40] If the already mentioned drugs fail to sufficiently lower the heart rate, amiodarone or atrioventricular node ablation with implantation of a pacemaker may become necessary. In patients with overt heart failure, intravenous administration of digitalis or amiodarone is recommended.[41] Other class I or III antiarrhythmic drugs are not effective for rate control.

ATRIOVENTRICULAR NODE ABLATION

The American College of Cardiology/American Heart Association/European Society of Cardiology guidelines state that nonpharmacologic therapy should be considered when pharmacologic measures fail.[1] Atrioventricular node ablation together with permanent pacemaker implantation provides highly effective rate control and improves symptoms in selected patients.[42–45] In general,

Table 1
Heart rate control assessment during AF

Study	Study Design	Drugs	Number of Patients	Conditions in Patients	Follow-Up	End Point	Results: HR	Results: Exercise Time or LVEF
β-Blocker vs Placebo								
Lundström et al[28]	Randomized double-blind crossover study	Xamoterol vs verapamil vs placebo	21	Permanent AF	2 wk	Resting HR, exercise HR	HR decreased with both	No improvement of exercise capacity
Atwood et al[29]	Randomized crossover study	Betaxolol vs placebo	12	Permanent AF	NA	HR at rest and exercise, exercise capacity	Reduction of HR at rest and during exercise	Maximal oxygen uptake reduced with betaxolol
Joglar et al[30]	Randomized placebo-controlled, double-blind, retrospective analysis	Carvedilol vs placebo	136	AF and heart failure	6 mo	LVEF	NA	LVEF improved with carvedilol
Kochiadakis et al[31]	Randomized crossover single-blind study	Metoprolol vs sotalol vs placebo	23	Permanent AF	4 wk	Mean HR, HR during exercise	Both lower mean HR compared with placebo. Sotalol reduced HR more during moderate exercise	NA
β-Blocker vs Digoxin								
Lanas et al[32]	Randomized double-blind crossover study	Digoxin vs atenolol	13	Permanent AF	2 wk	Resting HR, exercise HR, exercise capacity, symptoms	Resting HR was similar. HR at maximal exercise was lower	Exercise time longer with atenolol

Study	Study design	Comparison	N	Population	Duration	Outcomes measured	Resting HR	Exercise capacity
Koh et al[27]	Randomized crossover study	Control vs betaxolol + digoxin vs diltiazem + digoxin	45	Permanent AF	4 wk	Resting HR, HR during exercise, exercise capacity	Resting HR was more reduced with betaxolol	Exercise capacity improved in both compared with control
Farshi et al[25]	Randomized crossover open-label study	Digoxin vs diltiazem vs atenolol vs digoxin + diltiazem vs digoxin + atenolol	12	Permanent AF, LVEF >35%, NYHA I or II	2 wk	Mean HR, HR during exercise	Digoxin + atenolol most effective for mean 24-h HR and exercise HR	NA
Khand et al[26]	Randomized controlled double-blind study	Digoxin vs digoxin + carvedilol	47	AF for >1 mo, LVEF <40% (mean 24%)	6 mo	HR, LVEF, NYHA class	Digoxin + carvedilol lowered mean HR and submaximal exercise improved symptoms	Improved LVEF, 6 MWT unaltered and not different
Calcium Channel Blocker vs Placebo								
Lewis et al,[33]	Open-label crossover study	Digoxin vs verapamil vs diltiazem, alone and in combination	6	Permanent AF	1 d	Resting HR, HR during exercise, exercise tolerance, cardiac output	Best reduction exercise HR by digoxin + diltiazem	No difference in exercise capacity or cardiac output
Atwood et al[24]	Open-label clinical trial	Diltiazem vs control	9	Permanent AF	1 wk	Resting HR, exercise HR, exercise capacity	Diltiazem reduced resting HR and exercise HR	No differences in exercise capacity
Lundström and Ryden[34]	Randomized placebo-controlled study	Diltiazem vs verapamil vs placebo	18	Permanent AF		Mean HR, exercise tolerance	Verapamil and diltiazem decreased HR	Modest improvement of exercise tolerance with both

(continued on next page)

Table 1
(continued)

Study	Study Design	Drugs	Number of Patients	Conditions in Patients	Follow-Up	End Point	Results: HR	Results: Exercise Time or LVEF
Calcium Channel Blocker vs Digoxin								
Lang et al[35]	Open-label crossover study	Verapamil vs digoxin	52	Permanent AF	4 mo	Exercise HR	Verapamil reduced resting HR and HR during exercise	Verapamil increased exercise capacity
Lewis et al[36]	Randomized double-blind crossover study	Digoxin, diltiazem, and digoxin + diltiazem	14	Permanent AF	1 d	Resting HR, HR during exercise	Resting HR and HR during exercise lower with combination treatment	No improvement of exercise tolerance
Botto et al[37]	Randomized crossover study	Gallopamil vs diltiazem vs verapamil vs digoxin	18	Permanent AF	1 wk	HR during exercise	Gallopamil, diltiazem, and verapamil are superior for rate control	NA
Farshi et al[25]	Randomized crossover open-label study	Digoxin vs diltiazem vs atenolol vs digoxin + diltiazem vs digoxin + atenolol	12	Permanent AF, LVEF >35%, NYHA I or II	2 wk	Mean HR, HR during exercise	Digoxin + atenolol most effective for mean 24-h HR and exercise. Digoxin and diltiazem are least effective	NA
Dronedarone								
Davy et al[20]	Randomized controlled trial	Dronedarone vs placebo on top of rate control medication	174	Symptomatic permanent AF for >6 mo	6 mo	Mean HR	Reduction of mean HR and at maximal exercise	NA

Abbreviations: HR, heart rate; LVEF, left ventricular ejection fraction; 6 MWT, 6-minute walking test; NA, not available; NYHA, New York Heart Association functional class.

patients most likely to benefit from this therapy are severely symptomatic patients, those with adverse effects, and those with uncontrollable heart rates despite the use of negative dromotropic drugs.[1,44] However, this approach has several limitations, including the need for pacemaker implantation and permanent loss of atrioventricular node conduction. In addition, recent studies have shown that right ventricular pacing may be associated with an increased risk of heart failure,[46–48] also after long-term (4–7 years of follow-up) right ventricular pacing after atrioventricular node ablation in patients with an initially normal left ventricular function.[49,50] It remains to be investigated whether this risk relates to right ventricular pacing or progression of the underlying heart disease. Recently, a small-scale randomized study showed that in patients with a normal left ventricular function, right ventricular pacing resulted in an impaired left ventricular function, which was prevented by biventricular pacing.[48]

SUMMARY

Rate control may now be adopted as a first-choice therapy in a variety of patients, especially older relatively asymptomatic patients with hypertension or other underlying heart diseases. The goal of rate control therapy is to minimize symptoms, improve quality of life, decrease the risk of development of heart failure, and prevent thromboembolic complications. A lenient rate control approach may be the initial therapeutic strategy. If symptoms persist, a stricter rate control approach may be adopted. Although long-term randomized studies are lacking, the evidence available suggests that a β-blocker with or without digoxin is the first-choice rate control therapy.

REFERENCES

1. Fuster V, Ryden LE, Cannom DS, et al. ACC/AHA/ESC 2006 Guidelines for the Management of Patients with Atrial Fibrillation: a report of the American College of Cardiology/American Heart Association Task Force on Practice Guidelines and the European Society of Cardiology Committee for Practice Guidelines (Writing Committee to Revise the 2001 Guidelines for the Management of Patients With Atrial Fibrillation): developed in collaboration with the European Heart Rhythm Association and the Heart Rhythm Society. Circulation 2006;114: e257–354.

2. Wyse DG, Waldo AL, DiMarco JP, et al. A comparison of rate control and rhythm control in patients with atrial fibrillation. N Engl J Med 2002; 347:1825–33.

3. Van Gelder IC, Hagens VE, Bosker HA, et al. A comparison of rate control and rhythm control in patients with recurrent persistent atrial fibrillation. N Engl J Med 2002;347:1834–40.

4. Boriani G, Diemberger I, Martignani C, et al. The epidemiological burden of atrial fibrillation: a challenge for clinicians and health care systems. Eur Heart J 2006;27:893–4.

5. Curtis AB, Gersh BJ, Corley SD, et al. Clinical factors that influence response to treatment strategies in atrial fibrillation: the Atrial Fibrillation Follow-up Investigation of Rhythm Management (AFFIRM) study. Am Heart J 2005;149:645–9.

6. Rienstra M, Van Veldhuisen DJ, Hagens VE, et al. Gender-related differences in rhythm control treatment in persistent atrial fibrillation: data of the Rate Control Versus Electrical Cardioversion (RACE) study. J Am Coll Cardiol 2005;46:1298–306.

7. Rienstra M, Van Veldhuisen DJ, Crijns HJGM, et al. RACE investigators. Enhanced cardiovascular morbidity and mortality during rhythm control treatment in persistant atrial fibrillation in hypertensives; data of the RACE study. Eur Heart J 2007;28: 741–51.

8. Dorian P, Guerra PG, Kerr CR, et al. Validation of a new simple scale to measure symptoms in atrial fibrillation: the Canadian Cardiovascular Society Severity in Atrial Fibrillation scale. Circ Arrhythm Electrophysiol 2009;2:218–24.

9. Kirchhof P, Auricchio A, Bax J, et al. Outcome parameters for trials in atrial fibrillation: executive summary. Eur Heart J 2007;28:2803–17.

10. Roy D, Talajic M, Nattel S, et al. Rhythm control versus rate control for atrial fibrillation and heart failure. N Engl J Med 2008;358:2667–77.

11. Corley SD, Epstein AE, DiMarco JP, et al. Relationships between sinus rhythm, treatment, and survival in the Atrial Fibrillation Follow-up Investigation of Rhythm Management (AFFIRM) Study. Circulation 2004;109:1509–13.

12. Rienstra M, Van Gelder IC, Hagens VE, et al. Mending the rhythm does not improve prognosis in patients with persistent atrial fibrillation: a subanalysis of the RACE study. Eur Heart J 2006;27: 357–64.

13. Hagens VE, Ranchor AV, Van Sonderen E, et al. Effect of rate or rhythm control on quality of life in persistent atrial fibrillation. Results from the Rate Control Versus Electrical Cardioversion (RACE) Study. J Am Coll Cardiol 2004;43:241–7.

14. Singh SN, Tang XC, Singh BN, et al. Quality of life and exercise performance in patients in sinus rhythm versus persistent atrial fibrillation: a Veterans Affairs Cooperative Studies Program Substudy. J Am Coll Cardiol 2006;48:721–30.

15. Van Gelder IC, Van Veldhuisen DJ, Crijns HJ, et al. RAte Control Efficacy in permanent atrial fibrillation:

a comparison between lenient versus strict rate control in patients with and without heart failure. Background, aims, and design of RACE II. Am Heart J 2006;152:420–6.

16. Van Gelder IC, Groenveld HF, Crijns HJ, et al. Lenient versus strict rate control in patients with atrial fibrillation. N Engl J Med 2010;362:1363–73.

17. Groenveld HF, Crijns HJ, Rienstra M, et al. Does intensity of rate control influence outcome in persistent atrial fibrillation? Data of the RACE study. Am Heart J 2009;158:785–91.

18. Rienstra M, Van Gelder IC, Van den Berg MP, et al. A comparison of low versus high heart rate in patients with atrial fibrillation and advanced chronic heart failure: effects on clinical profile, neurohormones and survival. Int J Cardiol 2006;109:95–100.

19. Van Gelder IC, Wyse DG, Chandler ML, et al. Does intensity of rate-control influence outcome in atrial fibrillation? An analysis of pooled data from the RACE and AFFIRM studies. Europace 2006;8:935–42.

20. Davy JM, Herold M, Hoglund C, et al. Dronedarone for the control of ventricular rate in permanent atrial fibrillation: the Efficacy and safety of dRonedArone for The cOntrol of ventricular rate during atrial fibrillation (ERATO) study. Am Heart J 2008;156:527–9.

21. Singh BN, Connolly SJ, Crijns HJ, et al. Dronedarone for maintenance of sinus rhythm in atrial fibrillation or flutter. N Engl J Med 2007;357:987–99.

22. Nikolaidou T, Channer KS. Chronic atrial fibrillation: a systematic review of medical heart rate control management. Postgrad Med J 2009;85:303–12.

23. Ahmad K, Dorian P. Rate control in atrial fibrillation: looking beyond the average heart rate. Curr Opin Cardiol 2006;21:88–93.

24. Atwood JE, Myers JN, Sullivan MJ, et al. Diltiazem and exercise performance in patients with chronic atrial fibrillation. Chest 1988;93:20–5.

25. Farshi R, Kistner D, Sarma JS, et al. Ventricular rate control in chronic atrial fibrillation during daily activity and programmed exercise: a crossover open-label study of five drug regimens. J Am Coll Cardiol 1999;33:304–10.

26. Khand AU, Rankin AC, Martin W, et al. Carvedilol alone or in combination with digoxin for the management of atrial fibrillation in patients with heart failure? J Am Coll Cardiol 2003;42:1944–51.

27. Koh KK, Kwon KS, Park HB, et al. Efficacy and safety of digoxin alone and in combination with low-dose diltiazem or betaxolol to control ventricular rate in chronic atrial fibrillation. Am J Cardiol 1995;75:88–90.

28. Lundström T, Moor E, Ryden L. Differential effects of xamoterol and verapamil on ventricular rate regulation in patients with chronic atrial fibrillation. Am Heart J 1992;124:917–23.

29. Atwood JE, Myers J, Quaglietti S, et al. Effect of betaxolol on the hemodynamic, gas exchange, and cardiac output response to exercise in chronic atrial fibrillation. Chest 1999;115:1175–80.

30. Joglar JA, Acusta AP, Shusterman NH, et al. Effect of carvedilol on survival and hemodynamics in patients with atrial fibrillation and left ventricular dysfunction: retrospective analysis of the US Carvedilol Heart Failure Trials Program. Am Heart J 2001;142:498–501.

31. Kochiadakis GE, Kanoupakis EM, Kalebubas MD, et al. Sotalol vs metoprolol for ventricular rate control in patients with chronic atrial fibrillation who have undergone digitalization: a single-blinded crossover study. Europace 2001;3:73–9.

32. Lanas F, Salvatici R, Castillo G, et al. [Comparison between digoxin and atenolol in chronic atrial fibrillation]. Rev Med Chil 1995;123:1252–62 [in Spanish].

33. Lewis RV, Irvine N, McDevitt DG. Relationships between heart rate, exercise tolerance and cardiac output in atrial fibrillation: the effects of treatment with digoxin, verapamil and diltiazem. Eur Heart J 1988;9:777–81.

34. Lundström T, Ryden L. Ventricular rate control and exercise performance in chronic atrial fibrillation: effects of diltiazem and verapamil. J Am Coll Cardiol 1990;16:86–90.

35. Lang R, Klein HO, Weiss E, et al. Superiority of oral verapamil therapy to digoxin in treatment of chronic atrial fibrillation. Chest 1983;83:491–9.

36. Lewis RV, Laing E, Moreland TA, et al. A comparison of digoxin, diltiazem and their combination in the treatment of atrial fibrillation. Eur Heart J 1988;9:279–83.

37. Botto GL, Bonini W, Broffoni T. Modulation of ventricular rate in permanent atrial fibrillation: randomized, crossover study of the effects of slow-release formulations of gallopamil, diltiazem, or verapamil. Clin Cardiol 1998;21:837–40.

38. Lechat P, Hulot JS, Escolano S, et al. Heart rate and cardiac rhythm relationships with bisoprolol benefit in chronic heart failure in CIBIS II Trial. Circulation 2001;103:1428–33.

39. Olshansky B, Rosenfeld LE, Warner AL, et al. The Atrial Fibrillation Follow-up Investigation of Rhythm Management (AFFIRM) study: approaches to control rate in atrial fibrillation. J Am Coll Cardiol 2004;43:1201–8.

40. Hallberg P, Lindback J, Lindahl B, et al. Digoxin and mortality in atrial fibrillation: a prospective cohort study. Eur J Clin Pharmacol 2007;63:959–71.

41. Hou ZY, Chang MS, Chen CY, et al. Acute treatment of recent-onset atrial fibrillation and flutter with a tailored dosing regimen of intravenous amiodarone. A randomized, digoxin-controlled study. Eur Heart J 1995;16:521–8.

42. Brignole M, Gianfranchi L, Menozzi C, et al. Influence of atrioventricular junction radiofrequency ablation in patients with chronic atrial fibrillation and flutter on quality of life and cardiac performance. Am J Cardiol 1994;74:242–6.

43. Kay GN, Ellenbogen KA, Giudici M, et al. The Ablate and Pace Trial: a prospective study of catheter ablation of the AV conduction system and permanent pacemaker implantation for treatment of atrial fibrillation. APT Investigators. J Interv Card Electrophysiol 1998;2:121–35.

44. Wood MA, Brown-Mahoney C, Kay GN, et al. Clinical outcomes after ablation and pacing therapy for atrial fibrillation: a meta-analysis. Circulation 2000;101:1138–44.

45. Ozcan C, Jahangir A, Friedman PA, et al. Long-term survival after ablation of the atrioventricular node and implantation of a permanent pacemaker in patients with atrial fibrillation. N Engl J Med 2001;344:1043–51.

46. Wilkoff BL, Cook JR, Epstein AE, et al. Dual-chamber pacing or ventricular backup pacing in patients with an implantable defibrillator: the Dual Chamber and VVI Implantable Defibrillator (DAVID) Trial. JAMA 2002;288:3115–23.

47. Smit MD, Van Dessel PF, Nieuwland W, et al. Right ventricular pacing and the risk of heart failure in implantable cardioverter-defibrillator patients. Heart Rhythm 2006;3:1397–403.

48. Yu CM, Chan JY, Zhang Q, et al. Biventricular pacing in patients with bradycardia and normal ejection fraction. N Engl J Med 2009;361:2123–34.

49. Vernooy K, Dijkman B, Cheriex EC, et al. Ventricular remodeling during long-term right ventricular pacing following his bundle ablation. Am J Cardiol 2006;97:1223–7.

50. Tops LF, Schalij MJ, Holman ER, et al. Right ventricular pacing can induce ventricular dyssynchrony in patients with atrial fibrillation after atrioventricular node ablation. J Am Coll Cardiol 2006;48:1642–8.

Acute Antiarrhythmic Therapy of Ventricular Tachycardia and Ventricular Fibrillation

Mohan N. Viswanathan, MD[a],*, Richard L. Page, MD, FHRS[b]

KEYWORDS

- Ventricular tachycardia • Ventricular fibrillation
- Antiarrhythmic drugs • Implantable cardioverter-defibrillator
- Sudden cardiac death • Electrical storm

Ventricular arrhythmias, including ventricular tachycardia (VT) and ventricular fibrillation (VF), continue to be the major cause of acute sudden cardiac death.[1,2] The annual incidence of sudden cardiac death is approximately 1 to 2 per 1000 people (0.1%–0.2%) in the United States and may be rising because of the epidemic of metabolic syndrome and its effects on the heart. Coronary artery disease is found as the underlying cause of heart disease in 80% of all episodes of sudden cardiac death.[3] The remaining 20% are from nonischemic cardiomyopathy; congenital lesions with a predilection to ventricular arrhythmias, including genetic ion channel mutations such as the long QT syndrome; and idiopathic VF.[2,4]

Percutaneous coronary angioplasty and stent placement for restoring coronary blood flow during a myocardial infarction have significantly reduced the incidence of acute ventricular arrhythmias, especially the VT/VF episodes associated with acute myocardial injury. However, VT and VF continue to present significant challenges in terms of optimal management, and despite the development of algorithms for acute management, often ventricular arrhythmias prove refractory to initial pharmacologic treatment.[5]

In addition to acute antiarrhythmic therapy of VT/VF, nonpharmacologic treatments have been developed. The development of the implantable cardioverter-defibrillator (ICD) by Mirowski and colleagues[6] ushered in a new era of treatment of ventricular arrhythmias. Initially ICDs were reserved only for individuals at high risk for recurrent sudden cardiac death after at least one aborted sudden cardiac death event from ventricular arrhythmias; however, in the 3 decades after the original report by Mirowski and colleagues,[6] several large randomized clinical trials have shown their efficacy and mortality benefit for both primary and secondary prevention of sudden cardiac death in individuals with ischemic and nonischemic cardiomyopathy.[7–10] This article discusses the role of adjunctive pharmacologic antiarrhythmic therapy directed at treatment of VT and VF in patients with ICDs. This topic has also been reviewed in a few recent publications.[11–14]

Disclosures: Dr Page has no financial conflicts but previously received support from Procter and Gamble Pharmaceuticals and has been a consultant for Berlex Laboratories, Reliant Pharmaceuticals, Astellas, and sanofi-aventis. Dr Viswanathan has received speaking honoraria from Boston Scientific and Biotronik, Inc, and has been a consultant for Medtronic, Inc.

[a] Division of Cardiology/Cardiac Electrophysiology, University of Washington, Box 356422, 1959 NE Pacific Street, A-506B, Seattle, WA 98195-6422, USA
[b] Department of Medicine, University of Wisconsin, School of Medicine & Public Health, J5/219 Clinical Science Center MC2454, 600 Highland Avenue, Madison, WI 53792, USA
* Corresponding author.
E-mail address: viswanam@u.washington.edu

Card Electrophysiol Clin 2 (2010) 429–441
doi:10.1016/j.ccep.2010.07.001
1877-9182/10/$ — see front matter © 2010 Published by Elsevier Inc.

Radiofrequency catheter ablation of ventricular arrhythmias in patients with structural heart disease, including and initially targeting those with a history of coronary artery disease, was also introduced in the early 1980s.[15–17] Catheter ablative strategies have provided acute success rates in the range of 75% with a recurrence rate of 21% to 50% based on data from several studies.[17–23] Catheter ablation has been limited by the requirement of a hemodynamically tolerated, stable VT that would allow mapping in the electrophysiology laboratory.[24,25] With current electroanatomic mapping systems, a substrate-based approach at ablation for patients with identifiable myocardial scar can be successfully undertaken.[26] Catheter ablation, combined with pharmacologic approaches and the implantation of an ICD for recurrent VT, constitute the modern three-pronged treatment approach for ventricular arrhythmias that occur in the setting of structural heart disease, although studies are needed for direct comparison of catheter ablation versus pharmacologic approaches.[27] Detailed discussion of catheter ablation of ventricular arrhythmias is beyond the scope of this article, which focuses on acute pharmacologic antiarrhythmic therapy of VT/VF.

DEFINITION AND DIAGNOSIS OF VT

VT is usually defined as more than three consecutive spontaneous ventricular impulses at a mean rate of more than 100 beats per minute. If the duration is less than 30 seconds, this is usually termed *nonsustained* VT, whereas *sustained* VT is defined as a series of ventricular impulses lasting longer than 30 seconds or VT that results in hemodynamic instability in less than 30 seconds. Immediate treatment is required for VT associated with hemodynamic compromise.

Most individuals with underlying cardiovascular disease who present with a wide complex tachycardia have VT as the cause of the arrhythmia. In some cases, differentiating VT from a supraventricular tachycardia with aberrant conduction can be difficult despite obtaining a 12-lead electrocardiogram and taking a detailed history. The presence of atrioventricular dissociation with clearly discernable P waves unrelated to ventricular activity; single QRS complexes (usually more narrow in relation to the VT) likely representing fusion complexes between a VT and a conducted supraventricular impulse or a purely conducted complex (fusion or capture beats, respectively); a QRS duration greater than 140 ms; and a concordantly positive or negative QRS complex across the precordial leads all favor the diagnosis of VT over supraventricular tachycardia with aberrant conduction.

The use of intravenous adenosine in the setting of wide complex tachycardia can provide some insight regarding the mechanism (ie, termination of a wide complex tachycardia with adenosine would favor a diagnosis of supraventricular tachycardia with aberrant conduction over VT). However, given that most wide complex tachycardias of unclear origin are in fact VT rather than supraventricular tachycardia with aberrancy, especially in the setting of structural heart disease, the use of adenosine in this circumstance is generally discouraged. Its use in differentiating VT from supraventricular tachycardia has some associated risks, such as the delay of definitive treatment, the potential degeneration of wide complex tachycardia to VF in the setting of ventricular preexcitation and transient hypotension.[28] Occasionally, intravenous verapamil is used to treat a wide complex tachycardia that is thought to be a supraventricular tachycardia; however, it is also strongly discouraged in this situation unless the arrhythmia is known with certainty to be a supraventricular tachycardia or an idiopathic left ventricular VT arising from the left fascicular system (fascicular VT).[29]

IMMEDIATE ASSESSMENT AND MANAGEMENT OF SUSTAINED VT/VF

Every patient who presents initially with unstable sustained VT or VF requires immediate stabilization, including basic life support involving cardiopulmonary resuscitation (CPR), mechanical ventilation, and acute defibrillation for a pulseless or unconscious patient with hemodynamic compromise.[5] Once the patient has been resuscitated and stabilized from the ventilatory and circulatory standpoint, if the clinical status permits, a 12-lead electrocardiogram should be performed and the serum electrolytes investigated. A brief history and physical examination should be undertaken with an eye toward identifying the possibility of precipitating angina, ischemia, or acute myocardial infarction. Any prior history of cardiovascular disease, use of illicit drugs, and circumstances surrounding the onset of the clinical arrhythmia should be investigated and documented. Sustained VT/VF may have various causes, and the most appropriate treatment algorithm will depend on the specific cause of the ventricular arrhythmia, if this can be identified. Thus, this article now focuses on the acute pharmacologic treatment of ventricular arrhythmias based on clinical presentation. This article uses the Vaughan Williams[30] classification of antiarrhythmic drugs, which is based on the site of action of these agents on membrane-bound ion channels and their subsequent effect on action potential duration and conduction velocity. Although this classification has inherent limitations, it remains the most useful system.[31]

ACUTE ANTIARRHYTHMIC THERAPY OF VT/VF
Ventricular Arrhythmias in Acute Myocardial Infarction

For patients presenting with VT in the setting of an acute myocardial infarction (usually manifesting as polymorphic VT secondary to ongoing ischemia and infarction), management should be focused on treating the underlying cause (ie, achieving acute reperfusion of the coronary artery). The American College of Cardiology/American Heart Association (ACC/AHA) 2007 guidelines for management of patients with acute ST-elevation myocardial infarction and the Canadian Cardiovascular Society Working group adaptation for Canada both provide a relatively current algorithm for managing patients with acute myocardial infarction and options for acute reperfusion therapy.[32–35]

β-Blockers (Vaughan Williams class II)
Even though no controlled trials have evaluated the use of β-blockers after the development of sustained VT or VF in the setting of acute myocardial infarction, a meta-analysis has shown that intravenous use of β-blockers during and after myocardial infarction reduces the relative risk of death (during myocardial infarction: relative risk [RR], 0.87; CI, 0.77–0.98; $P = .02$; after myocardial infarction: RR, 0.77; CI, 0.7–0.84; $P<.001$).[36,37] Furthermore, a few older studies suggest that intravenous atenolol or a combination of intravenous and oral metoprolol given in suspected acute myocardial infarction were both associated with a reduction in the incidence of VT or VF.[38–40] Data from the COMMIT (Clopidogrel and Metoprolol in Myocardial Infarction) trial, which randomized 45,852 patients to either a combination of intravenous and oral metoprolol or placebo within 24 hours of suspected acute myocardial infarction, showed that early use of β-blocker therapy reduced the risk of development of VF, but this was counterbalanced by the development of cardiogenic shock, especially during the first day after admission.[41] **Table 1** provides a summary of this and other key clinical studies referenced throughout this article. In one study, intravenous propranolol use reduced the incidence of VF

from 3.8% to 0.5% in the first 48 hours during acute myocardial infarction.[42]

In summary, intravenous followed by oral β-blockade is recommended for all patients after acute myocardial infarction, except those who have contraindications, independent of whether ventricular arrhythmias occur in this acute setting.

Lidocaine (class IB)
Evidence regarding the use of intravenous lidocaine for the primary prevention of VF in acute myocardial infarction has been mixed.[36] A randomized trial of 903 subjects and an associated meta-analysis showed that a 200-mg intravenous bolus of lidocaine followed by a 3-mg/min infusion may reduce the incidence of VF (from 5.7% to 2%).[43] However, this study confirmed the finding of prior meta-analyses of randomized trials that showed a statistically significant 62% increase in mortality associated with this treatment compared with placebo (odds ratio [OR], 1.12; 95% CI, 0.91–1.36).[44,45]

In contrast, nonrandomized data from GUSTO-I and GUSTO-IIb suggest that patients who received prophylactic lidocaine did not have an increase in mortality.[46] Nevertheless, the use of lidocaine for primary prophylaxis of VT in the setting of acute myocardial infarction is not recommended.

Flecainide, encainide, and moricizine (class IC)
The Cardiac Arrhythmia Suppression Trial (CAST) compared the action of the class IC antiarrhythmic drugs (oral flecainide and encainide) and placebo in suppressing the development of premature ventricular complexes after myocardial infarction in patients who had a reduced left ventricular ejection fraction (LVEF) less than 40% (or <55% if within 90 days of infarction).[47] This investigation was predicated on the finding that premature ventricular complexes were associated with increased risk in patients after myocardial infarction, and the hypothesis that reducing premature ventricular complexes would reduce mortality. However, an increased mortality was seen in the drug treatment arm compared with the placebo arm, and the study was terminated at 10 months of follow-up because of arrhythmic and nonarrhythmic cardiac death. CAST had also randomized patients to oral moricizine, and the trial continued with this agent as CAST II, although no benefit was observed in patients treated with this agent.

Other studies comparing class I agents with the class III agents oral amiodarone and sotalol showed the class III agents to be superior.[48,49] Therefore, class I agents do not seem to be safe

Table 1
Selective clinical studies cited in review summarizing various antiarrhythmic drug therapies for ventricular arrhythmias

Study	Agent Studied	Participants	Follow-up	Primary End Point	Secondary End Point
Chen et al[41] COMMIT	Metoprolol after myocardial infarction (oral)	45,852 total Metoprolol: 22,929 Placebo: 22,923	4 wk or first hospital discharge	Composite of death, reinfarction or cardiac arrest: Metoprolol: 9.4% Placebo: 9.9% (OR, 0.96; P = .1) Death from any cause during the scheduled treatment period: Metoprolol: 7.7% Placebo: 7.8% (OR, 0.99; P = .69)	Ventricular fibrillation: Metoprolol: 581 Placebo: 698 (OR, 0.83; P = .001); Reinfarction, cardiogenic shock
Echt et al[47] CAST	Encainide, flecainide, or moricizine after myocardial infarction (oral)	1498 total Encainide: 432 Flecainide: 323 Placebo: 743	10 mo (study halted early because of excess mortality)	Incidence of sudden death in patients after infarction with ventricular ectopy suppressible with antiarrhythmic agents Arrhythmic death: Encainide or flecainide: 5.7% Placebo: 2.2% (P = .0004)	Nonlethal disqualifying ventricular tachycardia, proarrhythmia, syncope, need for pacemaker, congestive heart failure, recurrent myocardial infarction, angina, need for coronary artery bypass surgery or angioplasty
Boutitie et al[55] EMIAT and CAMIAT (pooled analysis)	Amiodarone in setting of β-blocker use (oral)	2687 total (pooled) EMIAT: 1486 CAMIAT: 1201 Amiodarone: +β-blocker: 691 −β-blocker: 657 Placebo: +β-blocker: 682 −β-blocker: 657	1 y	All-cause mortality, cardiac death, arrhythmic cardiac death, nonarrhythmic cardiac death, arrhythmic death, and resuscitated cardiac arrest Cardiac death: +β-blocker ± amiodarone: 5.5% −β-blocker ± amiodarone: 15% (RR, 0.57; P = .03) Arrhythmic cardiac death: +β-blocker ± amiodarone: 3.4% −β-blocker ± amiodarone: 7.2% (RR, 0.43; P = .07)	Primary and secondary end points combined in the pooled analysis

Study	Description	Patients	Follow-up	Primary results	Secondary/adverse outcomes
Kudenchuk et al[71] ARREST	Amiodarone in cardiac arrest (intravenous)	504 total Amiodarone: 246 Placebo: 258	Variable: depending on resuscitation time and survival beyond hospital admission and discharge	Admission to the hospital with a spontaneously perfusing rhythm: Amiodarone: 44% Placebo: 34% (OR, 1.6; $P = .02$)	Adverse events, number of precordial shocks delivered after amiodarone or placebo infusion, total duration of resuscitative efforts, need for additional antiarrhythmic drugs
Pacifico et al[81]	Sotalol for prevention of ICD shocks (oral)	302 total Sotalol: 151 Placebo: 151	12 mo	All-cause mortality or delivery of a first ICD shock for any reason: Sotalol: 34% reached end point Placebo: 54% reached end point (HR, 0.52; $P<.001$)	Frequency of shocks due to any cause: Sotalol: 1.43 ± 3.53 shocks/y Placebo: 3.89 ± 10.65 shocks/y ($P = .008$)
Connolly et al[83] OPTIC	β-blocker versus amiodarone + β-blocker vs sotalol for prevention of ICD shocks (oral)	412 total β-blocker: 138 amiodarone + β-blocker: 140 Sotalol: 134	1 y	ICD shock for any reason: β-blocker alone: 38.5% Sotalol: 24.3% Amiodarone + β-blocker: 10.3% Amiodarone + β-blocker versus β-blocker alone (HR, 0.27; $P<.001$) vs sotalol (HR, 0.43; $P = .02$)	
Dorian et al[87] SHIELD	Azimilide for recurrent ventricular arrhythmias and ICD therapies (intravenous)	633 total Azimilide, 75 mg/d: 220 Azimilide, 125 mg/d: 199 Placebo: 214	1 y	All-cause ICD shocks plus symptomatic tachyarrhythmias terminated by ATP Azimilide, 75 mg: 52% (HR, 0.43; $P = .0006$) Azimilide, 125 mg: 50% (HR, 0.53; $P = .0053$) (both compared with placebo) Placebo: 58% All-cause ICD shocks: Azimilide, 75 mg, 28% RR reduction Azimilide, 125 mg, 17% RR reduction (not statistically significant)	Appropriate ICD therapies (shocks or ATP): Azimilide, 75 mg: 48% RR reduction (HR, 0.52; $P = .017$) Azimilide, 125 mg: 62% RR reduction (HR, 0.38; $P = .0004$) (both compared with placebo)

Abbreviations: ATP, antitachycardia pacing; HR, hazard ratio; ICD, implantable cardioverter-defibrillator; OR, odds ratio; RR, relative risk.

Data from Patel C, Yan GX, Kocovic D, et al. Should catheter ablation be the preferred therapy for reducing ICD shocks?: ventricular tachycardia ablation versus drugs for preventing ICD shocks: role of adjuvant antiarrhythmic drug therapy. Circ Arrhythm Electrophysiol 2009;2:705–11; discussion: 712.

or effective in preventing ventricular arrhythmias in this setting of acute myocardial infarction.

Amiodarone (class III)

Amiodarone is a unique antiarrhythmic agent in that it has ion channel effects from all four of the Vaughan Williams classes, although it is technically classified as a class III (K^+-channel blocker) agent. The efficacy of oral amiodarone in preventing sudden cardiac death was established by prior randomized trials,[50–52] and meta-analyses showed that compared with placebo, oral amiodarone was associated with a 10% to 19% reduction in total mortality in patients with acute myocardial infarction, congestive heart failure,[53] and cardiac arrest.[54]

The role of amiodarone in the primary prevention of sudden cardiac death was assessed in a pooled analysis of two similar studies of postinfarction patients: the European Amiodarone Myocardial Infarction Trial (EMIAT) and the Canadian Amiodarone Myocardial Infarction Trial (CAMIAT). In this analysis, the incidences of cardiac death, arrhythmic death, and resuscitated cardiac arrest were significantly lower in patients receiving oral β-blockers and oral amiodarone than in those not taking β-blockers with or without amiodarone (P = .05 and 0.03 for EMIAT and CAMIAT, respectively).[55]

Termination of Sustained Monomorphic Ventricular Tachycardia or Wide Complex Tachycardia

The most expeditious treatment of any hemodynamically unstable sustained ventricular arrhythmia is external defibrillation.[5] If the rhythm is a stable monomorphic VT that is nonsyncopal, many physicians still elect to perform immediate synchronized cardioversion, because it is very effective and often the best first-line therapy for this arrhythmia. Intravenous antiarrhythmic drugs may also be used to achieve chemical cardioversion in this setting, and reduce the likelihood of recurrent VT. Agents that have been used in this setting include lidocaine, procainamide, sotalol, quinidine, bretylium (no longer available), and amiodarone.

Procainamide (class IA)

In a small study of 29 randomized patients with sustained VT, intravenous procainamide infused at 100 mg/min for a total of 10 mg/kg was able to terminate 80% of stable VTs, whereas intravenous lidocaine at 1.5 mg/kg given over 2 minutes only terminated 22% of VTs.[56]

Lidocaine

Observational trials of intravenous lidocaine use also suggest an acute conversion rate from VT to normal sinus rhythm of 10% to 20%.[57–60]

Sotalol (class III)

Ho and colleagues[59] undertook a small study of 33 patients with spontaneous sustained VT and randomized them in a double-blinded fashion to receive either sotalol or lidocaine (both given as 100 mg intravenously). Sotalol was significantly more effective than lidocaine (69% vs 18%) in acute termination of the VT. Sotalol became available in the United States as an intravenous infusion in November 2009 (Bioniche Pharma, Lake Forest, IL, USA).

Amiodarone

Limited studies are available on the use of amiodarone to terminate stable monomorphic VT, but it is presumed to be effective based on data obtained in patients with unstable VT. The current 2005 AHA Emergency Cardiac Care guidelines recommend intravenous amiodarone for the control of hemodynamically stable VT, polymorphic VT with a normal QT interval, and wide complex tachycardia of uncertain origin (class IIb recommendation) based on a few small studies.[5] Amiodarone is believed to be safer than procainamide in patients with impaired left ventricular function, because it is not associated with the same degree of hypotension as can be seen with procainamide.

Secondary Prevention of VT/VF

β-Blockers

Sympathetic blockade, including the use of intravenous esmolol or propranolol, was compared with Advanced Cardiac Life Support–guided therapy for the secondary prevention of VT/VF in the state of electrical storm (defined as the recurrences of two or more episodes of hemodynamically unstable sustained VT or VF during a 24-hour period).[61] Although the analysis was nonrandomized, the markedly improved survival (78% vs 18% at 1 week, and 67% vs 5% at 1 year) seen with β-blocker therapy suggests it may have an important role in the acute treatment of recurrent or treatment-resistant sustained ventricular arrhythmias.[62]

Amiodarone

Amiodarone has been evaluated in multiple trials for the treatment of frequent sustained VT or VF (electrical storm), with demonstrated efficacy ranging from 40% to 100% for mitigation of ventricular arrhythmias.[63] A dose of 1000 mg/d of intravenous amiodarone has efficacy and is not associated with an increase in serious adverse drug reaction or death.[61,64,65] Mooss and colleagues[66] noted that at higher doses (20–30 mg/kg/d, intravenously), amiodarone may have a greater ability to suppress ventricular arrhythmias, but that this came at the cost of increased serious side effects, such as hypotension, symptomatic bradycardia, and sinus arrest, occurring in up to 37% of patients.

Dofetilide (class III)

Dofetilide is a class III agent with selective blockade of the rapid delayed rectifier potassium current, I_{Kr}.[67] It is approved for rhythm control of atrial fibrillation and is only available in North America. One double-blinded, randomized, crossover trial of patients with ischemic heart disease and sustained VT showed that oral dofetilide was equally as effective as oral sotalol in the secondary prevention of ventricular arrhythmias and arrhythmic death after 1 year of follow up.[68]

Shock-Resistant VT or VF

Given that early defibrillation can be very effective at restoring a perfusing rhythm and resuscitate a marginal patient, the 2005 AHA Emergency Cardiac Care Guidelines advocate immediate CPR for five cycles, followed by a single external defibrillation and resumption of CPR, followed by another shock after five cycles of CPR if necessary. The guidelines also suggest the use of intravenous epinephrine and vasopressin before antiarrhythmic therapy is initiated.[5]

Bretylium (class III)

No clear evidence shows that bretylium is effective at suppressing shock-refractory VF. Two small randomized studies of intravenous lidocaine and bretylium showed no difference between the agents in restoring a perfusing rhythm in out-of-hospital cardiac arrest.[69,70] One large randomized, double-blinded, controlled study of intravenous amiodarone and bretylium in the treatment of patients with recurrent hemodynamically destabilizing VT or VF showed a significantly higher adverse event rate with bretylium compared with amiodarone.[61] However, bretylium is no longer available and or included as an option for treatment in the 2005 AHA Emergency Cardiac Care Guidelines.

Amiodarone

The ARREST (the Amiodarone and Out of Hospital Resuscitation of Refractory Sustained Ventricular Tachycardia) trial investigated the efficacy of intravenous amiodarone (as a single 300 mg dose)

versus placebo in a randomized, blinded, controlled trial of 504 individuals with out-of-hospital VF arrest resistant to defibrillation.[71] The primary end point of survival to hospital admission was reached in a higher percentage of patients (44%) in the amiodarone arm than in the placebo arm (34%, $P = .03$). The greatest survival to hospital admission was seen when amiodarone was given within 4 to 16 minutes from dispatch, and no significant difference was seen between amiodarone and placebo when a delay in drug administration of up to 55 minutes occurred after dispatch. In patients with return of spontaneous circulation before drug infusion, survival to hospital admission rose to 64% in the amiodarone group versus 41% with placebo.

Even though higher rates of survival to hospital admission seen with amiodarone did not translate into higher rates of survival to hospital discharge, this is the only study showing the efficacy of any pharmacologic agent in a randomized, blinded comparison to placebo or alternative therapy. Based on this study, intravenous amiodarone is recommended for treatment of defibrillation-resistant VF.

Polymorphic VT (Torsades de Pointes)

Polymorphic VT or torsades de pointes (TdP) occurs in the setting of prolonged repolarization (prolonged QT interval) and manifests as repeated salvos of nonsustained VT or sustained polymorphic VT that is triggered after a pause (often termed *pause-dependent* polymorphic VT). The preferred treatment is prompt defibrillation, as with any unstable VT/VF episodes, but immediate intravenous infusion of magnesium may be helpful.[72] Increasing the baseline heart rate with transvenous pacing or intravenous isoproterenol can reduce the incidence of the triggering pauses that may precede TdP. In addition, discontinuing any QT-prolonging agents and correcting hypokalemia, if present, is essential to the management of TdP.[73]

RECURRENT VENTRICULAR ARRHYTHMIAS IN PATIENTS WITH ICDS

Multiple studies have shown the considerable mortality benefit of the ICD as the primary treatment of patients with increased risk of life-threatening ventricular arrhythmias.[10,74–76] In some of these studies, ICD therapy was clearly shown to be superior to antiarrhythmic agents, such as amiodarone; however, the use of adjunctive therapy with antiarrhythmic drugs in those with an ICD is common, with data from various studies suggesting that between 16% and 70%

of patients who receive an ICD may ultimately be treated with antiarrhythmic drugs.[9,77,78]

The primary goal of adding antiarrhythmic therapy to the ICD is to reduce the incidence of ICD shocks, whether appropriate for ventricular arrhythmias or inappropriate for supraventricular arrhythmias. In addition, the Sudden Cardiac Death in Heart Failure Trial (SCD-HeFT) showed that ICD shocks, either appropriate or inappropriate, were associated with a marked increased risk of death, primarily because of worsening heart failure.[79] Thus, reducing clinical shocks may be associated with mortality benefit, in addition to increasing patient comfort. Even though ventricular arrhythmias in patients with an ICD may fall outside of the focus of this article on acute pharmacologic therapy of VT/VF, a few key studies are mentioned that assess the use of antiarrhythmic drug therapy for VT/VF in the ICD recipient, because this is being encountered clinically on an increasing basis.

β-Blockers

β-Blockers have been established as a mainstay of therapy in the post-MI patient as well as in congestive heart failure for mortality benefit. Even though no randomized controlled trials have studied β-blockers in patients with an ICD, β-blockers reduce the incidence of arrhythmias and sudden death in this group of patients. The Cardiac Insufficiency Bisoprolol Study II (CIBIS II) showed that oral bisoprolol reduced all-cause mortality by 34% (P<.0001) and sudden cardiac death by 44% in patients with congestive heart failure.[80]

Sotalol

Pacifico and colleagues[81] were the first to show the efficacy of oral sotalol in preventing appropriate and inappropriate ICD shocks. In this study, 302 patients with ICDs were randomized to receive either oral d,l-sotalol (160–320 mg/d) or placebo and then followed up for 1 year. The primary end point of all-cause death or delivery of a first shock for any reason was reached in 34% of patients in the sotalol group and 54% of those in the placebo arm (RR reduction of 48%, P<.001). In this study, β-blocker use was suboptimal compared with current practice (only 23% of the sotalol arm and 37% of the placebo arm). In fact, in approximately 27% of patients in the sotalol group, treatment was halted early because of adverse events, most commonly because of the β-blocking effects of sotalol, but only one episode of TdP occurred.

In a similar study published in the same year, Kuhlkamp and colleagues[82] showed that the addition of oral d,l-sotalol to ICD patients' medical regimen led to a significant reduction in the incidence of recurrent VT/VF and ICD therapies. In this study, roughly 26% of patients in the ICD-only arm also required institution of additional antiarrhythmic drug therapy to suppress recurrent VT/VF or supraventricular tachyarrhythmias, a finding that was similar to that seen in the ICD arm of the AVID (Antiarrhythmics vs Implantable Defibrillators) trial.[77]

Amiodarone

The OPTIC (Optimal Pharmacologic Therapy in Cardioverter Defibrillator Patients) trial randomized patients with ICDs to receive either oral amiodarone (200 mg/d) and oral β-blocker, oral sotalol alone (240 mg/d), or oral β-blocker alone (bisoprolol, 10 mg/d, or equivalent). This study enrolled 412 patients who had received a dual-chamber ICD for inducible or spontaneous VT/VF and an LVEF of 40% or less or unexplained syncope with inducible VT/VF by programmed stimulation; all ICDs were programmed to avoid shocks with antitachycardia pacing up to a rate of 222 beats per minute and supraventricular tachycardia discriminators programmed on.[83] At 1 year of follow-up, ICD shocks occurred in only 12 patients (10.3%) in the amiodarone and β-blocker arm, 26 patients (24.3%) in the sotalol-alone arm, but in 41 patients (38.5%) of the β-blocker–only arm. Treatment with amiodarone and a β-blocker significantly reduced the risk of any shock compared with β-blocker alone (hazard ratio [HR], 0.27; 95% CI, 0.14–0.52; P<.001) or sotalol alone (HR, 0.43; 95% CI, 0.22–0.85; P = .02). A trend toward reduction in shocks was seen in the sotalol group compared with the group treated with β-blocker alone (HR, 0.61; 95% CI, 0.37–1.01; P = .055). Drug discontinuation rates were high: 18.2% for amiodarone, 23.5% for sotalol, and 5.3% for β-blocker alone. Side effects of bradycardia or adverse pulmonary or thyroid events were more common with amiodarone treatment.

Dronedarone (Class III)

A derivative of its parent compound amiodarone, dronedarone is also classified as a class III agent, but with class I, II, and IV activity. It has been studied in patients with atrial fibrillation and those with moderate to severe congestive heart failure, but not extensively in patients with ventricular arrhythmias.[84,85] In a small study, oral dronedarone was effective in reducing the rate of appropriate ICD therapies during a 30-day follow-up period.[86] This antiarrhythmic agent is now approved by the U.S. Food and Drug Administration (FDA) for patients with atrial fibrillation, and further studies would be necessary to evaluate its effectiveness in suppressing ventricular arrhythmias.

Azimilide (Class III)

Azimilide is an investigational class III agent that blocks the rapid and slow delayed rectifier potassium currents I_{Kr} and I_{Ks}, respectively. In the SHIELD (Shock Inhibition Evaluation with Azimilide) trial, oral azimilide reduced the recurrence of VT/VF terminated by ICD shocks or antitachycardia pacing in patients with ICDs compared with placebo treatment, with RR reductions of 57% ($P = .0006$) in the group treated with 75 mg, and 47% ($P = .0053$) in the group treated with 125 mg seen after 1 year of follow-up.[87] Azimilide has shown promise based on the results of this and other studies, but is not yet approved by the FDA.

RADIOFREQUENCY CATHETER ABLATION OF VENTRICULAR ARRHYTHMIAS (NONPHARMACOLOGIC TREATMENT)

Currently, no randomized, controlled trials have compared radiofrequency catheter ablation (RFCA) of VT with antiarrhythmic drugs for the acute treatment of recurrent VT or the reduction of device therapy for VT in patients with ICDs. However, two recently published randomized trials compared ICD implantation with ICD implantation plus prophylactic RFCA in the secondary prevention of ventricular arrhythmias in patients with a history of myocardial infarction. The SMASH-VT (Substrate Mapping and Ablation in Sinus Rhythm to Halt Ventricular Tachycardia) trial included patients with a history of prior myocardial infarction and spontaneous VT or VF for which an ICD was being implanted.[88] No antiarrhythmic drugs were used in this trial. Substrate-based catheter ablation led to a reduction in ICD shocks from 31% to 9% over a follow-up period of 22.5 ± 5 months ($P = .003$) and reduced VT episodes from 33% to 12% ($P = .007$). Even though substantial ablation-related complications, such as pericardial effusion, congestive heart failure exacerbation, or deep venous thrombosis, occurred in 5% of patients, the 30-day mortality rate after catheter ablation was zero.

The more recently published VTACH (Ventricular Tachycardia Ablation in Coronary Heart Disease) trial enrolled patients with a history of hemodynamically stable VT, previous myocardial infarction, and LVEF ≤50%.[89] Patients were randomized to RFCA + ICD or ICD only. At 2 years of follow-up, estimated survival free of VT or VF was 47% in the ablation group versus 29% in the

control group (HR, 0.61; 95% CI, 0.37−0.99; $P = .045$). Again, no deaths occurred at 30 days of acute follow-up post-ablation.

The results of these trials are promising; however, whether these positive findings will translate into similar results for those with VT and nonischemic cardiomyopathy, and whether this approach can be undertaken at less experienced centers, is currently unclear. RFCA currently is not recommended as a first-line therapy but should be considered in drug-resistant VT/VF or electrical storm.

ELECTRICAL STORM

Electrical storm is defined as frequent recurrences of unstable sustained VT or VF, usually two or more episodes during a 24-hour period. In patients with an ICD, this results in two or more separate device interventions.[90,91] VT rather than VF underlies most cases of electrical storm, and up to 30% of patients with secondary prevention ICDs will have electrical storm at some point after implantation.[90–94] Intravenous amiodarone can be an effective first-line treatment in those who present with electrical storm.[61,64]

One large double-blinded study enrolled 302 patients with two or more episodes of sustained VT or VF and randomized them to either intravenous amiodarone at a high (1.8 g) or low (0.2 g) dose or intravenous bretylium.[61] An approximately 50% recurrence rate was seen within the first 24 hours after drug therapy in both groups. Overall, these agents were equally effective in the intention-to-treat analysis, but significantly more patients treated with bretylium had serious adverse effects (58% vs 42%; $P = .01$).

In the SHIELD study, oral azimilide at 125 mg/d reduced the risk of recurrent electrical storm by 55% versus placebo ($P = .018$).[94] In general, the origin of electrical storm has not been elucidated, but identifiable precipitants such as ongoing ischemia, worsening congestive heart failure, proarrhythmia from antiarrhythmic drugs, and electrolyte derangements should be investigated and corrected.

SUMMARY

The acute treatment of ventricular arrhythmias will depend largely on the origin, hemodynamic stability, long-term prognosis, and associated clinical conditions. Immediate goals involve emergency resuscitation, stabilization, and cardioversion/defibrillation in states of hemodynamic instability. The possible causes of the acute arrhythmic decompensation and the precipitating and contributing factors to the development of VT or VF should be considered to identify and treat the underlying cause. Antiarrhythmic drug therapy can be essential in achieving acute stabilization of the rhythm disturbance so that further decisions can be made regarding long-term antiarrhythmic therapy and ICD implantation given the potential high risk of recurrence in secondary prevention of SCD. Adjunctive therapy with antiarrhythmic drugs has become the mainstay of treatment for individuals with recurrent episodes of ventricular arrhythmias resulting in ICD shocks.

REFERENCES

1. Bayes de Luna A, Coumel P, Leclercq JF. Ambulatory sudden cardiac death: mechanisms of production of fatal arrhythmia on the basis of data from 157 cases. Am Heart J 1989;117:151–9.

2. Myerburg RJ, Interian A Jr, Mitrani RM, et al. Frequency of sudden cardiac death and profiles of risk. Am J Cardiol 1997;80:10F–9F.

3. Myerburg RJ. Sudden cardiac death: exploring the limits of our knowledge. J Cardiovasc Electrophysiol 2001;12:369–81.

4. Priori SG, Aliot E, Blomstrom-Lundqvist C, et al. Task Force on Sudden Cardiac Death of the European Society of Cardiology. Eur Heart J 2001;22:1374–450.

5. ECC Committee, Subcommittees and Task Forces of the American Heart Association. 2005 American Heart Association guidelines for cardiopulmonary resuscitation and emergency cardiovascular care. Circulation 2005;112:IV1–203.

6. Mirowski M, Reid PR, Mower MM, et al. Termination of malignant ventricular arrhythmias with an implanted automatic defibrillator in human beings. N Engl J Med 1980;303:322–4.

7. DiMarco JP. Implantable cardioverter-defibrillators. N Engl J Med 2003;349:1836–47.

8. Reiffel JA. Drug and drug-device therapy in heart failure patients in the post-COMET and SCD-HeFT era. J Cardiovasc Pharmacol Ther 2005;10(Suppl 1):S45–58.

9. Moss AJ, Zareba W, Hall WJ, et al. Prophylactic implantation of a defibrillator in patients with myocardial infarction and reduced ejection fraction. N Engl J Med 2002;346:877–83.

10. Bardy GH, Lee KL, Mark DB, et al. Amiodarone or an implantable cardioverter-defibrillator for congestive heart failure. N Engl J Med 2005;352:225–37.

11. Van Herendael H, Pinter A, Ahmad K, et al. Role of antiarrhythmic drugs in patients with implantable cardioverter defibrillators. Europace 2010;12:618–25.

12. Patel C, Yan GX, Kocovic D, et al. Should catheter ablation be the preferred therapy for reducing ICD shocks?: ventricular tachycardia ablation versus drugs for preventing ICD shocks: role of adjuvant antiarrhythmic drug therapy. Circ Arrhythm Electrophysiol 2009;2:705–11 [discussion: 712].

13. Reiffel JA. Adjunctive therapy for recurrent ventricular tachycardia in patients with implantable cardioverter defibrillators. Curr Cardiol Rep 2007;9:381–6.

14. Rajawat YS, Patel VV, Gerstenfeld EP, et al. Advantages and pitfalls of combining device-based and pharmacologic therapies for the treatment of ventricular arrhythmias: observations from a tertiary referral center. Pacing Clin Electrophysiol 2004;27:1670–81.

15. Hartzler GO. Electrode catheter ablation of refractory focal ventricular tachycardia. J Am Coll Cardiol 1983;2:1107–13.

16. Evans GT Jr, Scheinman MM, Zipes DP, et al. Catheter ablation for control of ventricular tachycardia: a report of the percutaneous cardiac mapping and ablation registry. Pacing Clin Electrophysiol 1986;9:1391–5.

17. Gursoy S, Chiladakis I, Kuck KH. First lessons from radiofrequency catheter ablation in patients with ventricular tachycardia. Pacing Clin Electrophysiol 1993;16:687–91.

18. Morady F, Harvey M, Kalbfleisch SJ, et al. Radiofrequency catheter ablation of ventricular tachycardia in patients with coronary artery disease. Circulation 1993;87:363–72.

19. Stevenson WG, Khan H, Sager P, et al. Identification of reentry circuit sites during catheter mapping and radiofrequency ablation of ventricular tachycardia late after myocardial infarction. Circulation 1993;88:1647–70.

20. Gonska BD, Cao K, Schaumann A, et al. Catheter ablation of ventricular tachycardia in 136 patients with coronary artery disease: results and long-term follow-up. J Am Coll Cardiol 1994;24:1506–14.

21. Kim YH, Sosa-Suarez G, Trouton TG, et al. Treatment of ventricular tachycardia by transcatheter radiofrequency ablation in patients with ischemic heart disease. Circulation 1994;89:1094–102.

22. Wilber DJ, Kopp DE, Glascock DN, et al. Catheter ablation of the mitral isthmus for ventricular tachycardia associated with inferior infarction. Circulation 1995;92:3481–9.

23. Stevenson WG, Friedman PL, Kocovic D, et al. Radiofrequency catheter ablation of ventricular tachycardia after myocardial infarction. Circulation 1998;98:308–14.

24. Bogun F, Kim HM, Han J, et al. Comparison of mapping criteria for hemodynamically tolerated, postinfarction ventricular tachycardia. Heart Rhythm 2006;3:20–6.

25. de Chillou C, Lacroix D, Klug D, et al. Isthmus characteristics of reentrant ventricular tachycardia after myocardial infarction. Circulation 2002;105:726–31.

26. Marchlinski FE, Callans DJ, Gottlieb CD, et al. Linear ablation lesions for control of unmappable ventricular tachycardia in patients with ischemic and nonischemic cardiomyopathy. Circulation 2000;101: 1288–96.

27. Kuck KH. Should catheter ablation be the preferred therapy for reducing ICD shocks?: ventricular tachycardia in patients with an implantable defibrillator warrants catheter ablation. Circ Arrhythm Electrophysiol 2009;2:713–20 [discussion: 720].

28. Sharma AD, Klein G, Yee R. Intravenous adenosine triphosphate during wide complex tachycardia: safety, therapeutic efficacy, and diagnostic utility. Br Heart J 1989;62:195–203.

29. Nogami A. Idiopathic left ventricular tachycardia: assessment and treatment. Card Electrophysiol Rev 2002;6:448–57.

30. Vaughan Williams EM. Classification of antiarrhythmic drugs. In: Flensted-Jensen E, Sandfte E, Olesen KH, editors. Symposium on cardiac arrhythmias. Sodertalje (Sweden): AB Astra; 1970. p. 449–72.

31. The Sicilian gambit. A new approach to the classification of antiarrhythmic drugs based on their actions on arrhythmogenic mechanisms. Task Force of the Working Group on Arrhythmias of the European Society of Cardiology. Circulation 1991;84:1831–51.

32. Antman EM, Anbe DT, Armstrong PW, et al. ACC/AHA guidelines for the management of patients with ST-elevation myocardial infarction; a report of the American College of Cardiology/American Heart Association Task Force on Practice Guidelines (Committee to Revise the 1999 Guidelines for the Management of patients with acute myocardial infarction). J Am Coll Cardiol 2004;44:E1–211.

33. Armstrong PW, Bogaty P, Buller CE, et al. The 2004 ACC/AHA Guidelines: a perspective and adaptation for Canada by the Canadian Cardiovascular Society Working Group. Can J Cardiol 2004;20:1075–9.

34. Antman EM, Hand M, Armstrong PW, et al. 2007 Focused Update of the ACC/AHA 2004 Guidelines for the Management of Patients With ST-Elevation Myocardial Infarction: a report of the American College of Cardiology/American Heart Association Task Force on Practice Guidelines: developed in collaboration With the Canadian Cardiovascular Society endorsed by the American Academy of Family Physicians: 2007 Writing Group to Review New Evidence and Update the ACC/AHA 2004 Guidelines for the Management of Patients With ST-Elevation Myocardial Infarction, Writing on Behalf of the 2004 Writing Committee. Circulation 2008; 117:296–329.

35. Welsh RC, Travers A, Huynh T, et al. Canadian Cardiovascular Society Working Group: Providing a perspective on the 2007 focused update of the American College of Cardiology and American Heart Association 2004 guidelines for the management of ST elevation myocardial infarction. Can J Cardiol 2009;25:25–32.

36. Hennekens CH, Albert CM, Godfried SL, et al. Adjunctive drug therapy of acute myocardial infarction—evidence from clinical trials. N Engl J Med 1996;335:1660–7.

37. Teo KK, Yusuf S, Furberg CD. Effects of prophylactic antiarrhythmic drug therapy in acute myocardial infarction. An overview of results from randomized controlled trials. JAMA 1993;270:1589–95.

38. Rossi PR, Yusuf S, Ramsdale D, et al. Reduction of ventricular arrhythmias by early intravenous atenolol in suspected acute myocardial infarction. Br Med J (Clin Res Ed) 1983;286:506–10.

39. Ryden L, Ariniego R, Arnman K, et al. A double-blind trial of metoprolol in acute myocardial infarction. Effects on ventricular tachyarrhythmias. N Engl J Med 1983;308:614–8.

40. Yusuf S, Peto R, Lewis J, et al. Beta blockade during and after myocardial infarction: an overview of the randomized trials. Prog Cardiovasc Dis 1985;27: 335–71.

41. Chen ZM, Pan HC, Chen YP, et al. Early intravenous then oral metoprolol in 45,852 patients with acute myocardial infarction: randomised placebo-controlled trial. Lancet 2005;366:1622–32.

42. Norris RM, Barnaby PF, Brown MA, et al. Prevention of ventricular fibrillation during acute myocardial infarction by intravenous propranolol. Lancet 1984;2: 883–6.

43. Sadowski ZP, Alexander JH, Skrabucha B, et al. Multicenter randomized trial and a systematic overview of lidocaine in acute myocardial infarction. Am Heart J 1999;137:792–8.

44. MacMahon S, Collins R, Peto R, et al. Effects of prophylactic lidocaine in suspected acute myocardial infarction. An overview of results from the randomized, controlled trials. JAMA 1988;260: 1910–6.

45. Hine LK, Laird N, Hewitt P, et al. Meta-analytic evidence against prophylactic use of lidocaine in acute myocardial infarction. Arch Intern Med 1989; 149:2694–8.

46. Alexander JH, Granger CB, Sadowski Z, et al. Prophylactic lidocaine use in acute myocardial infarction: incidence and outcomes from two international trials. The GUSTO-I and GUSTO-IIb Investigators. Am Heart J 1999;137:799–805.

47. Echt DS, Liebson PR, Mitchell LB, et al. Mortality and morbidity in patients receiving encainide, flecainide, or placebo. The Cardiac Arrhythmia Suppression Trial. N Engl J Med 1991;324:781–8.

48. Greene HL. The CASCADE Study: randomized antiarrhythmic drug therapy in survivors of cardiac arrest in Seattle. CASCADE Investigators. Am J Cardiol 1993;72:70F–4F.

49. Mason JW. A comparison of seven antiarrhythmic drugs in patients with ventricular tachyarrhythmias. Electrophysiologic Study versus Electrocardiographic Monitoring Investigators. N Engl J Med 1993;329:452–8.

50. Garguichevich JJ, Ramos JL, Gambarte A, et al. Effect of amiodarone therapy on mortality in patients with left ventricular dysfunction and asymptomatic complex ventricular arrhythmias: Argentine Pilot Study of Sudden Death and Amiodarone (EPAMSA). Am Heart J 1995;130:494–500.

51. Burkart F, Pfisterer M, Kiowski W, et al. Effect of antiarrhythmic therapy on mortality in survivors of myocardial infarction with asymptomatic complex ventricular arrhythmias: Basel Antiarrhythmic Study of Infarct Survival (BASIS). J Am Coll Cardiol 1990; 16:1711–8.

52. Doval HC, Nul DR, Grancelli HO, et al. Randomised trial of low-dose amiodarone in severe congestive heart failure. Grupo de Estudio de la Sobrevida en la Insuficiencia Cardiaca en Argentina (GESICA). Lancet 1994;344:493–8.

53. Effect of prophylactic amiodarone on mortality after acute myocardial infarction and in congestive heart failure: meta-analysis of individual data from 6500 patients in randomised trials. Amiodarone Trials Meta-Analysis Investigators. Lancet 1997;350: 1417–24.

54. Sim I, McDonald KM, Lavori PW, et al. Quantitative overview of randomized trials of amiodarone to prevent sudden cardiac death. Circulation 1997; 96:2823–9.

55. Boutitie F, Boissel JP, Connolly SJ, et al. Amiodarone interaction with beta-blockers: analysis of the merged EMIAT (European Myocardial Infarct Amiodarone Trial) and CAMIAT (Canadian Amiodarone Myocardial Infarction Trial) databases. The EMIAT and CAMIAT Investigators. Circulation 1999;99: 2268–75.

56. Gorgels AP, van den Dool A, Hofs A, et al. Comparison of procainamide and lidocaine in terminating sustained monomorphic ventricular tachycardia. Am J Cardiol 1996;78:43–6.

57. Armengol RE, Graff J, Baerman JM, et al. Lack of effectiveness of lidocaine for sustained, wide QRS complex tachycardia. Ann Emerg Med 1989;18: 254–7.

58. Griffith MJ, Linker NJ, Garratt CJ, et al. Relative efficacy and safety of intravenous drugs for termination of sustained ventricular tachycardia. Lancet 1990; 336:670–3.

59. Ho DS, Zecchin RP, Richards DA, et al. Double-blind trial of lignocaine versus sotalol for acute termination of spontaneous sustained ventricular tachycardia. Lancet 1994;344:18–23.

60. Nasir NJ, Taylor A, Doyle TK, et al. Evaluation of intravenous lidocaine for the termination of sustained monomorphic ventricular tachycardia in patients with coronary artery disease with or without healed myocardial infarction. Am J Cardiol 1994;74: 1183–6.

61. Kowey PR, Levine JH, Herre JM, et al. Randomized, double-blind comparison of intravenous amiodarone and bretylium in the treatment of patients with recurrent, hemodynamically destabilizing ventricular tachycardia or fibrillation. The Intravenous Amiodarone Multicenter Investigators Group. Circulation 1995;92:3255–63.

62. Nademanee K, Taylor R, Bailey WE, et al. Treating electrical storm: sympathetic blockade versus advanced cardiac life support-guided therapy. Circulation 2000;102:742–7.

63. Desai AD, Chun S, Sung RJ. The role of intravenous amiodarone in the management of cardiac arrhythmias. Ann Intern Med 1997;127:294–303.

64. Scheinman MM, Levine JH, Cannom DS, et al. Dose-ranging study of intravenous amiodarone in patients with life-threatening ventricular tachyarrhythmias. The Intravenous Amiodarone Multicenter Investigators Group. Circulation 1995;92:3264–72.

65. Levine JH, Massumi A, Scheinman MM, et al. Intravenous amiodarone for recurrent sustained hypotensive ventricular tachyarrhythmias. Intravenous Amiodarone Multicenter Trial Group. J Am Coll Cardiol 1996;27:67–75.

66. Mooss AN, Mohiuddin SM, Hee TT, et al. Efficacy and tolerance of high-dose intravenous amiodarone for recurrent, refractory ventricular tachycardia. Am J Cardiol 1990;65:609–14.

67. Carmeliet E. Voltage- and time-dependent block of the delayed K+ current in cardiac myocytes by dofetilide. J Pharmacol Exp Ther 1992;262:809–17.

68. Boriani G, Lubinski A, Capucci A, et al. A multicentre, double-blind randomized crossover comparative study on the efficacy and safety of dofetilide vs sotalol in patients with inducible sustained ventricular tachycardia and ischaemic heart disease. Eur Heart J 2001;22:2180–91.

69. Haynes RE, Chinn TL, Copass MK, et al. Comparison of bretylium tosylate and lidocaine in management of out of hospital ventricular fibrillation: a randomized clinical trial. Am J Cardiol 1981;48:353–6.

70. Olson DW, Thompson BM, Darin JC, et al. A randomized comparison study of bretylium tosylate and lidocaine in resuscitation of patients from out-of-hospital ventricular fibrillation in a paramedic system. Ann Emerg Med 1984;13:807–10.

71. Kudenchuk PJ, Cobb LA, Copass MK, et al. Amiodarone for resuscitation after out-of-hospital cardiac arrest due to ventricular fibrillation. N Engl J Med 1999;341:871–8.

72. Tzivoni D, Banai S, Schuger C, et al. Treatment of torsade de pointes with magnesium sulfate. Circulation 1988;77:392–7.

73. Ahmad K, Dorian P. Drug-induced QT prolongation and proarrhythmia: an inevitable link? Europace 2007;9(Suppl 4):iv16–22.

74. Connolly SJ, Hallstrom AP, Cappato R, et al. Meta-analysis of the implantable cardioverter defibrillator secondary prevention trials. AVID, CASH and CIDS studies. Antiarrhythmics vs Implantable Defibrillator study. Cardiac Arrest Study Hamburg. Canadian Implantable Defibrillator Study. Eur Heart J 2000; 21:2071–8.

75. Bokhari F, Newman D, Greene M, et al. Long-term comparison of the implantable cardioverter defibrillator versus amiodarone: eleven-year follow-up of a subset of patients in the Canadian Implantable Defibrillator Study (CIDS). Circulation 2004;110: 112–6.

76. Lee KL, Hafley G, Fisher JD, et al. Effect of implantable defibrillators on arrhythmic events and mortality in the multicenter unsustained tachycardia trial. Circulation 2002;106:233–8.

77. Steinberg JS, Martins J, Sadanandan S, et al. Antiarrhythmic drug use in the implantable defibrillator arm of the Antiarrhythmics Versus Implantable Defibrillators (AVID) Study. Am Heart J 2001;142:520–9.

78. Gradaus R, Block M, Brachmann J, et al. Mortality, morbidity, and complications in 3344 patients with implantable cardioverter defibrillators: results from the German ICD Registry EURID. Pacing Clin Electrophysiol 2003;26:1511–8.

79. Poole JE, Johnson GW, Hellkamp AS, et al. Prognostic importance of defibrillator shocks in patients with heart failure. N Engl J Med 2008;359:1009–17.

80. The Cardiac Insufficiency Bisoprolol Study II (CIBIS-II): a randomised trial. Lancet 1999;353:9–13.

81. Pacifico A, Hohnloser SH, Williams JH, et al. Prevention of implantable-defibrillator shocks by treatment with sotalol. d, l-Sotalol Implantable Cardioverter-Defibrillator Study Group. N Engl J Med 1999;340: 1855–62.

82. Kuhlkamp V, Mewis C, Mermi J, et al. Suppression of sustained ventricular tachyarrhythmias: a comparison of d, l-sotalol with no antiarrhythmic drug treatment. J Am Coll Cardiol 1999;33:46–52.

83. Connolly SJ, Dorian P, Roberts RS, et al. Comparison of beta-blockers, amiodarone plus beta-blockers, or sotalol for prevention of shocks from implantable cardioverter defibrillators: the OPTIC Study: a randomized trial. JAMA 2006;295:165–71.

84. Hohnloser SH, Crijns HJ, van Eickels M, et al. Effect of dronedarone on cardiovascular events in atrial fibrillation. N Engl J Med 2009;360:668–78.

85. Kober L, Torp-Pedersen C, McMurray JJ, et al. Increased mortality after dronedarone therapy for severe heart failure. N Engl J Med 2008;358: 2678–87.

86. Kowey PR, Singh BN. Late breaking clinical trials oral presentation: dronedarone in patients with implantable defibrillators. Heart Rhythm Society Scientific Sessions 2004 [abstract chair]. San Francisco (CA): Heart Rhythm; 2004.

87. Dorian P, Borggrefe M, Al-Khalidi HR, et al. Placebo-controlled, randomized clinical trial of azimilide for prevention of ventricular tachyarrhythmias in patients with an implantable cardioverter defibrillator. Circulation 2004;110:3646–54.

88. Reddy VY, Reynolds MR, Neuzil P, et al. Prophylactic catheter ablation for the prevention of defibrillator therapy. N Engl J Med 2007;357:2657–65.

89. Kuck KH, Schaumann A, Eckardt L, et al. Catheter ablation of stable ventricular tachycardia before defibrillator implantation in patients with coronary heart disease (VTACH): a multicentre randomised controlled trial. Lancet 2007;375:31–40.

90. Credner SC, Klingenheben T, Mauss O, et al. Electrical storm in patients with transvenous implantable cardioverter-defibrillators: incidence, management and prognostic implications. J Am Coll Cardiol 1998;32:1909–15.

91. Exner DV, Pinski SL, Wyse DG, et al. Electrical storm presages nonsudden death: the antiarrhythmics versus implantable defibrillators (AVID) trial. Circulation 2001;103:2066–71.

92. Villacastin J, Almendral J, Arenal A, et al. Incidence and clinical significance of multiple consecutive, appropriate, high-energy discharges in patients with implanted cardioverter-defibrillators. Circulation 1996;93:753–62.

93. Greene M, Newman D, Geist M, et al. Is electrical storm in ICD patients the sign of a dying heart? Outcome of patients with clusters of ventricular tachyarrhythmias. Europace 2000;2:263–9.

94. Hohnloser SH, Al-Khalidi HR, Pratt CM, et al. Electrical storm in patients with an implantable defibrillator: incidence, features, and preventive therapy: insights from a randomized trial. Eur Heart J 2006;27: 3027–32.

Chronic Suppression of Ventricular Tachyarrhythmias in Patients with ICDs

Michael S. Zawaneh, MD[a,b], Bruce S. Stambler, MD[c],*

KEYWORDS

- Antiarrhythmic drug • Ventricular tachycardia
- Ventricular fibrillation • Implantable cardioverter-defibrillator
- ICD shock

Ventricular arrhythmias, ranging from asymptomatic ventricular premature beats to sustained ventricular tachycardia (VT) or ventricular fibrillation (VF), are common in patients with heart failure. VT and VF are the most common causes of sudden cardiac death (SCD). SCD accounts for up to two-thirds of all deaths in patients with heart failure.[1]

Implantable cardioverter-defibrillators (ICDs) effectively terminate VT or VF with a success rate close to 100%.[2] This high antiarrhythmic effectiveness, combined with low ICD-associated morbidity and mortality, renders ICD therapy the treatment of choice and the dominant therapy for improving survival in patients who have suffered a cardiac arrest or symptomatic sustained VT. Three major randomized clinical trials (Cardiac Arrest Study Hamburg [CASH], Canadian Implantable Defibrillator Study [CIDS], and Antiarrhythmics versus Implantable Defibrillators [AVID]) and several meta-analyses comparing ICD to pharmacologic therapy in survivors of SCD or patients with sustained VT demonstrated a significant reduction in mortality with ICD therapy.[3–7] A clear role for ICD implantation in the primary prevention of SCD in patients with heart failure and both ischemic and nonischemic cardiomyopathy also has been established by multiple randomized clinical trials in high-risk patients, including

Multicenter Automatic Defibrillator Implantation Trial (MADIT), Multicenter UnSustained Tachycardia Trial, MADIT-II, and Sudden Cardiac Death in Heart Failure Trial (SCD-HeFT). The current indications for ICD implantation are derived from inclusion criteria of these major clinical trials.[8–11]

The trials cited in the preceding paragraph demonstrated that ICD therapy is superior to antiarrhythmic drugs (AADs) in reducing mortality among SCD survivors.[3–7] Randomized clinical trials do not support the use of prophylactic, Vaughan Williams class I or III AAD therapy in place of the ICD for primary prevention of SCD in high-risk patients.[8–11] Moreover, use of AAD therapy (except for beta-blockers) has never been conclusively demonstrated to result in a reduction in SCD or all-cause mortality. This lack of benefit is thought, at least in part, to be attributable to incomplete suppression of ventricular arrhythmias, risk of proarrhythmia, and/or negative inotropic properties of AADs.[12–15]

Despite the superiority of ICD therapy, this device is not without its limitations. Patients most commonly treated with ICDs are patients with significant left ventricular (LV) dysfunction and heart failure. This group of patients is at substantially increased risk for developing recurrent atrial and ventricular tachyarrhythmias. This increased risk of tachyarrhythmias frequently will result in

[a] Department of Cardiovascular Medicine, Cleveland Clinic, Cleveland, OH 44195, USA
[b] Arizona Arrhythmia Consultants, 7283 East Earll Road, Scottsdale, AZ 85251, USA
[c] Division of Cardiology, Cardiac Electrophysiology, University Hospitals Case Medical Center, Case Western Reserve University, 11100 Euclid Avenue, Cleveland, OH 44106, USA
* Corresponding author.
E-mail address: bss4@cwru.edu

Card Electrophysiol Clin 2 (2010) 443–457
doi:10.1016/j.ccep.2010.06.008

an increased risk for ICD shocks. In the SCD-HeFT, the occurrence of shocks (both appropriate and inappropriate) was associated with a markedly increased risk of death, mainly because of progressive heart failure.[16] Whether ICD shocks possibly increase risk of death or simply are a marker of increased risk of death remains uncertain.

ICD shocks are uncomfortable, create significant psychological stress, and diminish quality of life. Virtually all studies have consistently demonstrated a significant decrease in the quality of life of patients with ICDs receiving shocks (both appropriate and inappropriate) compared with those who do not.[17–20] Fear of being shocked is an almost universal experience among patients with ICDs and can lead to avoidance behaviors, limitation of activities of daily living, and inability to exercise.[17] ICD shocks often trigger the need for recurrent hospitalizations and increased health care costs and use. In both primary and secondary prevention trials of ICD therapy, patients who received an ICD were more likely to require hospital readmissions than those initially treated with AADs. In AVID, 60% of patients in the ICD group were rehospitalized by 1 year and patients with ICDs were rehospitalized sooner than those treated with AADs.[21] The primary indication for rehospitalization was for recurrent arrhythmias and defibrillator shocks. In the European Registry of Implantable Defibrillators observational German ICD registry, 1691 hospital readmissions were required among 3344 patients and more than 60% of admissions were for ventricular arrhythmias.[22] Antitachycardia pacing (ATP) is capable of terminating some episodes of VT painlessly and reducing the burden of painful and potentially harmful ICD shocks, but ATP does not always eliminate shocks. If shocks are repetitive or frequent, premature ICD battery depletion can result.

In this review, we examine the data evaluating the role of adjuvant AAD therapy in chronic suppression of ventricular tachyarrhythmias in the patient with an ICD. It must be noted that all uses of AADs for this indication represent "off-label" prescription. No AAD is approved by the Food and Drug Administration (FDA) specifically as a therapy to reduce ICD shocks.

THE POTENTIAL ROLE OF ADJUVANT ANTIARRHYTHMIC DRUG THERAPY IN THE PATIENT WITH AN ICD

These aforementioned reasons maintain an important role for adjuvant pharmacologic therapy to suppress ICD therapies (**Box 1**). AADs are administered to suppress both atrial and ventricular

---

Box 1
Potential Benefits of Adjuvant Antiarrhythmic Drug Therapy in a Patient with an ICD

- Decreasing incidence of appropriate ICD shocks attributable to suppression of VT and VF
- Decreasing incidence of inappropriate ICD shocks attributable to reduced frequency and improved ventricular rate control of supraventricular tachyarrhythmias
- Preventing electrical storm
- Slowing ventricular tachycardia rate to improve hemodynamic tolerance
- Improving symptomatic status from arrhythmias and shocks
- Improving quality of life
- Lowering defibrillation thresholds
- Enhancing ATP efficacy
- Prolonging ICD battery life
- Reducing hospitalization and emergency room visits
- Preventing sudden cardiac death
- Improving mortality

---

tachyarrhythmias in a patient with an ICD to subsequently reduce the frequency of both appropriate ICD shocks for ventricular arrhythmias and inappropriate shocks for supraventricular arrhythmias.[23,24] Prevention of supraventricular arrhythmias with drug therapy also may reduce the burden and frequency of ventricular tachyarrhythmias and shocks in a patient with an ICD. Interestingly at least one retrospective study has suggested that in up to 10% of cases, VT or VF is preceded by an episode of supraventricular tachycardia.[25] Beyond prevention of frequent ICD therapies (shocks and ATP), the potential additional clinical benefits of prophylactic AAD therapy in a patient with an ICD might include improving symptomatic status and quality of life, slowing the rate of VT thereby making the arrhythmia better tolerated hemodynamically, lowering of defibrillation thresholds (DFTs), enhancing the efficacy of ATP, reducing need for rehospitalization, and possibly preventing SCD and improving overall survival.

It is estimated that at least 30% of patients who receive an ICD are also treated with a class I or III AAD at some point during follow-up.[21,22,26] In the AVID trial, 26% of patients randomized to the ICD arm required AADs after 2 years of follow-up.[21] In the MADIT-II, 16% of patients in the ICD arm received treatment with AADs at last follow-up (average 20 months).[26] The apparently more frequent use of AADs in the AVID versus the MADIT-II populations is consistent with the notion that patients who undergo ICD implantation for secondary prevention are at considerably higher risk of ICD shocks than patients who undergo ICD implantation for primary prevention. Furthermore, secondary prevention ICD recipients who have VT as their presenting arrhythmia are more likely to receive appropriate ICD therapy than those who undergo ICD implantation after an episode of VF (76% vs 47% during 3 years of follow-up in AVID).[27] Likewise in another prospective study, the relative risk for ICD therapy in patients presenting with sustained monomorphic VT versus cardiac arrest was 2.57 (range, 1.32 to 5.01). In addition, in the study by Freedberg and colleagues,[28] patients with a left ventricular ejection fraction less than 25% were at almost twofold increased risk for a first ICD therapy (ATP or shock).[29] Furthermore, if AAD therapy was not changed or initiated after a first ICD therapy, 80% of patients received additional ICD therapy within 1 year. Subsequent device therapy (ATP and shock) occurred sooner (66 ± 93 days for second therapy compared with 138 ± 168 days for first therapy) and was unpredictable.

Thus, concomitant use of AAD therapy in a patient with an ICD, especially in those who experience frequent shocks or potentially in those who are identified at implantation as being at high risk of receiving ICD shocks, makes intuitive sense and is a common clinical practice. Unfortunately, however, the relative risks versus benefits of adjunctive AAD therapy in patients who have an ICD have been evaluated prospectively in only a few randomized, clinical trials. Many questions in this regard remain unanswered, including when AADs should be started in a patient with an ICD (routinely as prophylactic therapy to prevent ICD shocks or only after ICD therapies occur to prevent future events); which drug should be used first; when catheter ablation should be considered (before or after AADs fail); and should AADs be continued or stopped after successful catheter ablation in a patient with an ICD? It must be appreciated that use of this type of adjunct pharmacologic therapy exposes the patient to potential drug-related side effects and adverse drug–device interactions (**Box 2**). AADs could interact with the ICD in ways that might be potentially harmful such as producing AAD side effects, including proarrhythmia (especially torsades de pointes [TdP]); making monomorphic VTs more easily provoked or incessant; prolonging VT cycle length below the ICD rate cutoff, making ventricular tachyarrhythmias undetected and untreated; interfering with proper ICD sensing function by decreasing the amplitude or prolonging the duration of sensed electrograms; elevating DFTs; slowing the heart rate or impairing

---

Box 2
Potential Adverse Effects of Adjuvant Antiarrhythmic Drug Therapy in a Patient with an ICD

- Producing antiarrhythmic drug side effects, toxicities, and adverse events
- Provoking ventricular proarrhythmia including torsades de pointes
- Making monomorphic VTs more easily provoked or incessant
- Slowing ventricular tachycardia rate below the ICD rate cutoff making ventricular tachyarrhythmias undetected and untreated
- Interfering with ICD sensing function by decreasing the amplitude or prolonging the duration of sensed electrograms
- Slowing sinus rate or ventricular rate during atrial fibrillation
- Elevating defibrillation thresholds
- Elevating pacing thresholds
- Impairing atrioventricular conduction, thereby increasing frequency and cumulative percentage of right ventricular pacing
- Impairing myocardial contractility
- Increasing hospitalization and emergency room visits for drug initiation or toxicities
- Increasing mortality

---

atrioventricular conduction thereby increasing the frequency and cumulative percentage of right ventricular pacing; and elevating pacing thresholds. Furthermore, AADs can impair myocardial contractility, may cause extracardiac side effects and toxicities, and potentially may increase mortality. In a long-term, follow-up observational study of 1382 patients who received ICDs at a single institution from 1980 to 2003, AAD use at the time of ICD implantation was independently associated with increased mortality.[29]

CLINICAL TRIALS EVALUATING THE ROLE OF ADJUNCTIVE ANTIARRHYTHMIC DRUG THERAPY IN THE PATIENT WITH AN ICD

In this section, we examine the clinical trials that have assessed the efficacy and safety of adjunctive AADs for preventing ICD therapies. We focus on class III AADs and discuss use of sotalol, dofetilide, amiodarone, and azimilide, as the randomized trials designed to guide therapy with AADs in patients with ICDs have evaluated these specific AADs. The role of conventional beta-blockers (class II) for VT/VF suppression is not discussed in detail because beta-blocker therapy has an established role and should be used at appropriate doses in patients with an ICD for heart failure or cardioprotection after myocardial infarction.

Sotalol

Sotalol, a class III AAD, consists of a racemic mixture of d and I isomers in an approximate 1:1 ratio. The d isomer prolongs repolarization by blocking the rapid component of the delayed rectifier potassium channel (IKr). The I isomer prolongs repolarization and has beta-blocking activity (class II effect), which is dose-dependent. The beta-blocker component is not cardio-selective and is not associated with membrane-stabilizing activity or intrinsic sympathomimetic activity.[30–32] Sotalol is renally excreted and dosing needs to be adjusted in patients with impaired renal function.

Sotalol therapy for VT and VF is primarily considered for use in the current era as adjunctive therapy to an ICD to reduce the frequency of appropriate or inappropriate shocks. The role for sotalol in suppression of ventricular tacharrhythmias in patients with ICDs has been examined in 3 prospective, randomized, placebo-controlled studies.

In the study by Pacifico and colleagues,[33] 302 patients who received ICDs for documented ventricular arrhythmias were randomized to receive either d,I-sotalol (160–320 mg/d) or placebo. Treatment with sotalol was associated with a 48% reduction in the composite end point of time to first ICD shock or death compared with placebo during 1 year of follow-up (P<.001). Thirty-four percent of patients in the sotalol group and 54% of patients in the placebo group met the primary end point. Sotalol was effective in reducing frequency of both appropriate and inappropriate shocks. Shock frequency was reduced from 3.9 ± 10.6 per year to 1.4 ± 3.5 per year with sotalol (P = .008). The impressive benefit of sotalol in this study, however, must be interpreted in the context of the suboptimal treatment with conventional beta-blockers in the study population. Only 28% and 37% of patients in the placebo arm were receiving beta-blockers at the start and end of the study, respectively.

The finding that sotalol reduces recurrences of sustained ventricular arrhythmias in patients with ICDs also was demonstrated in a smaller study by Kuhlkamp and colleagues.[34] Ninety-three patients with an ICD who had ventricular arrhythmia inducibility during programmed stimulation were randomized to long-term d,I-sotalol or no antiarrhythmic therapy. The 46 patients who received sotalol had significantly fewer arrhythmia recurrences (33% vs 53%) than the 47 patients who received no antiarrhythmic (P = .023).

The randomized controlled Optimal Pharmacologic Therapy in Cardioverter Defibrillator Patients (OPTIC) trial examined the frequency of ICD shock therapy in 412 patients with ICDs for inducible or spontaneously occurring VT or VF.[35] Patients were randomized to 1 of 3 treatment arms: amiodarone (200 mg) plus beta blocker, sotalol alone (240 mg, adjusted for renal function), or beta-blocker alone (bisoprolol 10 mg or equivalent). ICDs were optimally programmed to avoid shocks (ATP up to a rate of 222 beats/min; SVT discriminators enabled), yet the risk of an ICD shock during follow-up remained high in the control group given beta-blocker alone.

Fig. 1 shows the cumulative risk of a shock for the 3 different treatment groups in the OPTIC study. During 1 year of follow-up, shocks (appropriate and inappropriate) occurred in 41 patients (38.5%) assigned to beta-blocker alone, 26 (24.3%) assigned to sotalol alone, and 12 (10.3%) assigned to amiodarone plus beta-blocker. There was a nonsignificant trend for sotalol to reduce risk of shocks compared with beta-blocker therapy alone (hazard ratio [HR], 0.61; 95% confidence interval [CI], 0.37–1.01; log-rank P = .055). Amiodarone plus beta-blocker was more effective than sotalol in reducing the risk of an ICD shock (HR, 0.43; 95% CI, 0.22–0.85; log-rank P = .02). As summarized in Table 1, these findings also were found for appropriate (for VT or VF) as well as inappropriate shocks (for atrial fibrillation, atrial flutter, and SVT). Thus, in OPTIC, sotalol was inferior to amiodarone and was not significantly better than a conventional beta-blocker in preventing ICD shocks. Furthermore, sotalol therapy had the highest discontinuation rates among the 3 adjuvant drug therapies tested. Kaplan-Meier estimates of rates of drug discontinuation at 1 year were 18.2% for amiodarone, 23.5% for sotalol, and 5.3% for beta-blocker alone.

The finding that sotalol is no better than a conventional beta-blocker in reducing ICD shocks likewise was demonstrated in at least 2 other studies in patients with ICDs, both of which used metoprolol as the control group.[36,37] Similarly, a systematic review of adjunctive AAD therapy in patients with ICDs found that the risk of shocks was reduced when comparing sotalol with placebo (HR 0.55; 95% CI 0.4–0.78), but sotalol's efficacy was not conclusive when comparing it with other beta-blockers (HR 0.61; 95% CI 0.37–1.00).[38]

An observational study in ICD recipients with arrhythmogenic right ventricular cardiomyopathy/dysplasia (ARVC/D) evaluated the efficacy of empiric AAD therapy on the subsequent occurrence of VT/VF.[39] Interestingly, similar to the OPTIC study, but in a different patient population, empiric sotalol therapy (median dose, 240 mg) did not improve VT/VF outcomes during follow-up,

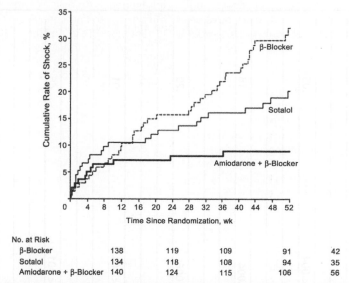

Fig. 1. Cumulative risk of a shock for the 3 treatment groups by time since randomization in the OPTIC study. Amiodarone plus beta-blocker significantly reduced the risk of shock compared with beta-blocker alone (HR, 0.27; *P* < .001) and sotalol (HR, 0.43; *P* = .02). (*Reproduced from* Connolly SJ, Dorian P, Roberts RS, et al. Comparison of beta-blockers, amiodarone plus beta-blockers, or sotalol for prevention of shocks from implantable cardioverter defibrillators: the OPTIC Study: a randomized trial. JAMA 2006;295(2):165–71; with permission.)

whereas amiodarone significantly decreased follow-up VT/VF. Also of note, in the population of patients with ARVC/D who had an ICD, standard beta-blockers neither increased nor decreased follow-up VT/VF.

The dose of sotalol is an important determinant of its efficacy and safety and is likely a confounding factor that may partly explain the variability of its antiarrhythmic efficacy. A relatively high dose of sotalol is required to achieve the class III drug effect. As in the OPTIC study and ARVC/D registry, the most commonly prescribed dosage of sotalol in clinical practice is 240 mg/d in patients with preserved renal function, but the dosage typically ranges from 160 to 320 mg/d. However, these dosages may be insufficient in their antiarrhythmic efficacy, as the successful experience with sotalol often involves dosages of 320 to 480 mg/d and up to 640 mg/d in some cases. The use of sotalol at optimal, therapeutic dosages, however, is frequently limited because of side effects, especially fatigue, as well as excessive QT prolongation. Furthermore, ICD patients usually are already receiving appropriate beta-blocker therapy. Sotalol has significant beta-blocking activity and excessive adrenergic blockade may result in hypotension, bradycardia, and increased RV pacing, which can in turn lead to hemodynamic compromise in patients with heart failure. Avoiding the consequent hemodynamic side effects of these agents often calls for decreasing the recommended effective dosage of sotalol.

Dofetilide

Dofetilide is a pure class III AAD that selectively blocks IKr. Blocking IKr prolongs action potential duration, effective refractory period, and QT interval in a dose-dependent manner. This is responsible for the drug's antiarrhythmic effect as well as its increased risk of TdP. Dofetilide administration requires in-hospital initiation and loading, potentially allowing early detection of TdP and dose adjustment based on QTc interval and creatinine clearance.[40] In contrast with d,l-sotalol, dofetilide does not have beta-blocking properties. This may be a clinical advantage of dofetilide over sotalol, allowing attainment of class III antiarrhythmic actions without troublesome beta-blocker side effects (eg, excessive bradycardia, fatigue, hypotension). A concomitantly administered beta-blocker can be given safely along with dofetilide and the beta-blocker dosage can be titrated on an individualized basis. Dofetilide currently is available only in North America.

Although the FDA has approved the use of dofetilide only in atrial fibrillation and atrial flutter, this drug may have a role in the suppression of VT and VF. A double-blind, randomized crossover trial in patients with coronary artery disease and sustained VT in the pre-ICD era showed similar efficacy for oral dofetilide and sotalol in preventing ventricular arrhythmia recurrence and arrhythmic death during 1 year of follow-up.[41] Dofetilide was better tolerated than sotalol.

Table 1
Outcome events of the 3 treatment groups in the Optimal Pharmacologic Therapy in Cardioverter Defibrillator Patients (OPTIC) study

Outcome	β-Blocker (n = 138)	Amiodarone + β-Blocker (n = 140)	Sotalol (n = 134)	P Value	
				Amiodarone + β-Blocker versus β-Blocker	Sotalol versus β-Blocker
Any shock					
No. of events	41	12	26		
Annual event rate, %	38.5	10.3	24.3		
HR (95% CI)	1.00	0.27 (0.14–0.52)	0.61 (0.37–1.01)	<.004	.055
Appropriate shock					
No. of events	25	8	17		
Annual event rate, %	22.0	6.7	15.1		
HR (95% CI)	1.00	0.30 (0.14–0.68)	0.65 (0.36–1.24)	.004	.18
Inappropriate shock					
No. of events	18	4	11		
Annual event rate, %	15.4	3.3	9.4		
HR (95% CI)	1.00	0.22 (0.07–0.64)	0.61 (0.29–1.30)	.006	.20
Any shock, censoring first 21 d					
No. of events	41	8	23		
Annual event rate, %	33.2	6.6	20.8		
HR (95% CI)	1.00	0.18 (0.08–0.37)	0.52 (0.31–0.88)	<.001	.01
Appropriate shock or ATP					
No. of events	45	15	38		
Annual event rate, %	45.0	13.0	38.9		
Hr (95% CI)	1.00	0.30 (0.17–0.53)	0.85 (0.55–1.31)	<.001	.46
Appropriate shock or arrhythmic death					
No. of events	25	9	18		
Annual event rate, %	22.0	7.5	16.0		
HR (95% CI)	1.00	0.34 (0.16–0.74)	0.69 (0.37–1.28)	.006	.24

Shown are observed annual event rates and treatment effects (relative to beta-blockers) for the primary outcome of first occurrence of any shock delivered by the ICD and secondary outcomes including appropriate and inappropriate shocks, appropriate shock or ATP, and appropriate shock or arrhythmic death. Both appropriate and inappropriate shocks were significantly reduced by amiodarone plus beta-blocker but not significantly reduced by sotalol.

Abbreviations: ATP, antitachycardia pacing therapy; CI, confidence Interval; HR, hazard ratio.

Data from Connolly SJ, Dorian P, Roberts RS, et al. Comparison of beta-blockers, amiodarone plus beta-blockers, or sotalol for prevention of shocks from implantable cardioverter defibrillators: the OPTIC Study: a randomized trial. JAMA 2006;295(2):165–71.

Virtually all the published information available regarding the efficacy of dofetilide as adjuvant therapy in patients with ICDs comes from a single, small-size study published only as an abstract by O'Toole and colleagues.[42] Oral dofetilide (500 μg twice daily) was evaluated in patients with ICDs in a randomized, placebo-controlled trial. In this study, dofetilide (n = 87) did not change the incidence of ICD shocks for VT or VF compared with placebo (n = 87) and there was no effect on the time to first ICD intervention (ATP or shock) for VT or VF with dofetilide. Treatment with dofetilide tended to prolong the median time to all-cause shock (290 vs 83 days, $P = .07$).

An analysis of ICD electrograms from dofetilide- and placebo-treated patients in the O'Toole and colleagues'[42] study was performed by Mazur and colleagues.[43] The incidence and cycle length of monomorphic VT occurring during follow-up was similar in the dofetilide and placebo groups. However, interestingly, therapy with dofetilide was associated with significantly higher ATP efficacy: ATP successfully terminated 97 of 98 (99%) episodes of monomorphic VT in the dofetilide group compared with 116 of 127 (91%) in the placebo group ($P<.02$).

Mazur and colleagues[43] also demonstrated a worrisome incidence of TdP during long-term therapy with dofetilide, occurring both early and late after drug initiation in the ICD population. The incidence of pause-dependent polymorphic VT or TdP was significantly higher with dofetilide than placebo (17% vs 6%). Of the 15 events on dofetilide therapy, 5 occurred early (<3 days on therapy); however, 10 were late events and occurred after 3 days or longer on dofetilide. Of the patients with late events, the median time on therapy was 22 days (range, 6 to 107 days) for dofetilide-treated patients. A case report also has been published of late dofetilide-associated ventricular proarrhythmia occurring 6 months after drug initiation for atrial fibrillation in a patient with an ICD.[44]

In summary, definitive conclusions regarding the utility of dofetilide for suppression of VT/VF in the ICD population cannot be made because of lack of available data. Dofetilide may have potential advantages over other AADs, such as sotalol and amiodarone, including the ability to individually titrate beta-blocker dose, lack of extracardiac toxicity and side effects, and neutral mortality effect in patients with heart failure. On the other hand, the risk of TdP with this drug even in ICD patients is concerning, availability of this drug worldwide is limited and in-patient initiation of this drug is required.

Amiodarone

Amiodarone is thought by many to be the most effective AAD. Initially evaluated in the 1960s as an antianginal agent, it was later discovered to have antiarrhythmic properties. Amiodarone has little negative inotropic activity and a low rate of proarrhythmia.[45] Oral amiodarone is classified as a class III AAD, but mechanistically combines antiarrhythmic properties from Vaughan Williams classes I, II, III, and IV.[46,47] It prolongs action potential duration (phase 3) and refractory period of both atrial and ventricular tissue by blockade of IKr. Although amiodarone prolongs the QT interval, in contrast with other class III agents it has a very low potential to cause TdP. The activity of amiodarone on myocardial tissue is not limited to IKr blockade. It affects multiple channels and receptors. Amiodarone binds to and inhibits inactivated (phase 0) sodium channels in a use-dependent fashion. It inhibits sympathetic activity via noncompetitive beta receptor blockade and also blocks L-type (slow) calcium channels.

Although clinical experience with amiodarone for ventricular arrhythmias is extensive, the evidence to support its use for this indication is sparse, especially in the patient with an ICD. Most data examining the role of amiodarone in patients with ICDs are observational and nonrandomized. In the AVID trial, amiodarone was the most common AAD used in patients with ICDs. After addition of AADs, there were 1.4 ± 3.7 fewer ICD therapies and time to first ICD therapy was extended from 4 to 11 months.[21]

Two older studies investigated the role of AAD therapy in patients with ICDs implanted for VT/VF. In both studies, the most commonly used antiarrhythmic therapy was amiodarone. In the first, by Kou and colleagues,[48] 74 patients were either treated with an AAD (n = 33) or not (n = 41). There was no significant difference between both groups in the number of patients who experienced at least one ICD shock. Time to first appropriate shock in both groups was 5 ± 5 months. In another study by Anderson and colleagues,[49] 34 patients were randomized to either AAD therapy (n = 17) or no therapy (n = 17). The number of patients who had a first event as well as time to first event did not differ between groups.

As discussed previously, the OPTIC study examined the frequency of ICD shock therapy in patients randomized to treatment with oral amiodarone plus beta-blocker, sotalol alone, or beta-blocker alone.[35] Amiodarone plus beta-blocker significantly reduced the risk of shock compared with beta-blocker alone (HR, 0.27; 95% CI, 0.14–0.52; $P<.001$) and sotalol (HR, 0.43; 95% CI, 0.22–0.85;

$P = .02$) (see **Fig. 1**). As summarized in **Table 1**, the beneficial effects of amiodarone over the other 2 adjunctive agents were also demonstrated for prevention of appropriate shocks as well as inappropriate shocks.

The OPTIC study also examined the incidence of adverse outcomes associated with use of the 3 adjunctive ICD therapies.[38] As detailed in **Table 2**, there were no differences in rates of death, arrhythmic death, heart failure, or myocardial infarction between treatment groups. However, there were higher rates of adverse thyroid and pulmonary effects and symptomatic bradycardia during amiodarone plus beta-blocker treatment. There were no cases of TdP identified in any patient in the study.

A systematic review of adjunctive AAD therapy in patients with ICDs concluded that there is clearly a beneficial effect of amiodarone (in contrast to other AADs in which the data were inconclusive) in reducing the risk of overall ICD shock therapies, risk of appropriate ICD shocks, and antitachycardia pacing therapies.[38] However, this conclusion regarding amiodarone was entirely based on the results of the only available randomized trial in this patient population (ie, OPTIC).

Despite its overall efficacy, it is difficult to recommend oral amiodarone as first-line therapy to be used routinely for chronic suppression of VT/VF in patients with ICDs because of its poor tolerability and risk of extracardiac toxicity. However, because of the lack of availability of other suitable, efficacious, and safe AADs to prevent recurrent ICD shocks, especially in patients with heart failure and advanced structural heart disease, amiodarone often becomes in reality the agent of choice after optimized beta-blocker therapy does not work or cannot be tolerated. For ventricular arrhythmias, amiodarone usually is initiated at a higher dosage, from 300 to 600 mg/d, but attempts should be made to reduce the dosage to 200 mg/d once the arrhythmia stabilizes over several months of follow-up.

Intravenous amiodarone along with beta-blockade has an important role in stabilizing the patient who experiences electrical storm. Electrical storm constitutes a medical emergency and almost always requires hospitalization. In the patient with an ICD, it is defined as recurrent VT or VF resulting in 3 or more separate device interventions during a single 24-hour period.[50] A combination of intravenous (IV) beta-blocker and amiodarone (bolus of 150–300 mg/1 hour and 1–1.2 g/24 hours) can be highly effective in preventing frequent ICD shocks even in those chronically receiving beta-blockers or amiodarone.

Azimilide

Azimilide is a novel nonselective class III antiarrhythmic agent. Its mechanism of action consists of blocking both rapid and slow components of the delayed rectifier cardiac potassium channels (IKr and IKs), which prolongs action potential and refractory periods. These unique blocking properties of both components rather than just the rapid component of the delayed rectifier potassium current are believed to contribute to the lower incidence of TdP with this agent as compared with selective IKr blockers.[51,52] Azimilide has no known effect on cardiac hemodynamics. It has been shown to be effective and generally well tolerated in patients with supraventricular arrhythmia.[53,54]

The first trial to investigate the role of azimilide in reducing ventricular arrhythmias randomized 172 patients with ICDs to treatment with placebo or oral azimilide (35 mg, 75 mg, or 125 mg) in a dose-ranging pilot study.[55] Sixty-two percent of patients enrolled had an LV ejection fraction less than 35% and most had class II or III heart failure. At a mean follow-up of 257 ± 158 days, the frequency of appropriate ICD therapies (shocks and ATPs) was significantly lower among azimilide-treated compared with placebo-treated patients. The incidence of ICD therapies per patient-year in the placebo group was 36% compared with 10%, 12%, and 9% among 35 mg, 75 mg, and 125 mg azimilide-treated patients, respectively (HR = 0.31, $P = .0001$). There was no significant difference in adverse events, deaths, or episodes of TdP in the azimilide-treated group when compared with placebo.

The largest clinical trial of azimilide in patients with ICDs conducted to date was the Shock Inhibition Evaluation with Azimilide (SHIELD) trial.[56] A total of 633 patients with ICDs were enrolled in a randomized, double-blind, placebo-controlled study to evaluate the effect of daily dosages of 75 or 125 mg of azimilide on recurrent symptomatic ventricular arrhythmias and ICD therapies. Importantly, azimilide was added to optimal medical therapy, as more than 86% of patients were receiving beta-blockers and 75% were on ACE inhibitor therapy. At a median follow-up of 367 days, the primary end point of total all-cause shocks plus symptomatic tachyarrhythmias terminated by ATP was reduced significantly by both dosages of azimilide, with relative risk reductions of 57% (HR = 0.43, 95% CI 0.26 to 0.69, $P = .0006$) and 47% (HR = 0.53, 95% CI 0.34 to 0.83, $P = .0053$) at 75- and 125-mg/d dosages, respectively (**Fig. 2**A). The secondary end point of appropriate ICD therapies (shocks or ATP-terminated VT) was reduced significantly among

Table 2
Adverse events for the 3 treatment groups in the Optimal Pharmacologic Therapy in Cardioverter Defibrillator Patients (OPTIC) study

	No. of Patients (%)			
Adverse Event	β-Blocker (n = 138)	Amiodarone + β-Blocker (n = 140)	Sotalol (n = 134)	P Value[a]
Death	2 (1.4)	6 (4.3)	4 (3.0)	.36
Arrhythmic death	1 (0.7)	2 (1.4)	1 (0.8)	.60
Myocardial infarction	1 (0.7)	1 (0.7)	0	.62
Heart failure	9 (6.5)	12 (8.6)	14 (13.4)	.14
Atrial fibrillation	6 (4.4)	1 (0.7)	6 (4.5)	.13
Pulmonary adverse event	0	7 (5.0)	4 (3.0)	.03
Hypothyroidism	0	6 (4.3)	1 (0.8)	.01
Hypothyroidism	0	2 (1.4)	0	.14
Symptomatic bradycardia	1 (0.7)	8 (6.4)	2 (1.5)	.009
Torsades de pointes	0	0	0	>.99
Skin adverse event	2 (1.5)	4 (2.9)	3 (2.2)	.72
Device infection	1 (0.7)	2 (1.4)	4 (3.0)	.34
Hospitalized during follow-up	60 (43.3)	49 (34.9)	40 (30.1)	.32

The mortality rate was not significantly different among treatment groups. In the amiodarone plus beta-blocker group, there were higher rates of adverse thyroid and pulmonary effects and of symptomatic bradycardia.

[a] For any difference among 3 treatment assignments.

Data from Connolly SJ, Dorian P, Roberts RS, et al. Comparison of beta-blockers, amiodarone plus beta-blockers, or sotalol for prevention of shocks from implantable cardioverter defibrillators: the OPTIC Study: a randomized trial. JAMA 2006;295(2):165–71.

patients taking 75 mg of azimilide by 48% (HR = 0.52, 95% CI 0.30 to 0.89, P<.017) and those taking 125 mg of azimilide by 62% (HR = 0.38, 95% CI 0.22 to 0.65, P<.0004) (see **Fig. 2**B). The reduction in all-cause shocks with neither azimilide dosage achieved statistical significance.

The efficacy of azimilide in suppressing electrical storm was assessed in the SHIELD trial.[57] Azimilide did not significantly reduce the number of patients with electrical storm: of the 148 patients who experienced electrical storm, 58 (27%) were on placebo, 51 (23%) were on 75 mg, and 39 (20%) were on 125 mg azimilide. However ,compared with placebo, the risk of recurrent electrical storm was reduced significantly by azimilide (by 37% in the 75-mg group and 55% in the 125-mg group). Consistent with the efficacy of azimilide in reducing symptomatic ventricular arrhythmias and ICD therapies, azimilide reduced arrhythmic-related emergency department visits and hospitalizations by 47% at the 75 mg/d dosage and 31% at the 125 mg/d dosage in the SHIELD study population.[58]

Azimilide was well tolerated with an adverse event profile similar to placebo in SHIELD. Notably, 5 patients in the azimilide groups and 1 in the placebo group experienced TdP. One

patient taking azimilide (75 mg) had severe but reversible neutropenia.[56]

In summary, azimilide is an investigational AAD that reduces recurrent symptomatic VT or VF episodes terminated by ICD shocks or ATP therapies. Azimilide is the first-ever drug submitted to the FDA for this indication and currently is under review to be used in ICD recipients. It seems to have a lower risk of TdP than sotalol or dofetilide and has a low incidence of extracardiac toxicity and side effects. An additional phase 3 confirmatory clinical trial with this agent in patients with ICDs is being contemplated. If approved, this AAD would be the first drug that would be labeled for adjunctive use in patients with ICDs.

NOVEL ADJUVANT PHARMACOLOGIC OPTIONS FOR SUPPRESSING REFRACTORY VT AND VF IN THE PATIENT WITH AN ICD

Some patients with recurrent VT or VF will not respond to or will not tolerate the AADs discussed previously and alternative therapies must be considered. After optimization of beta-blocker therapy, revascularization in the setting of ischemic heart disease, and aggressive ICD programming to

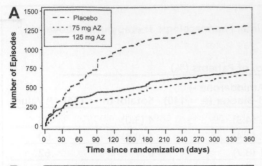

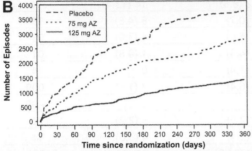

Fig. 2. Effects of azimilide (AZ) on prevention of ventricular tachyarrhythmias and ICD therapies in the SHIELD trial. (*A*) Cumulative number of arrhythmia episodes as primary end point (all-cause shocks plus symptomatic tachyarrhythmias terminated by ATP). Treatment with 75 mg/d and 125 mg/d azimilide significantly reduced risk of all-cause shocks and symptomatic tachyarrhythmia by 57% and 47%, respectively. (*B*) Cumulative number of episodes of VT or VF (all appropriate therapies). Treatment with 75 mg/d and 125 mg/d of azimilide significantly reduced the risk of all appropriate ICD therapies by 48% and 62%, respectively. (*Reproduced from* Dorian P, Borggrefe M, Al-Khalidi HR, et al Placebo-controlled, randomized clinical trial of azimilide for prevention of ventricular tachyarrhythmias in patients with an implantable cardioverter defibrillator. Circulation 2004;110(24): 3646–54; with permission.)

avoid shocks as much as possible with algorithms that include long detection times and multiple ATP trains before shocks, catheter ablation is usually considered or attempted. However, when catheter ablation is contraindicated or not successful in reducing or eliminating shocks, then additional alternatives need to be sought. Few clinical trials are available to guide AAD therapy in such cases.

Monotherapy with class I AADs for prevention of ventricular arrhythmias and shocks in patients with ICDs is not recommended because these agents generally are not safe and increase the risk of SCD and all-cause mortality in patients with advanced structural heart disease; however, occasionally a class I drug can be combined with a class III drug for enhanced antiarrhythmic

efficacy. The combination of mexiletine with amiodarone or sotalol or, alternatively, procainamide with amiodarone or sotalol may be considered for controlling refractory VT or VF.[59,60] These combination AAD regimens may be lifesaving for intractable arrhythmias and in some cases, may permit lower dosages of each of the AADs to be used and still remain effective but better tolerated.

Dronedarone is a noniodinated derivative of amiodarone with a similar electropharmacological profile that includes multiple cardiac ion channel blockade.[61] The FDA has approved dronedarone for use in patients with atrial fibrillation. Based on clinical experience with amiodarone, there is interest in whether dronedarone is safe and effective for suppression of ventricular arrhythmias; however, dronedarone is contraindicated in class IV heart failure and class II and III heart failure with recent decompensation. In a clinical trial involving high-risk patients with heart failure who were hospitalized with symptomatic heart failure and severe LV systolic dysfunction, dronedarone use was associated with an increase in mortality.[62] In preclinical studies, dronedarone had similar AAD efficacy as amiodarone in suppression of ventricular arrhythmias after myocardial infarction and during acute ischemia.[63,64] In a small study in patients with ICDs, dronedarone was effective in reducing the rate of appropriate ICD therapies during a 30-day follow-up.[65] Sixty-seven percent of placebo-treated patients had an appropriate ICD therapy compared with 39% of patients treated with dronedarone.

Celivarone is an investigational AAD with electrophysiological effects similar to dronedarone and amiodarone.[66] In a phase 2 study in patients with ICDs, 2 dosages of celivarone (100 and 300 mg daily) were compared with placebo over 6 months.[67] A 46% reduction in sustained ventricular arrhythmia episodes requiring ICD therapy that did not achieve statistical significance was noted in the 300-mg group. Future clinical trials testing the efficacy of this AAD for prevention of ICD interventions are expected.

Ranolazine is an agent approved for use in treating chronic stable angina that also has antiarrhythmic properties mediated via inhibition of cardiac late sodium currents.[68] The efficacy and safety of this drug as an antiarrhythmic agent for suppression of ventricular arrhythmias in ICD recipients has not yet been demonstrated. The Metabolic Efficiency with Ranolazine for Less Ischemia in Non–ST-Elevation Acute Coronary Syndromes–Thrombolysis in Myocardial Infarction 36 (MERLIN-TIMI 36) trial enrolled patients with a non–ST-elevation acute coronary syndrome who were randomly assigned to either ranolazine (intravenous initiation, then 1000 mg twice daily) or placebo.[69] A significant decrease in frequency of nonsustained VT during the first 7 days of therapy in the ranolazine group was observed. A few isolated case reports describing the efficacy of ranolazine in suppression of refractory ventricular arrhythmias also have been published.[70]

In patients with inherited cardiac arrhythmia syndromes (ie, channelopathies), AAD use should be tailored to the specific underlying syndrome. Specific drug therapy can prevent episodes of VT/VF in congenital long QT syndrome (beta-blockers in LQTS 1, 2; mexitine, flecainide, or ranolazine in LQTS 3; verapamil or ranolazine in LQTS 8 [Timothy syndrome]), short QT syndrome (quinidine or disopyramide), idiopathic VF (quinidine or verapamil), Brugada syndrome (quinidine, hydroquinidine, or verapamil), and catecholaminergic polymorphic VT (beta-blockers, verapamil, or flecainide).

Because of the disappointing efficacy and safety of conventional ion channel AAD therapy for prevention of ventricular arrhythmias and SCD, there is interest in "upstream" therapies that prevent development of an electrically vulnerable substrate. Drugs are available that are not classified as AADs, but can modify electrophysiological remodeling and produce an indirect antiarrhythmic effect. These nonantiarrhythmic drugs reduce the likelihood of VT/VF in patients with coronary artery disease or heart failure.

Lipid-lowering therapy (eg, statins) in ICD recipients with coronary artery disease was associated in the AVID (secondary prevention) and MADIT-II (primary prevention) trials with significant reductions in VT/VF recurrence, appropriate ICD therapy, arrhythmic death, or all-cause mortality.[71,72] The benefit with statins was also seen in patients with nonischemic cardiomyopathy in the Defibrillators in Non-Ischemic Cardiomyopathy Treatment Evaluation (DEFINITE) study in which statin use was associated with a significant reduction in total mortality in ICD recipients.[73]

Long-chain n-3 fatty acids in fish have antiarrhythmic properties in experimental models and prevent SCD in patients after myocardial infarction. Several studies have prospectively evaluated the potential benefit of fish oil supplementation (1.8–2.6 g per day) in patients with ICDs.[74–76] Conflicting results have been reported in studies with fish oil including a decrease, increase, and no effect on VT/VF events. Thus, present evidence does not support an antiarrhythmic role of fish oil in preventing VT/VF in patients with ICDs.

Aldosterone blockers are indicated in patients with class III/IV heart failure. These agents reduced SCD and all-cause mortality in patients with LV systolic dysfunction when added to standard medical therapies for heart failure that included beta-blockers and angiotensin-converting enzyme (ACE) inhibitors.[77,78] However, the efficacy of aldosterone blockers in reducing spontaneous ventricular tachyarrhythmias or shocks in patients with heart failure who have an ICD has not been investigated. In experimental heart failure, aldosterone blockade attenuated ventricular tachyarrhythmia vulnerability by inhibiting myocardial activation delays during premature excitation.[79] Prevention and reversal of electrical delays with aldosterone blockade were related to suppression of fibrosis and inflammatory mediators in this heart failure model.

SUMMARY

ICDs have had an enormous impact on the treatment of survivors of potentially life-threatening ventricular arrhythmias and in patients with heart failure and LV systolic dysfunction. The most profound disadvantage of ICD therapy is recurrent appropriate and inappropriate shocks, which can occur in a substantial proportion of ICD recipients. Although these ICD shocks can be lifesaving, they can be painful and emotionally traumatic. ICD shocks increase hospitalizations, risk of death, and premature ICD battery depletion. Antitachycardia pacing is often effective in terminating VT and thus reduces the incidence of ICD shocks; however, the role of ATP is often limited. It does not eliminate the need for shocks, as ATP can be ineffective for the termination of some monomorphic VT, polymorphic VT, or VF. Therefore, adjunctive AAD therapy often is necessary in many patients with ICDs for control of recurrent ventricular tachyarrhythmias and prevention of ICD shocks. However, given the scarcity of safe and effective AADs for this indication, the decision of when to start an AAD in the patient with an ICD must be individualized. The weight of evidence from clinical trials and experience indicates that the most effective, empiric AAD therapy in the ICD recipient is amiodarone in combination with a beta-blocker. If AAD therapy is initiated, the potential for drug-related toxicities and device interactions must be recognized and anticipated. Additional safe and effective options for this challenging clinical problem are clearly needed. Studies evaluating investigational AADs as well as novel and innovative agents as adjunctive therapies in patients with ICDs are eagerly anticipated. Hopefully, these newer agents will prove to have favorable effects on arrhythmic events and be better tolerated than existing therapies in patients with ICDs.

ACKNOWLEDGMENTS

Dr Stambler has received consulting fees, lecture fees, and research grant support from Sanofi-Aventis, Procter and Gamble, CV Therapeutics, Pfizer, Medtronic, St Jude Medical, Boston Scientific, and Biotronik.

REFERENCES

1. Narang R, Cleland JG, Erhardt L, et al. Mode of death in chronic heart failure. A request and proposition for more accurate classification. Eur Heart J 1996;17(9):1390–403.
2. DiMarco JP. Implantable cardioverter-defibrillators. N Engl J Med 2003;349(19):1836–47.
3. The Antiarrhythmics versus Implantable Defibrillators (AVID) Investigators. A comparison of antiarrhythmic-drug therapy with implantable defibrillators in patients resuscitated from near-fatal ventricular arrhythmias. N Engl J Med 1997;337(22):1576–83.
4. Connolly SJ, Gent M, Roberts RS, et al. Canadian implantable defibrillator study (CIDS): a randomized trial of the implantable cardioverter defibrillator against amiodarone. Circulation 2000;101(11):1297–302.
5. Desai AS, Fang JC, Maisel WH, et al. Implantable defibrillators for the prevention of mortality in patients with nonischemic cardiomyopathy: a meta-analysis of randomized controlled trials. JAMA 2004;292(23):2874–9.
6. Kuck KH, Cappato R, Siebels J, et al. Randomized comparison of antiarrhythmic drug therapy with implantable defibrillators in patients resuscitated from cardiac arrest: the Cardiac Arrest Study Hamburg (CASH). Circulation 2000;102(7):748–54.
7. Lee DS, Green LD, Liu PP, et al. Effectiveness of implantable defibrillators for preventing arrhythmic events and death: a meta-analysis. J Am Coll Cardiol 2003;41(9):1573–82.
8. Bardy GH, Lee KL, Mark DB, et al. Amiodarone or an implantable cardioverter-defibrillator for congestive heart failure. N Engl J Med 2005;352(3):225–37.
9. Buxton AE, Lee KL, Fisher JD, et al. A randomized study of the prevention of sudden death in patients with coronary artery disease. Multicenter Unsustained Tachycardia Trial Investigators. N Engl J Med 1999;341(25):1882–90.
10. Moss AJ, Hall WJ, Cannom DS, et al. Improved survival with an implanted defibrillator in patients with coronary disease at high risk for ventricular arrhythmia. Multicenter Automatic Defibrillator Implantation Trial Investigators. N Engl J Med 1996;335(26):1933–40.
11. Moss AJ, Zareba W, Hall WJ, et al. Prophylactic implantation of a defibrillator in patients with myocardial infarction and reduced ejection fraction. N Engl J Med 2002;346(12):877–83.
12. Hallstrom A, Pratt CM, Greene HL, et al. Relations between heart failure, ejection fraction, arrhythmia suppression and mortality: analysis of the Cardiac Arrhythmia Suppression Trial. J Am Coll Cardiol 1995;25(6):1250–7.
13. Pratt CM, Eaton T, Francis M, et al. The inverse relationship between baseline left ventricular ejection fraction and outcome of antiarrhythmic therapy: a dangerous imbalance in the risk-benefit ratio. Am Heart J 1989;118(3):433–40.
14. Ravid S, Podrid PJ, Lampert S, et al. Congestive heart failure induced by six of the newer antiarrhythmic drugs. J Am Coll Cardiol 1989;14(5):1326–30.
15. Slater W, Lampert S, Podrid PJ, et al. Clinical predictors of arrhythmia worsening by antiarrhythmic drugs. Am J Cardiol 1988;61(4):349–53.
16. Poole JE, Johnson GW, Hellkamp AS, et al. Prognostic importance of defibrillator shocks in patients with heart failure. N Engl J Med 2008;359:1009–17.
17. Schron EB, Exner DV, Yao Q, et al. Quality of life in the antiarrhythmics versus implantable defibrillators trial: impact of therapy and influence of adverse symptoms and defibrillator shocks. Circulation 2002;105:589–94.
18. Irvine J, Dorian P, Baker B, et al. Quality of life in the Canadian Implantable Defibrillator Study (CIDS). Am Heart J 2002;144:282–9.
19. Sears SF, Conti JB. Understanding implantable cardioverter defibrillator shocks and storms: Medical and psychosocial considerations for research and clinical care. Clin Cardiol 2003;26:107–11.
20. Piotrowicz K, Noyes K, Lyness JM, et al. Physical functioning and mental well-being in association with health outcome in patients Role of antiarrhythmic drugs enrolled in the Multicenter Automatic Defibrillator Implantation Trial II. Eur Heart J 2007;28:601–7.
21. Steinberg JS, Martins J, Sadanandan S, et al. AVID Investigators. Antiarrhythmic drug use in the implantable defibrillator arm of the Antiarrhythmics Versus Implantable Defibrillators (AVID) Study. Am Heart J 2001;142:520–9.
22. Gradaus R, Block M, Brachmann J, et al. German EURID Registry. Mortality, morbidity, and complications in 3344 patients with implantable cardioverter defibrillators: results from the German ICD Registry EURID. Pacing Clin Electrophysiol 2003;26:1511–8.
23. Bollmann A, Husser D, Cannom DS. Antiarrhythmic drugs in patients with implantable cardioverter-defibrillators. Am J Cardiovasc Drugs 2005;5(6):371–8.
24. Singh S, Murawski MM. Implantable cardioverter defibrillator therapy and the need for concomitant antiarrhythmic drugs. J Cardiovasc Pharmacol Ther 2007;12(3):175–80.

25. Stein KM, Euler DE, Mehra R, et al. Do atrial tachyarrhythmias beget ventricular tachyarrhythmias in defibrillator recipients? J Am Coll Cardiol 2002;40: 335–40.

26. Moss AJ, Zareba W, Hall WJ, et al. Prophylactic implantation of a defibrillator in patients with myocardial infarction and reduced ejection fraction. For the multicenter automatic defibrillator implantation trial II investigators. N Engl J Med 2002;346:877–83.

27. Raitt MH, Klein RC, Wyse DG, et al. Comparison of arrhythmia recurrence in patients presenting with ventricular fibrillation versus ventricular tachycardia in the Antiarrhythmics Versus Implantable Defibrillators (AVID) Trial. Am J Cardiol 2003;91:812–6.

28. Freedberg NA, Hill JN, Fogel RI, et al. Recurrence of symptomatic ventricular arrhythmias in patients with implantable cardioverter defibrillator after the first device therapy. J Am Coll Cardiol 2001;37:1910–5.

29. Tandri H, Griffith LS, Tang T, et al. Clinical course and long-term follow-up of patients receiving implantable-cardioverter defibrillators. Heart Rhythm 2006;3: 762–8.

30. Singh BN. Sotalol: current status and expanding indications. J Cardiovasc Pharmacol Ther 1999; 4(1):49–65.

31. Anderson JL, Prystowsky EN. Sotalol: an important new antiarrhythmic. Am Heart J 1999;137(3): 388–409.

32. Hohnloser SH, Woosley RL. Sotalol. N Engl J Med 1994;331(1):31–8.

33. Pacifico A, Hohnloser SH, Williams JH, et al. Prevention of implantable-defibrillator shocks by treatment with sotalol. d, l-Sotalol Implantable Cardioverter-Defibrillator Study Group. N Engl J Med 1999;340(24): 1855–62.

34. Kuhlkamp V, Mewis C, Mermi J, et al. Suppression of sustained ventricular tachyarrhythmias: a comparison of d, l-sotalol with no antiarrhythmic drug treatment. J Am Coll Cardiol 1999;33(1):46–52.

35. Connolly SJ, Dorian P, Roberts RS, et al. Comparison of beta-blockers, amiodarone plus beta-blockers, or sotalol for prevention of shocks from implantable cardioverter defibrillators: the OPTIC Study: a randomized trial. JAMA 2006;295(2): 165–71.

36. Kettering K, Mewis C, Dornberger V, et al. Efficacy of metoprolol and sotalol in the prevention of recurrences of sustained ventricular tachyarrhythmias in patients with an implantable cardioverter defibrillator. Pacing Clin Electrophysiol 2002;25: 1571–6.

37. Seidl K, Hauer B, Schwick NG, et al. Comparison of metoprolol and sotalol in preventing ventricular tachyarrhythmias after the implantation of a cardioverter/defibrillator. Am J Cardiol 1998;82:744–8.

38. Ferreira-González I, Dos-Subirá L, Guyatt GH. Adjunctive antiarrhythmic drug therapy in patients with implantable cardioverter defibrillators: a systematic review. Eur Heart J 2007;28:469–77.

39. Marcus GM, Glidden DV, Polonsky B, et al. Efficacy of antiarrhythmic drugs in arrhythmogenic right ventricular cardiomyopathy: a report from the North American ARVC Registry. J Am Coll Cardiol 2009; 54:609–15.

40. Mounsey JP, DiMarco JP. Cardiovascular drugs. Dofetilide. Circulation 2000;102(21):2665–70.

41. Boriani G, Lubinski A, Capucci A, et al. A multicentre, double blind randomized crossover comparative study on the efficacy and safety of dofetilide vs sotalol in patients with inducible sustained ventricular tachycardia and ischemic heart disease. Eur Heart J 2001;22:2180–91.

42. O'Toole M, O'Neill G, Kluger J, et al. Efficacy and safety of oral dofetilide in patients with an implanted defibrillator: a multicenter study [abstract]. Circulation 1999;100:I–794.

43. Mazur A, Anderson ME, Bonney S, et al. Pause-dependent polymorphic ventricular tachycardia during long-term treatment with dofetilide: a placebo-controlled, implantable cardioverter-defibrillator-based evaluation. J Am Coll Cardiol 2001;37(4):1100–5.

44. Kolb C, Ndrepepa G, Zrenner B. Late dofetilide-associated life-threatening proarrhythmia. Int J Cardiol 2008;127(2):e54–6.

45. Goldschlager N, Epstein AE, Naccarelli GV, et al. A practical guide for clinicians who treat patients with amiodarone: 2007. Heart Rhythm 2007;4(9):1250–9.

46. Kodama I, Kamiya K, Toyama J. Cellular electropharmacology of amiodarone. Cardiovasc Res 1997;35(1):13–29.

47. Kamiya K, Nishiyama A, Yasui K, et al. Short- and long-term effects of amiodarone on the two components of cardiac delayed rectifier K(+) current. Circulation 2001;103(9):1317–24.

48. Kou WH, Kirsh MM, Bolling SF, et al. Effect of antiarrhythmic drug therapy on the incidence of shocks in patients who receive an implantable cardioverter defibrillator after a single episode of sustained ventricular tachycardia/fibrillation. Pacing Clin Electrophysiol 1991;14(11 Pt 1): 1586–92.

49. Anderson JL, Karagounis LA, Roskelley M, et al. Effect of prophylactic antiarrhythmic therapy on time to implantable cardioverter-defibrillator discharge in patients with ventricular tachyarrhythmias. Am J Cardiol 1994;73(9):683–7.

50. Credner SC, Klingenheben T, Mauss O, et al. Electrical storm in patients with transvenous implantable cardioverter-defibrillators: incidence, management and prognostic implications. J Am Coll Cardiol 1998;32(7):1909–15.

51. Busch AE, Eigenberger B, Jurkiewicz NK, et al. Blockade of HERG channels by the class III

antiarrhythmic azimilide: mode of action. Br J Pharmacol 1998;123(1):23–30.

52. Karam R, Marcello S, Brooks RR, et al. Azimilide dihydrochloride, a novel antiarrhythmic agent. Am J Cardiol 1998;81(6A):40D–6D.

53. Cannom DS, Gidney B. Azimilide: another effort to prevent implantable cardioverter-defibrillator shocks and their sequelae why it is important and how it works. J Am Coll Cardiol 2008;52(13):1084–5.

54. Pritchett EL, Page RL, Connolly SJ, et al. Antiarrhythmic effects of azimilide in atrial fibrillation: efficacy and dose-response. Azimilide Supraventricular Arrhythmia Program 3 (SVA-3) Investigators. J Am Coll Cardiol 2000;36(3):794–802.

55. Singer I, Al-Khalidi H, Niazi I, et al. Azimilide decreases recurrent ventricular tachyarrhythmias in patients with implantable cardioverter defibrillators. J Am Coll Cardiol 2004;43(1):39–43.

56. Dorian P, Borggrefe M, Al-Khalidi HR, et al. Placebo-controlled, randomized clinical trial of azimilide for prevention of ventricular tachyarrhythmias in patients with an implantable cardioverter defibrillator. Circulation 2004;110(24):3646–54.

57. Hohnloser SH, Al-Khalidi HR, Pratt CM, et al. Electrical storm in patients with an implantable defibrillator: incidence, features, and preventive therapy: insights from a randomized trial. Eur Heart J 2006;27:3027–32.

58. Dorian P, Al-Khalidi HR, Hohnloser SH, et al. Azimilide reduces emergency department visits and hospitalizations in patients with an implantable cardioverter-defibrillator in a placebo-controlled clinical trial. J Am Coll Cardiol 2008;52(13):1076–83.

59. Waleffe A, Mary-Rabine L, Legrand V, et al. Combined mexiletine and amiodarone treatment of refractory recurrent ventricular tachycardia. Am Heart J 1980;100:788–93.

60. Lee SD, Newman D, Ham M, et al. Electrophysiologic mechanisms of antiarrhythmic efficacy of a sotalol and class Ia drug combination: elimination of reverse use dependence. J Am Coll Cardiol 1997;29:100–5.

61. Patel C, Yan GX, Kowey PR. Dronedarone. Circulation 2009;120:636–44.

62. Kober L, Torp-Pedersen C, McMurray JJV, et al. Increased mortality after dronedarone therapy for severe heart failure. N Engl J Med 2008;358:2678–87.

63. Finance O, Manning A, Chatelain P. Effects of a new amiodarone-like agent, SR 33589, in comparison to amiodarone, D, L-sotalol, and lignocaine, on ischemia-induced ventricular arrhythmias in anesthetized pigs. J Cardiovasc Pharmacol 1995;26:570–6.

64. Agelaki MG, Pantos C, Korantzopoulos P, et al. Comparative antiarrhythmic efficacy of amiodarone and dronedarone during acute myocardial infarction in rats. Eur J Pharmacol 2007;564:150–7.

65. Kowey PR, Singh BN. Dronedarone in patients with implantable defibrillators. Heart Rhythm Society

2004 Scientific Session, Late breaking Clinical Trials Oral Presentation. San Francisco, May 22, 2004.

66. Gautier P, Serre M, Cosnier-Pucheu S, et al. In vivo and in vitro antiarrhythmic effects of SSR149744C in animal models of atrial fibrillation and ventricular arrhythmias. J Cardiovasc Pharmacol 2005;45:125–35.

67. Kowey PR, Aliot E, Cappucci A, et al. Placebo-controlled double-blind dose-ranging study of the efficacy and safety of celivarone for the prevention of ventricular arrhythmia-triggered ICD interventions [abstract]. J Am Coll Cardiol 2008;51:A2.

68. Antzelevitch C, Belardinelli L, Wu L, et al. Electrophysiologic and antiarrhythmic actions of a novel antianginal agent. J Cardiovasc Pharmacol Ther 2004;9(Suppl 1):S65–83.

69. Scirica BM, Morrow DA, Hod H, et al. Effect of ranolazine, an antianginal agent with novel electrophysiological properties, on the incidence of arrhythmias in patients with non-ST elevation acute coronary syndrome: result from the Metabolic Efficiency with Ranolazine for Less Myocardial Ischemia in Non-ST-Elevation Acute Coronary Syndrome-Thrombolysis in Myocardial Infarction 36 (MERLIN-TIMI 36) randomized controlled trial. Circulation 2007;116:1647–52.

70. Murdock DK, Kaliebe J, Overton N. Ranolazine-induced suppression of ventricular tachycardia in a patient with non-ischemic cardiomyopathy: a case report. Pacing Clin Electrophysiol 2008;31:765–8.

71. Mitchell LB, Powell JL, Gillis AM, et al. AVID Investigators. Are lipid-lowering drugs also antiarrhythmic drugs? An analysis of the Antiarrhythmics versus Implantable Defibrillators (AVID) trial. J Am Coll Cardiol 2003;42:81–7.

72. Vyas A, Guo H, Moss A, et al. Reduction in ventricular tachyarrhythmias with statins in the Multicenter Automatic Defibrillator Implantation Trial (MADIT)-II. J Am Coll Cardiol 2006;47:769–73.

73. Goldberger J, Subacius H, Schaechter A, et al. Effects of statin therapy on arrhythmic events and survival in patients with nonischemic dilated cardiomyopathy. J Am Coll Cardiol 2006;48:1228–33.

74. Leaf A, Albert C, Johnson D, et al. Prevention of fatal arrhythmias in high risk subjects by fish oil n-3 fatty acid intakes. Circulation 2005;112:2762–8.

75. Brouwer I, Zock P, Camm A, et al. Effect of fish oil on ventricular tachyarrhythmia and death in patients with implantable cardioverter defibrillators. J Am Coll Cardiol 2006;295:2613–9.

76. Raitt M, Connor W, Morris C, et al. Fish oil supplementation and risk of ventricular tachycardia and ventricular fibrillation in patients with implantable defibrillators: a randomized controlled trial. JAMA 2005;293:2884–91.

77. Pitt B, Zannad F, Remme WJ, et al. The effect of spironolactone on morbidity and mortality in patients with severe heart failure. Randomized Aldactone Evaluation Study Investigators. N Engl J Med 1999;341:709–17.

78. Pitt B, Remme W, Zannad F, et al. Eplerenone, a selective aldosterone blocker, in patients with left ventricular dysfunction after myocardial infarction. N Engl J Med 2003;348:1309–21.

79. Stambler BS, Laurita KR, Shroff SC, et al. Aldosterone blockade attenuates development of an electrophysiological substrate associated with ventricular tachyarrhythmias in heart failure. Heart Rhythm 2009;6:776–83.

Aggravation of Arrhythmia by Antiarrhythmic Drugs (Proarrhythmia)

Philip J. Podrid, MD

KEYWORDS

- Antiarrhythmic drugs • Aggravation of arrhythmic
- Proarrhythmia • Prolonged QT interval
- Torsade des pointes

Although intended to prevent or suppress arrhythmia, antiarrhythmic drugs may actually cause an unexpected and unpredictable worsening or aggravation of arrhythmia.[1] This complication is commonly referred to as proarrhythmia, and was first recognized with the use of quinidine. The condition was termed "quinidine syncope," and the mechanism was subsequently found to be an atypical polymorphic ventricular tachycardia now termed torsade des pointes.[2] Although this adverse effect was most commonly reported with quinidine, it is now clear that proarrhythmia may occur with any antiarrhythmic drug.

DEFINITION OF ARRHYTHMIA AGGRAVATION

Arrhythmia aggravation by antiarrhythmic drugs is defined as follows[3]:

1. Worsening or a change of a preexisting arrhythmia
   Statistically significant increase in the frequency of premature ventricular complexes (PVCs), ventricular couplets, runs of nonsustained ventricular tachycardia, or episodes of sustained ventricular tachycardia not previously observed
   Conversion from nonsustained to sustained ventricular tachycardia
   Arrhythmia that becomes incessant and cannot be terminated
   Ventricular tachycardia that occurs at a more rapid rate and which is associated with hemodynamic instability
   Arrhythmia that is more easily inducible during electrophysiologic study
2. Development of a new arrhythmia
   Sustained monomorphic ventricular tachycardia
   Polymorphic ventricular tachycardia
   QT prolongation and torsade des pointes
   Ventricular fibrillation
   Supraventricular tachyarrhythmia
3. Development of a bradyarrhythmia
   Depression of sinus node function
   Abnormalities of atrioventricular (AV) nodal function.

Whether the aggravation, change, or induction of an arrhythmia is derived from the direct effects of an antiarrhythmic agent may be difficult to determine because these changes may be a result of the natural history of the arrhythmia or of random variability in arrhythmia frequency. One clear proarrhythmic effect, however, is the development of a new arrhythmia temporally related to the initiation of an antiarrhythmic drug. Proarrhythmia is also probable if a significant change in the arrhythmia occurs in relation to the initiation of drug therapy or a change in dose. Proarrhythmia may also be established when there is development of marked QT prolongation and the occurrence of torsade des pointes.

The author has nothing to disclose.

Section of Cardiology, West Roxbury Veterans Administration Hospital, 1400 VFW Parkway, West Roxbury, MA 02132, USA

E-mail address: Philip.Podrid@va.gov

Card Electrophysiol Clin 2 (2010) 459–470

doi:10.1016/j.ccep.2010.06.006

Aggravation of arrhythmia usually occurs within several days of beginning an antiarrhythmic drug or increasing the dose of the drug. The time of occurrence is based on the particular drug and its pharmacokinetic properties.[1,4] In one study of 26 patients treated with quinidine, procainamide or disopyramide the first episode of ventricular fibrillation occurred within a mean of 3 days of the initiation of drug therapy.[4] However, the Cardiac Arrhythmia Suppression Trial (CAST), which initiated antiarrhythmic drug therapy in patients with a recent acute myocardial infarction, showed that arrhythmia aggravation may also occur as a late complication of antiarrhythmic drugs.[5] In this study of 2309 patients treated with encainide, flecainide, or moricizine, arrhythmia aggravation occurred throughout the entire follow-up period (mean follow-up 10 months). Although the mechanism for arrhythmia aggravation in this study is not clear, one possible reason is that patients with a recent myocardial infarction are not stable. Ongoing or even transient overt or silent myocardial ischemia or ventricular remodeling may modify the underlying myocardial substrate, and convert a stable myocardium into an unstable and potentially arrhythmogenic tissue.

The degree of arrhythmic increase can also suggest a proarrhythmic effect. For example, in one report of 155 patients undergoing evaluation with various antiarrhythmic drugs (total of 722 drugs studies), arrhythmia aggravation occurred in 53 patients and in 11.1% of studies.[1] In this report it was concluded that the arrhythmic events were proarrhythmic because the extent of arrhythmia increase was far in excess of what could be expected from the established random variability of arrhythmia in these patients. The criteria for arrhythmia aggravation in this trial were:

1. A fourfold increase in the frequency of PVCs
2. A tenfold increase in the frequency of repetitive forms (couplets or nonsustained ventricular tachycardia)
3. A new sustained ventricular tachyarrhythmia not previously observed in the patient (**Fig. 1**).

It has been established that there is significant random variability of spontaneous arrhythmia, particularly in patients without a history of serious heart disease or those who have never experienced a sustained ventricular tachyarrhythmia. However, variability of arrhythmia is less and reproducibility of arrhythmia frequency is greater in such patients when the hourly frequency of arrhythmia increases. Criteria have therefore been proposed for the definition of arrhythmia

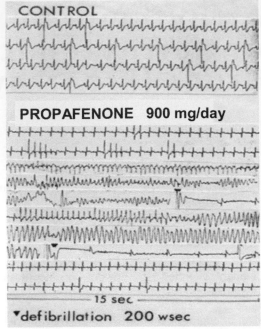

Fig. 1. Aggravation of arrhythmia with propafenone as evaluated with Holter monitoring. The patient was a 55-year-old woman without structural heart disease. She did have frequent premature ventricular complexes (PVCs) that were associated with symptoms of palpitations and lightheadedness. As a result of symptoms she was started on propafenone, titrated up to 900 mg/d. On the second day of this dose she began complaining of worsening lightheadedness. As a result she was admitted to the hospital and placed on telemetry. Two hours later she was noted to have rapid ventricular tachycardia that degenerated into ventricular fibrillation. Normal sinus rhythm was established after 2 defibrillation shocks.

aggravation based on the density of underlying arrhythmia[6]:

1. Tenfold increase in PVCs if baseline frequency is 10 to 50 PVCs per hour
2. Fivefold increase in PVCs if baseline is 51 to 100 PVCs per hour
3. Fourfold increase in PVCs if baseline is 100 to 300 PVCs per hour
4. Threefold increase in PVCs if baseline is more than 300 PVCs per hour
5. Tenfold increase in the episodes of nonsustained ventricular tachycardia independent of the baseline frequency of this arrhythmia.

Despite these definitions, the discontinuation of the implicated agent followed by a drug rechallenge is the only definitive method of determining arrhythmia aggravation. However, this may be hazardous and is not recommended.

INCIDENCE OF ARRHYTHMIA AGGRAVATION IN PATIENTS WITH A HISTORY OF VENTRICULAR ARRHYTHMIA

Several studies have found that arrhythmia aggravation as detected noninvasively (ambulatory monitoring or exercise testing) in patients being treated for the suppression of ventricular arrhythmia can occur with any antiarrhythmic drug. The reported incidence of arrhythmia aggravation with an individual agent varies from 6% to 23%.[1,7] Overall, arrhythmic aggravation occurred during 11% of all drugs studies. In patients undergoing serial drugs evaluation, up to 34% of patients experienced arrhythmia aggravation with at least one administered agent.[7] In the majority of cases, the proarrhythmic event was the development of a new sustained ventricular tachyarrhythmia.[7,8] Up to one-third of events occurred during an exercise test, even though ambulatory monitoring demonstrated suppression of arrhythmia.

Arrhythmia aggravation has also been reported in patients undergoing evaluation using electrophysiologic testing.[9–11] One study of 63 patients undergoing 216 drugs studies reported arrhythmia aggravation in 16% of tests involving 30% of patients.[9] Another study of 314 patients undergoing 801 drug studies found that conversion from nonsustained ventricular tachycardia to ventricular tachycardia occurred in 18% of studies involving 28% of patients (**Fig. 2**).[10] An arrhythmia that was more difficult to terminate occurred in 7% of studies in 13% of patients, whereas in 20% of patients arrhythmia was induced with a less aggressive protocol. Lastly, a spontaneous or incessant ventricular tachycardia occurred in only 1% of drugs studies.

Aggravation of arrhythmia may also be seen in patients with an implantable cardioverter defibrillator (ICD) who are receiving antiarrhythmic agents to prevent the frequent recurrences of arrhythmia resulting in ICD therapy (such as antitachycardia pacing or defibrillation), to aid in the effectiveness of antitachycardia pacing, or as therapy for associated atrial arrhythmias.[12,13] Aggravation of arrhythmia in this situation may be manifest as more frequent episodes of arrhythmia resulting in more frequent device therapies or the occurrence of a ventricular tachycardia, previously terminated with antitachycardia pacing, which can no longer be terminated with antitachycardia pacing (ie, it is incessant) (**Fig. 3**).

BRADYARRHYTHMIA

Potentially serious bradyarrhythmias may also occur as a proarrhythmic effect. However, the incidence of this complication is unknown.

Sinus Node Effects

Sinus pauses or sinus node arrest may develop because many of the antiarrhythmic drugs have a depressive effect on the automaticity of the sinus node. This effect is more common with drugs that block the sympathetic inputs into the sinus node (β-blockers and amiodarone) or those that interfere with slow action potential generation, which is mediated by calcium currents (calcium channel blockers and amiodarone). However, other classes of antiarrhythmic drugs may also directly depress the sinus node and membrane automaticity.

Atrioventricular Node Effects

Perhaps more common than sinus node slowing is depression of AV nodal conduction, resulting in the development of second- or third-degree (complete) AV block. This effect may occur with any antiarrhythmic drugs, although it is more common with the β-blockers and calcium channel blockers.

His and Distal Bundle Effects

Heart block caused by conduction slowing within the bundle of His or the distal bundle branches is less frequently observed and requires the use of electrophysiologic testing for this to be established. However, the development of an intraventricular conduction delay (QRS complex widening)

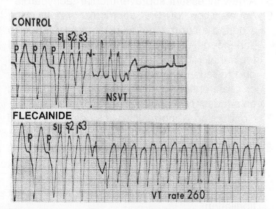

Fig. 2. Aggravation of arrhythmia with flecainide as evaluated with electrophysiologic testing. The patient is a 65-year-old man with a history of nonsustained ventricular tachycardia associated with dizziness. He underwent electrophysiologic testing. At baseline, 3 extrastimuli provoked nonsustained ventricular tachycardia. During therapy with flecainide, 3 extrastimuli induced sustained monomorphic ventricular tachycardia at a rate of 260 beats per minute (bpm). Termination required electric cardioversion.

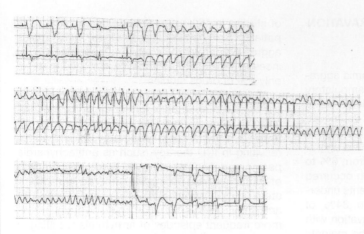

Fig. 3. Aggravation of arrhythmia in a patient with an ICD. The patient had an ICD placed for recurrent episodes of ventricular tachycardia. Several months after ICD placement, telemetric interrogation of the ICD showed very frequent episodes of ventricular tachycardia that were successfully terminated with antitachycardia pacing (burst pacing). Given the frequency of the episodes, therapy with sotalol was begun in order to decrease the frequency of the ventricular tachycardia and the need for antitachycardia pacing. However, the patient began complaining of palpitation and episodes of loss of consciousness. Device interrogation demonstrated episodes of ventricular tachycardia that were not terminated with overdrive pacing. In contrast overdrive pacing provoked ventricular fibrillation resulting in device discharge with a high-energy shock (defibrillation).

or a bundle branch block with antiarrhythmic agents is more commonly observed. Conduction abnormalities involving the His-Purkinje system are more frequently seen with the class I antiarrhythmic agents, as they interfere with the sodium channel, fast action potential generation, and impulse propagation.

His-Purkinje or intraventricular conduction block with the class I agents, especially class IC, may be observed more frequently only at higher heart rates. As heart rate increases the depressive effects of these agents becomes progressively more profound, a property referred to as the "use-dependent" effect.[14–16] The class I agents bind to a receptor in the sodium channel during systole. By blocking the channel, the rate of sodium influx during phase 0 is decreased and this results in a decrease in the conduction velocity. In diastole, the drug dissociates from the receptor. However, when the heart rate increases and diastole is shortened, there is less time for the drug to dissociate and hence the number of sodium channel receptors that are blocked increases. As a result the rate of sodium influx during phase 0 is further decreased, resulting in a more marked slowing of impulse conduction and hence further widening of the QRS complex. Although uncertain, it is likely that such conduction abnormalities are more common in patients with advanced heart disease who have underlying abnormalities of the conduction system.

ARRHYTHMIA AGGRAVATION IN PATIENTS TREATED FOR ATRIAL ARRHYTHMIA

Aggravation of arrhythmia caused by antiarrhythmic drugs may also occur in patients receiving drug therapy for an atrial arrhythmia,[17,18] which may involve a new or worsened atrial arrhythmia or the provocation of a new ventricular arrhythmia. Proposed criteria for this form of arrhythmia aggravation include[19]:

1. Atrial tachycardia with or without AV block (as with digoxin toxicity)
2. Conversion of paroxysmal atrial fibrillation to atrial flutter
3. Increased frequency of paroxysmal atrial arrhythmia
4. Conversion from paroxysmal to a sustained atrial tachyarrhythmia
5. A new incessant supraventricular tachycardia
6. Acceleration of the ventricular rate during a during a supraventricular tachycardia due to enhanced AV nodal conduction, slowing of the atrial rate (increasing the ventricular rate due to less concealed AV nodal conduction), or preferential conduction to the ventricle via an accessory pathway (**Fig. 4**)
7. Conduction abnormalities including AV nodal block and sinus node dysfunction
8. A new ventricular tachyarrhythmia including QT prolongation and torsade des pointes, polymorphic ventricular tachycardia, monomorphic ventricular tachycardia, or ventricular fibrillation.

Unfortunately the incidence of any one form of arrhythmia aggravation in patients being treated for an atrial arrhythmia is uncertain, although the risk of a new ventricular tachyarrhythmia is generally considered to be low (1%–3%), and is more common in those subjects with structural heart disease than in those with a structurally normal heart.[18–20]

A

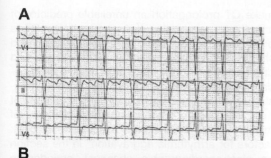

B

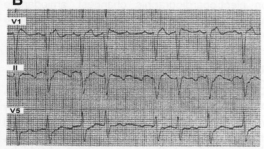

C

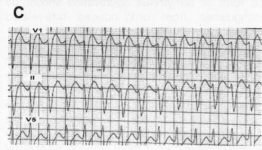

Fig. 4. Aggravation of arrhythmia during propafe-none therapy for atrial flutter. (*A*) Before therapy the patient presented with atrial flutter, with a flutter rate of 240 bpm and varying AV conduction (2:1 and 3:1). (*B*) Three days after beginning propafenone therapy (450 mg/d), atrial flutter was still present, but the atrial flutter rate slowed to 150 bpm. Varying AV block was still present. (*C*) One hour after the elec-trocardiogram (ECG) in *B* was recorded, the patient went to the bathroom. There was an acceleration of the heart rate to 150 bpm, the same rate as the atrial flutter seen in *B*. The QRS complex widened from 0.12 to 0.18 seconds. Hence the patient developed atrial flutter with 1:1 AV conduction and a widening of the QRS complex as a result of the "use-dependent" effect of propafenone.

QT Prolongation and Torsade des Pointes

The most frequent and most serious proarrhythmic event in patients with atrial arrhythmias is the occurrence of torsade des pointes, which occurs with drugs in class IA (quinidine, procainamide, disopyramide) and class III (sotalol, amiodarone, dofetilide, and ibutilide).[21,22] Torsade des pointes is defined as a polymorphic ventricular tachy-cardia with a changing QRS complex morphology

and axis (twisting of points) associated with QT interval prolongation (**Fig. 5**). When torsade des pointes is drug related, it is usually associated with a bradycardia or is pause dependent, that is, it is initiated by a long, followed by a short RR interval (**Fig. 6**).[23–27]

There are several risk factors for the develop-ment of drug-induced torsade des pointes[23,26,28,29]:

1. Female gender, as females tend to have longer QT intervals at baseline compared with males[30–32]
2. Hyopokalemia or hypomagnesemia
3. Bradycardia
4. Diuretic use
5. Higher doses or blood levels of the drug
6. Recent conversion from atrial fibrillation
7. Heart failure or cardiac hypertrophy
8. Rapid intravenous infusion
9. Baseline electrocardiogram (ECG) showing marked QT prolongation and T-wave lability
10. ECG during drug therapy that shows marked QT prolongation, T-wave lability, T-wave mor-phologic changes, increased T-wave dispersion
11. Congenital long QT syndrome.

The proposed mechanism for torsade des pointes is the development of early afterdepolar-izations and the occurrence of triggered activity resulting from prolonged repolarization.[33,34] Because time for repolarization is rate dependent

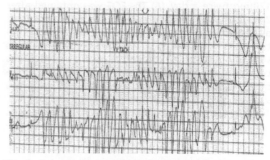

Fig. 5. Torsade des pointes associated with QT prolon-gation resulting for ibutilide therapy for atrial fibrilla-tion. The patient developed atrial fibrillation with a rapid ventricular rate after aortic valve surgery. Therapy with a β-blocker, verapamil, and diltiazem was ineffective for rate slowing. As a result it was decided to attempt chemical reversion with ibutilde. Five minutes after the administration of ibutilide (1 mg over 10 minutes), the atrial fibrillation termi-nated and sinus rhythm was restored. Significant QT interval prolongation was noted. Several minutes later an episode of polymorphic ventricular tachy-cardia, termed torsade des pointes occurred.

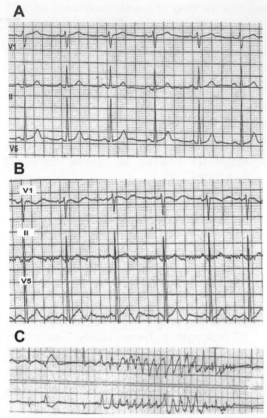

Fig. 6. Drug-induced QT prolongation associated with pause-dependent torsade des pointes. (*A*) Baseline ECG in a patient with a history of paroxysmal atrial fibrillation. As a result of symptoms, drug therapy with sotalol was initiated, at an initial dose of 80 mg twice a day. On day 3, the dose was increased to 120 mg twice a day. (*B*) The ECG was obtained after 2 days of sotalol therapy at a dose of 120 mg twice a day. Noted is significant QT/QTc interval prolongation to 580 milliseconds. In addition, the T wave is very abnormal. (*C*) Although a dose of sotalol was withheld and the dose reduced, 2 hours later the patient was noted to have occasional PVC, with the sudden onset of an episode of torsade des pointes. Torsade was pause dependent, that is, it occurred as a result of the compensatory pause following the PVC.

and is more pronounced at slower heart rates, torsade des points usually occurs in association with bradycardia or is pause dependent, that is, when there are long-short intervals as may be seen with single ectopic complexes.

Many of the class IA and class III antiarrhythmic agents that cause torsade des pointes have a property of "reverse use dependency," that is, there is an inverse correlation between the heart rate and the degree of repolarization or refractoriness (ie, the QT interval).[35,36] This property may

make QT prolongation an unreliable predictor of arrhythmic aggravation.[37] As a result, the QT is prolonged further with slow heart rates and shortens at faster heart rates. Amiodarone and dronedarone, a noniodinated derivative of amiodarone, are exceptions in that they do not demonstrate reverse use dependency.[38,39] As a result of this, among other factors, including blockade of multiple ionic channels (as discussed in "Risk factors for arrhythmia aggravation" in the section on electrocardiographic changes), amiodarone and dronedarone do not generally produce torsade des pointes.[40–44]

Rate-Related Aberration of Ventricular Conduction

Although antiarrhythmic drugs may provoke new ventricular tachyarrhythmia in patients being treated for a supraventricular tachyarrhythmia, this form of arrhythmia aggravation should be distinguished from drug-induced rate-related aberration of ventricular conduction or prolongation of the QRS complex duration during a supraventricular tachyarrhythmia (see **Fig. 4**).[45–47] In this situation the wide complex tachycardia may be confused with a new ventricular tachyarrhythmia. As previously indicated, the wide QRS complex results from the use-dependent effects of the antiarrhythmic drug, that is, the effect on slowing of conduction is more pronounced at faster heart rates.

Enhancement of AV Nodal Conduction and Acceleration of Ventricular Rate

Enhancement of AV nodal conduction and acceleration of the ventricular rate may occur during therapy with some of the antiarrhythmic drugs, especially the class I agents. This enhancement is especially more common in patients being treated for atrial flutter (see **Fig. 4**). Acceleration of the ventricular rate results from the depressive effect of the antiarrhythmic drug on atrial myocardium. This effect causes a slowing of the rate of the atrial flutter and results in a decrease in the amount of concealed conduction within the AV node. Concealed conduction means that at a rapid atrial rate some of the atrial impulses may not completely penetrate the AV node, but rather are extinguished within the node (concealed); but by making the AV node partially refractory, they can affect the rate of conduction of a subsequent impulse. With the acceleration of the ventricular rate, the QRS complex may become widened as the result of the use-dependent effect of the antiarrhythmic agent. In this situation it may be difficult to distinguish this arrhythmia from ventricular tachycardia.[45,46]

These agents may also organize atrial activity and may convert atrial fibrillation to atrial flutter. In this situation, the atrial flutter rate may be slow and hence the ventricular response rate may be more rapid.

Patients with a preexcitation syndrome, particularly Wolff-Parkinson-White syndrome, may also experience an acceleration in the ventricular rate, especially during atrial fibrillation, as a result of an antiarrhythmic agent. In this situation drugs that block the AV node, including digoxin, β-blockers, and calcium channel blockers, may cause an increase in impulse conduction to the ventricles via the accessory pathway.[48,49] This process occurs through a loss of any modulating effect of AV nodal impulse conduction on the His-Purkinje system and the ventricular myocardium. If the accessory pathway has a short refractory period and is capable of very rapid conduction, there could be an acceleration of the ventricular response rate during atrial fibrillation and the potential precipitation of ventricular fibrillation (**Fig. 7**).[50]

RISK FACTORS FOR ARRHYTHMIA AGGRAVATION

An important concern in the use of antiarrhythmic drugs is identification of the patient at risk and recognition of factors associated with aggravation of arrhythmia. Although some risk factors have been identified, most proarrhythmic events occur in the absence of any recognized risk factors. Moreover, most risk factors apply in relatively circumscribed clinical situations. Aggravation with one antiarrhythmic drug does not predict this complication with any other drug, even if it is of the same class or subclass.[1]

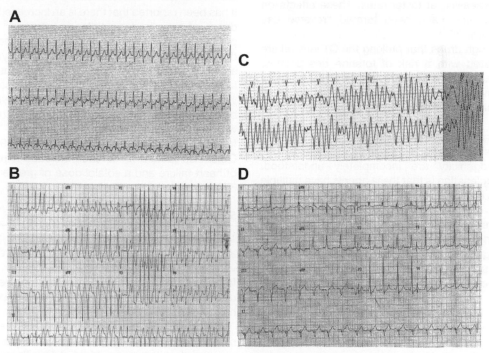

Fig. 7. Verapamil-induced ventricular fibrillation in a patient with atrial fibrillation associated with Wolff-Parkinson-White syndrome. (*A*) The patient initially presented with a rapid supraventricular tachycardia at a rate of 280 bpm. Adenosine was administered, as the etiology of the arrhythmia was not certain, although with a rate of 280 bpm the etiology can only be atrial flutter with 1:1 AV conduction. (*B*) Shortly after the administration of adenosine the rhythm became irregular, with an average rate of 250 bpm, although there were rates that were more than 300 bpm; this is atrial fibrillation. Noted is variability of the QRS complex duration and morphology. Of importance, there is no relationship between rate and QRS complex width. Therefore, this is not atrial fibrillation with rate-related aberration but is rather atrial fibrillation associated with Wolff-Parkinson-White. However, this was not recognized. (*C*) As it was not recognized that the atrial fibrillation was associated with Wolff-Parkinson-White, the patient was treated with intravenous verapamil in an attempt to slow the ventricular response rate. Within 5 minutes of initiation of this drug, the patient developed ventricular fibrillation that required cardiopulmonary resuscitation and defibrillation. (*D*) After successful resuscitation, a 12-lead ECG was obtained showing a typical pattern of Wolff-Parkinson-White syndrome.

Risk factors for the development of arrhythmia aggravation that have been defined include QT interval prolongation, elevated serum drug levels, electrolyte abnormalities, left ventricular dysfunction especially when there is clinical heart failure, structural heart disease, a history of a sustained ventricular tachyarrhythmia, and the presence of myocardial ischemia.

Electrocardiographic Changes

Torsade des pointes resulting from class IA or class III antiarrhythmic drugs is defined as polymorphic ventricular tachycardia associated with marked prolongation of the QT interval as well as increased homogeneity of repolarization, resulting in QT dispersion. With the use of antiarrhythmic drugs, that is, an acquired prolonged QT syndrome, the prolongation of repolarization and the QT interval is rate related, being more pronounced at slower heart rates or with pauses, and decreasing at faster rates. These effects on repolarization have been termed "reverse use dependent."[35,36]

Although drugs that prolong the QT interval are associated with a risk of torsade des pointes, amiodarone[40–42] and dronedarone,[51,52] class III antiarrhythmic agents, are an exception because the incidence of torsade des pointes with these agents is exceptionally low, despite the fact that they significantly prolong the QT interval. The electrophysiologic effects responsible for the low arrhythmogenicity are incompletely understood. One explanation is that these agents have multiple effects in the heart, including potassium, sodium, β, and calcium channel blockade. As previously indicated these agents do not exhibit reverse use dependency. Another explanation is that the heterogeneity of action potential duration and ventricular repolarization or QT dispersion is considerably less in patients treated with these agents, especially at slow heart rates.[43] It has been observed that the only cases of torsade des pointes with amiodarone occur whenever another drug that prolongs the QT interval is given along with amiodarone.[40,41]

There are, however, no changes on the surface ECG that predict other types of arrhythmia aggravation. Many antiarrhythmic drugs alter the QRS or QT intervals to some degree, but this represents a pharmacologic effect of these drugs and not toxicity. The class I agent slows conduction and therefore can prolong the QRS duration. As indicated earlier, this is more obvious at higher heart rates due to the use-dependent effects of these agents, that is, the slowing of conduction is more pronounced at higher heart rates.

Serum Drug Levels

Toxic blood levels of the antiarrhythmic drugs may be associated with the occurrence of a new tachyarrhythmia or bradyarrhythmia. However, the majority of proarrhythmic events occur with therapeutic blood levels.

Electrolyte Abnormalities

Electrolyte abnormalities, especially hypokalemia and perhaps hypomagnesemia (especially when associated with significant bradycardia), may be responsible for arrhythmia aggravation under certain conditions. These abnormalities have been associated with an increased tendency of patients taking quinidine to develop torsade des pointes. However, serum electrolyte levels are normal in the majority of cases of drug-induced arrhythmia aggravation.

Possible Importance of Gender

It has been reported that there is an increased incidence of torsade des pointes in women.[30–32] In one study of 322 cases of torsade des pointes due to therapy with a class IA or III antiarrhythmic agent, women constituted 70% of the cases,[30] independent of the type of heart disease, left ventricular function, or nature of the arrhythmia being treated. In a review of 3135 patients treated with sotalol, torsade des pointes was more frequent in women than men (4.1% vs 1.9%).[31] Other risk factors for torsade included a history of heart failure and a sotalol dose of greater than 320 mg/d.

Structural Heart Disease

There is a strong correlation between arrhythmic aggravation and a significantly reduced left ventricular function, a history of clinical heart failure (risk ratio 2.3), a history of sustained ventricular tachyarrhythmia (risk ratio 3.4), and structural heart disease (risk ratio 2–3).[7,53,54]

The presence of heart failure can alter the myocardial distribution of antiarrhythmic agents, resulting in inhomogeneity of drug effects.[55] In addition, heart failure and diastolic dysfunction lead to an increase in myocardial wall stress, resulting in stretch of myocardial fibers.[56] This process causes a reduction in action potential duration and refractoriness, and an increase in automaticity. These factors can interact with antiarrhythmic drug action.

Patients with coronary artery disease and active ischemia may also be at an increased risk for arrhythmia aggravation, as suggested by the result of the CAST trial.[5] This trial evaluated antiarrhythmic drug therapy (encainide, flecainide, or moricizine) in 2309 patients with a recent myocardial infarction who had asymptomatic or mild symptomatic PVC. Compared with placebo, encainide and flecainide were associated with a significant increase in arrhythmic death or nonfatal sudden cardiac arrest (1.5% vs 4.5%, relative risk 3.6). The increase in mortality associated with these 2 agents was observed in all patient groups. However, it was especially high in patients with a previous myocardial infarction and in those presenting with a subendocardial infarction (risk ratio 3.4). The increased risk in this group was equivalent to that observed in those with more severe disease, substantial left ventricular dysfunction, and a history of serious ventricular arrhythmia.

The increased mortality and late proarrhythmia observed with these agents has been hypothesized to result from the interactions between these drugs and myocardial ischemia.[7,57] Ongoing or even transient overt or silent myocardial ischemia may modify the underlying myocardial substrate and convert stable myocardium into unstable and potentially arrhythmogenic tissue, capable of generating and supporting reentrant arrhythmia. The use of an antiarrhythmic drug may further enhance this potential and increase the possibility of arrhythmia aggravation.

Although the most likely cause of the increased number of sudden deaths seen in CAST was a ventricular tachyarrhythmia, another possible explanation is the occurrence of a serious bradyarrhythmia, a result of the potent effects of these agents on the conduction system.

Proarrhythmia and Ischemia

Complex interactions among myocardial ischemia, metabolic abnormalities, and antiarrhythmic drugs provide the ideal milieu for proarrhythmic initiation.[58]

Alteration in blood flow. Ischemia results in spatial heterogeneity of blood flow between ischemic and nonischemic tissue.[59] The net effect is a marked heterogeneity of oxygen supply to all areas of the myocardium, including the ischemic area. The disparity in blood flow to even small areas causes marked differences in the degree of myocardial ischemia, and the resultant effects on local tissue pH (which decreases with ischemia) and on extracellular potassium levels (which increase with ischemia). Ischemia also produces a disparity of blood flow to the epicardial, myocardial, and endocardial layers within a region.[60] Blood flow to the endocardium is most significantly impaired. As a result, the degree of ischemia and its effect are more pronounced in this layer. Because the Purkinje fiber network is located within the endocardium, ischemia at this site is more likely to disrupt impulse conduction and myocardial activation.

Cellular and electrophysiologic alterations. Alterations of tissue potassium concentration and pH resulting from ischemia each independently produce changes in local myocardial electrophysiologic properties.[58] As ischemia is nonuniform, these changes are heterogeneous:

1. The resting membrane potential becomes less negative
2. Myocardial conduction velocity slows
3. Activation time of the ventricular myocardium lengthens.

The concentration of extracellular potassium in the center of the ischemic zone is significantly higher than the concentration at the margins of this zone. There is also significant inhomogeneity in extracellular potassium levels at different tissue depths within the ischemic myocardium.[61] The magnitude of the electrophysiologic changes parallel the changes in the potassium concentrations.

Interaction between ischemia and antiarrhythmic drugs. The interaction between the physiologic effects of antiarrhythmic drugs and the electrophysiologic, metabolic, and drug distribution changes resulting from ischemia may enhance the initiation and maintenance of ventricular arrhythmia.[62,63] The nonuniform reductions in blood flow produce differences in regional distribution, clearance, and resultant tissue concentrations of antiarrhythmic drugs, producing an inhomogeneity of electrophysiologic properties even in the absence of ischemia. Moreover, there is further augmentation of this inhomogeneity in the presence of ischemia, which may enhance the potential for arrhythmia aggravation.

Therefore, the electrophysiologic characteristics of the myocardium are altered by an interaction between differences in the regional concentration of antiarrhythmic drugs and regional differences in pH and potassium concentrations as a result of ischemic heterogeneity. These various influences can affect membrane conduction properties and refractoriness.

Sympathetic Stimulation and Antiarrhythmic Drugs

An additional factor that can further affect the action of antiarrhythmic drugs and enhance the potential for arrhythmic aggravation is sympathetic stimulation and the action of circulating catecholamines.[64] Sympathetic stimulation can offset or negate the action of antiarrhythmic drugs by enhancing impulse conduction velocity and shortening membrane refractoriness. The changes resulting from sympathetic stimulation may be disparate between normal and ischemic tissue, particularly when there are differences in local drug concentration and differences in tissue pH and local potassium levels. This process can further alter the membrane inhomogeneity, enhancing the potential for arrhythmic aggravation.

REFERENCES

1. Velebit V, Podrid PJ, Cohen B, et al. Aggravation and provocation of ventricular arrhythmia by antiarrhythmic drugs. Circulation 1982;65:886.
2. Keren A, Tzivoni D, Gavish D, et al. Etiology and warning signs and therapy of torsade des pointes—a study of ten patients. Circulation 1961; 54:1167.
3. Zipes DP. Proarrhythmic effects of antiarrhythmic drugs. Am J Cardiol 1967;59:26E.
4. Minardo JD, Heger JJ, Miles WM, et al. Clinical characteristics of patients with ventricular fibrillation during antiarrhythmic drug therapy. N Engl J Med 1986;319:257.
5. Echt DS, Liebson PR, Mitchell LB, et al. Mortality and morbidity in patients receiving encainide, flecainide, or placebo. The cardiac arrhythmia suppression trial. N Engl J Med 1991;324:781.
6. Morganroth S, Horowitz LN. Flecainide—its proarrhythmic effect and expected changes on the surface electrocardiogram. Am J Cardiol 1984;53:893.
7. Podrid PJ, Lampert S, Graboys TB, et al. Aggravation of arrhythmia by antiarrhythmic drugs—incidence and predictors. Am J Cardiol 1987;59:38E.
8. Stanton MS, Prystowsky EN, Fineberg NS, et al. Arrhythmogenic effects of antiarrhythmic drugs. A study of 506 patients treated for ventricular tachycardia or fibrillation. J Am Coll Cardiol 1989;14:209.
9. Poser RF, Podrid PJ, Lombardi F, et al. Aggravation of arrhythmia induced with antiarrhythmic drugs during electrophysiologic testing. Am Heart J 1985;110:9—16.
10. Rae AP, Kay HR, Horowitz LN, et al. Proarrhythmic effects of antiarrhythmic drugs in patients with malignant ventricular arrhythmias evaluated by electrophysiologic testing. J Am Coll Cardiol 1988;12: 131—9.
11. Rinkenberger RL, Prystowsky EN, Jackman WN, et al. Drug conversion of nonsustained ventricular tachycardia to sustained ventricular tachycardia during serial electrophysiologic studies: identification of drugs that exacerbate tachycardia and potential mechanisms. Am Heart J 1982;103:177.
12. Bollmann A, Husser D, Cannom DS. Antiarrhythmic drugs in patients with implantable cardioverter-defibrillators. Am J Cardiovasc Drugs 2005;5:371—8.
13. Santini M, Pandozi C, Ricci R. Combining antiarrhythmic drugs and implantable devices therapy: benefits and outcome. J Interv Card Electrophysiol 2000;4(Suppl 1):65—8.
14. Takanaka C, Lee JK, Nonokawa M, et al. Frequency dependent effects of class I antiarrhythmic agents studied in patients with implanted pacemakers. Pacing Clin Electrophysiol 1994;17:2100.
15. Sadanaga T, Ogawa S, Okada Y, et al. Clinical evaluation of the use-dependent QRS prolongation and the reverse use-dependent QT prolongation of class I and class III antiarrhythmic agents and their value in predicting efficacy. Am Heart J 1993;126:114.
16. Kidwell GA, Greenspon AJ, Greenberg RM, et al. Use-dependent prolongation of ventricular tachycardia cycle length by type I antiarrhythmic drugs in humans. Circulation 1993;87:118.
17. Berns E, Rinkenberger PL, Jeany M, et al. Clinical efficacy and safety of flecainide acetate on the treatment of primary atrial tachycardias. Am J Cardiol 1987;59:1337.
18. Falk RH. Flecainide induced ventricular tachycardia and fibrillation in patient treated for atrial fibrillation. Ann Intern Med 1989;111:107.
19. Falk RH. Proarrhythmic responses to atrial antiarrhythmic therapy. In: Falk RH, Podrid PJ, editors. Atrial fibrillation: mechanisms and management. 2nd edition. Philadelphia: Lippincott Raven; 1997. p. 371—96.
20. Podrid PJ, Anderson JL. Safety and tolerability of long-term propafenone therapy for supraventricular tachyarrhythmias. The Propafenone Multicenter Study Group. Am J Cardiol 1996;78:430.
21. McKibbin JW, Pocock N, Barlow JM, et al. Sotalol, hypokalemia, syncope and torsade de pointes. Br Heart J 1984;51:157.
22. Shantsila E, Watson T, Lip GY. Drug induced QT-interval prolongation and proarrhythmic risk in the treatment of atrial arrhythmias. Europace 2007;9: 37—44, iv.
23. El-Sherif N, Turitto G. Torsade de pointes. Curr Opin Cardiol 2003;18:6.
24. Moss AJ. Long QT syndrome. JAMA 2003;289:2041.
25. Kurita T, Ohe T, Marui N, et al. Bradycardia-induced abnormal QT prolongation in patients with complete atrioventricular block with torsades de pointes. Am J Cardiol 1992;69:628.
26. Furushima H, Niwano S, Chinushi M, et al. Relation between bradycardia dependent long QT syndrome and QT prolongation by disopyramide in humans. Heart 1998;79:56.
27. Halkin A, Roth A, Lurie I, et al. Pause-dependent torsade de pointes following acute myocardial

infarction. A variant of the acquired long QT syndrome. J Am Coll Cardiol 2001;38:1168.

28. Roden DM. Drug-induced prolongation of the QT interval. N Engl J Med 2004;350:1013.

29. Roden DM. Taking the "idio" out of "idiosyncratic": Predicting torsade des pointes. Pacing Clin Electrophysiol 1998;21:1029.

30. Wolbrette DL. Risk of proarrhythmia with class III antiarrhythmic agents: sex-based differences and other issues. Am J Cardiol 2003;91:39D–44D.

31. Makkar R, Fromm B, Steihman R, et al. Female gender as a risk factor for torsades de pointes associated with cardiovascular drugs. JAMA 1993;270: 2590.

32. Hreiche R, Morissette P, Turgeon J. Drug-induced long QT syndrome in women: review of current evidence and remaining gaps. Gend Med 2008;5: 124–35.

33. Tan H, Hou C, Lauer M, et al. Electrophysiologic mechanisms of the long QT interval syndromes and torsades de pointes. Ann Intern Med 1995; 122:701.

34. Yan GX, Wu Y, Liu T, et al. Phase 2 early afterdepolarization as a trigger of polymorphic ventricular tachycardia in acquired long-QT syndrome: direct evidence from intracellular recordings in the intact left ventricular wall. Circulation 2001;103:2851.

35. Hondeghem LM, Snyders DJ. Class III antiarrhythmic agents have a lot of potential but a long way to go. Reduced effectiveness and dangers of reverse use dependence. Circulation 1990;81:686.

36. Bárándi L, Virág L, Jost N, et al. Reverse rate-dependent changes are determined by baseline action potential duration in mammalian and human ventricular preparations. Basic Res Cardiol 2010; 105:315.

37. Hondeghem LM. QT prolongation is an unreliable predictor of ventricular arrhythmia. Heart Rhythm 2008;8:1210.

38. Singh BN. Antiarrhythmic actions of amiodarone: a profile of a paradoxical agent. Am J Cardiol 1996;78(4A):41.

39. Sun W, Sarma JS, Singh BN. Chronic and acute effects of dronedarone on the action potential of rabbit atrial muscle preparations: comparison with amiodarone. J Cardiovasc Pharmacol 2002;39(5): 677–84.

40. Hohnloser SH, Klingenheben T, Singh BN. Amiodarone-associated proarrhythmic effects. A review with special reference to torsades de pointes tachycardia. Ann Intern Med 1994;121:529.

41. Brown MA, Smith WM, Cubbe WF, et al. Amiodarone induced torsade de pointes. Eur Heart J 1986;7:234.

42. van Opstal JM, Schoenmakers M, Verduyn SC, et al. Chronic amiodarone evokes no torsade de pointes arrhythmias despite QT lengthening in an animal model of acquired long-QT syndrome. Circulation 2001;104:2722.

43. Drouin E, Lande G, Charpentier F. Amiodarone reduces transmural heterogeneity of repolarization in the human heart. J Am Coll Cardiol 1998;32:1063.

44. Tafreshi MJ, Rowles J. A review of the investigational antiarrhythmic agent dronedarone. J Cardiovasc Pharmacol Ther 2007;12(1):15–26.

45. Murduck CJ, Kyles AE, Yeung-Lai-Wah JA, et al. Atrial flutter in patients treated for atrial fibrillation with propafenone. Am J Cardiol 1990;66:755–7.

46. Feld GK, Chen PS, Nicod P, et al. Possible atrial proarrhythmic effects of class IC antiarrhythmic agents. Am J Cardiol 1990;66:378–83.

47. Marcus FI. The hazards of using type IC antiarrhythmic drugs for the treatment of paroxysmal atrial fibrillation. Am J Cardiol 1990;66:366–7.

48. McGovern B, Garan H, Ruskin JN. Precipitation of cardiac arrest by verapamil in patients with Wolff-Parkinson-White syndrome. Ann Intern Med 1986; 104:791–4.

49. Garratt C, Antionio A, Ward D, et al. Misuse of verapamil in pre-excited atrial fibrillation. Lancet 1989;1: 367–9.

50. Klein GJ, Bashore TM, Sellers TD, et al. Ventricular fibrillation in the Wolff-Parkinson-White syndrome. N Engl J Med 1979;301:1080–5.

51. Davy JM, Herold M, Hoglund C, et al. ERATO Study Investigators. Dronedarone for the control of ventricular rate in permanent atrial fibrillation: the Efficacy and safety of dRonedArone for the cOntrol of ventricular rate during atrial fibrillation (ERATO) study. Am Heart J 2008;156:527, e1–9.

52. Hohnloser SH, Crijns HJ, van Eickels M, et al. Effect of dronedarone on cardiovascular events in atrial fibrillation. N Engl J Med 2009;360:668–78.

53. Slater WS, Lampert S, Podrid PJ, et al. Clinical predictors of arrhythmia worsening by antiarrhythmic drugs. Am J Cardiol 1988;61:349–53.

54. Pratt CM, Eaton T, Frances M, et al. The inverse relationship between baseline left ventricular ejection fraction and outcome of antiarrhythmic drug therapy. A dangerous imbalance in the risk-benefit ratio. Am Heart J 1989;118:433–40.

55. Woosley RL, Echt DS, Roden DM. Effects of congestive heart failure on the pharmacokinetics and pharmacodynamics of antiarrhythmic drugs. Am J Cardiol 1986;57:25B–33B.

56. Dean JW, Lab MJ. Arrhythmia in heart failure. Role of mechanically induced changes in electrophysiology. Lancet 1989;1(98650):1309–12.

57. Podrid PJ, Fogel RI. Aggravation of arrhythmia by antiarrhythmic drugs and the important role of underlying ischemia. Am J Cardiol 1992;70:100–2.

58. Kagiyama Y, Hill JL, Gettes LS. Interaction of acidosis and increased extracellular potassium on action potential characteristics and conduction in

guinea pig ventricular muscle. Circ Res 1982;51: 614–23.

59. Marcus ML, Kerber RE, Erhardt JC, et al. Spatial and temporal heterogeneity of left ventricular perfusion in awake dogs. Am Heart J 1977;94:748–54.

60. Coggins DL, Flynn AE, Austin RE, et al. Nonuniform loss of regional flow reserve during myocardial ischemia in dogs. Circ Res 1990;67:253–64.

61. Hill JL, Gettes LS. Effects of acute coronary occlusion on local myocardial extracellular K+ activity in swine. Circulation 1980;61:768–78.

62. Nattel S, Pedersen DH, Zipes DP. Alterations in regional myocardial distribution and arrhythmogenic effects of aprindine produced by coronary occlusion in the dog. Cardiovasc Res 1981;15:80–5.

63. Elharrar V, Gaum WE, Zipes D. Effects of drugs on conduction delay and incidence of ventricular arrhythmias induced by acute occlusion in dogs. Am J Cardiol 1977;39:544–9.

64. Podrid PJ, Fuchs T, Candinas R. Role of the sympathetic nervous system in the genesis of ventricular arrhythmia. Circulation 1990;82(Suppl I):I103–13.

Advances in Antiarrhythmic Drug Therapy: New and Emerging Therapies

Arnold Pinter, MD, Paul Dorian, MD, MSc*

KEYWORDS

- Dronedarone • Vernakalant • Celivarone
- Upstream therapy • Gap junction

Despite major advances in nonpharmacologic therapy for arrhythmias in the past decades, there is still a substantial role for antiarrhythmic drug therapy, especially in the treatment of atrial fibrillation and ventricular tachycardia. The most effective antiarrhythmic drug is amiodarone, but its use is limited by extracardiac toxicity. One approach to the development of new antiarrhythmic drugs is to modify the amiodarone molecule, thus retaining its multichannel blocking action but reducing its toxicity. One such agent, dronedarone, was approved by the Food and Drug Administration (FDA) in 2009 for the reduction of cardiovascular hospitalization in patients with paroxysmal or persistent atrial fibrillation or atrial flutter, and associated cardiovascular risk factors. Another similar drug, celivarone, is being studied in a phase 3 clinical trial in patients with ventricular tachyarrhythmia and an implantable cardioverter defibrillator (ICD).

Another approach to the treatment of atrial fibrillation is to develop drugs that act primarily on atrial tissue by targeting ion channels that exist primarily in the atrium. Most of the recently approved antiarrhythmic drugs are potassium channel blockers (dofetilide, ibutilide), which have an important safety concern as they can cause torsade de pointes ventricular tachyarrhythmia due to prolongation of the QT interval. An atrially selective potassium channel blocker would overcome this

safety problem. One such agent, vernakalant, is being studied for the conversion of acute and persistent atrial fibrillation and flutter, and has been the subject of several phase 3 trials.

While ion channel blockers that exert their antiarrhythmic effect at the cellular level are still the mainstream of research, modification of cell-to-cell interaction (gap junctions) and the substrate of arrhythmias are other strategies being tested for arrhythmia management. For example, the development of atrial fibrillation potentially could be reduced by the prevention of atrial electroanatomic remodeling, the substrate of atrial fibrillation, with the use of so-called upstream therapies such as rennin-angiotensin system antagonists, statins, and n-3 polyunsaturated fatty acids.

This article reviews dronedarone, which is already approved and available; antiarrhythmic agents that are the most advanced in development; and upstream therapy for atrial fibrillation.

NEW ANTIARRHYTHMIC DRUG THERAPY
Dronedarone

General overview

Dronedarone is a noniodinated benzofuran derivative that was approved in 2009 by the United States FDA and by the European Medicines Agency for the treatment of patients with atrial fibrillation. Dronedarone is a modified amiodarone

Disclosure: Arnold Pinter: No conflict of interest; Paul Dorian: Received consulting fees and research grants from Sanofi-Aventis, Boehringer Ingelheim, Astellas, Cardiome, and Astra Zeneca.
Division of Cardiology, St Michael's Hospital, University of Toronto, 30 Bond Street, Toronto, ON M5B 1W8, Canada
* Corresponding author.
E-mail address: dorianp@smh.toronto.on.ca

Card Electrophysiol Clin 2 (2010) 471–478
doi:10.1016/j.ccep.2010.06.005
1877-9182/10/$ — see front matter © 2010 Publsiched by Elsevier Inc.

molecule without the iodine, which is considered the main cause of the thyroid side effect and pulmonary toxicity of amiodarone, and with the addition of a methane-sulfonyl group. Similarly to amiodarone, dronedarone blocks multiple ion channels including both the rapidly activating and the slowly activating delayed-rectifier potassium currents, the inward rectifier potassium current, the acetylcholine-activated potassium current, the sodium current, and the L-type calcium current, and has an antiadrenergic effect.[1]

Dronedarone absorption increases 2- to 3-fold when it is taken with food. Therefore, it is recommended that it is taken with meals. Dronedarone undergoes first-pass metabolism that reduces its bioavailability to 15%. Because it is less lipophilic than amiodarone, it does not require loading doses and has a shorter half-life of approximately 24 hours. The recommended daily dose of 400 mg twice a day results in steady-state plasma concentrations of 85 to 150 ng/mL in 7 days.[2] Elimination is mostly non-renal. Dronedarone partially inhibits the tubular transportation of creatinine, hence it can increase the serum creatinine level by 10% to 20%, but does not reduce glomerular filtration.[3]

Dronedarone is both an inhibitor of and a substrate for CYP3A4. It should not be coadministered with potent CYP3A4 inhibitors such as macrolide antibiotics, ketoconazole, and other antifungals or protease inhibitors because the dronedarone exposure may increase by as much as 25-fold.[2] If dronedarone is used in combination with verapamil or diltiazem, which are moderate inhibitors of CYP3A4, lower doses of concomitant drugs should be considered to avoid bradycardia or conduction block.[2] Through the inhibition of CYP3A4, dronedarone can increase simvastatin levels by 2- to 4-fold, increasing the risk of statin-induced myopathy. Dronedarone also increases digoxin level by 1.7- to 2.5-fold, therefore close monitoring of the digoxin level, and possible dose reduction is suggested.[2]

Clinical trials with dronedarone

Rhythm control The dose-finding study of the Dronedarone Atrial Fibrillation Study after Electrical Cardioversion (DAFNE) randomized 270 patients with persistent atrial fibrillation to dronedarone versus placebo 400 mg twice a day, 600 mg twice a day, or 800 mg twice a day.[4] There was a dose-dependent conversion to sinus rhythm in 5.8%, 8.2%, and 14.8% of patients in the 3 treatment groups, compared with 3.1% in the placebo group. During the 6 months follow-up, dronedarone 400 mg twice a day but not the other 2 doses delayed the time to first recurrence of atrial fibrillation. At the end of follow-up, 35% of patients taking dronedarone 400 mg twice a day were in sinus rhythm compared with 10% in the placebo group. Based on this dose-ranging study, the 400 mg twice a day dronedarone dose was used in later studies.

The identical trials of the American-Australian-African Trial with Dronedarone in Atrial Fibrillation or Flutter Patients for the Maintenance of Sinus Rhythm (ADONIS) and the European Trial in Atrial Fibrillation or Flutter Patients Receiving Dronedarone for the Maintenance of Sinus Rhythm (EURIDIS) used the first recurrence of atrial fibrillation as their primary end point. The 2 trials were reported together.[5] Overall, 1237 patients were randomized in a 2:1 ratio to receive dronedarone 400 mg twice a day or placebo. Although the majority of the patients had a history of structural heart disease, the mean left ventricular function was preserved (58%), 83% of the patients had no history of heart failure, and no patient had a history of severe heart failure. The mean age in the 2 studies was 63 years. The prespecified pooled analysis showed that dronedarone was more effective than placebo in maintaining sinus rhythm, with a median time to first recurrence of atrial fibrillation of 116 days versus 53 days in the placebo group. This measure of drug efficacy, though commonly used, has an uncertain clinical importance. A post hoc analysis showed a 27% relative risk reduction of hospitalization or death in the dronedarone group compared with the placebo group.

Rate control During atrial fibrillation recurrences in the ADONIS and EURIDIS trials, the ventricular rate was reduced by 10 to 15 beats per minute (bpm) by dronedarone compared with placebo.[5] The Efficacy and Safety of Dronedarone for Control of Ventricular Rate (ERATO) study randomized 174 elderly patients with permanent atrial fibrillation and a resting heart rate of 80 bpm or more despite rate control therapy using conventional atrioventricular node blocking agents.[6] The addition of dronedarone to conventional rate-controlling agents reduced the ventricular rate by a mean of 11.7 bpm at rest and 24.5 bpm during exercise, but it did not translate into improved exercise tolerance.

Mortality and morbidity The Assess the Efficacy of Dronedarone for the Prevention of Cardiovascular Hospitalization or Death from Any Cause in Patients with Atrial Fibrillation/Atrial Flutter (ATHENA) trial used first hospitalization due to cardiovascular causes or death as the primary end points.[7] The ATHENA trial was a large study of 4628 elderly (mean age 72 years) moderate- to high-risk patients (all patients had at least one cardiovascular risk factor) with paroxysmal or persistent atrial fibrillation and without severe heart failure. Patients were randomized to drone-darone 400 mg twice daily or placebo, and were followed for a mean of 21 months. Dronedarone significantly reduced the primary end point by 24% (31.9% in the dronedarone group vs 39.4% in the placebo group, $P<.001$). The difference was mainly a result of reduced hospitalization for atrial fibrillation, but dronedarone also significantly reduced nonatrial fibrillation—related cardiovascular hospitalizations by 14%. Also, dronedarone reduced the primary end point by 26% in "perma-nent" atrial fibrillation patients. There was a signifi-cant reduction in cardiovascular mortality (2.7% in the dronedarone group vs 3.9% in the placebo group, $P = .03$), but no significant difference in total mortality was observed (5.0% in the drone-darone group vs 6.0% in the placebo group, $P = .18$). Of note, dronedarone reduced the incidence of stroke by 34% ($P = .027$), which cannot be completely attributed to the reduction of atrial fibrillation because the trend was observed in patients with atrial fibrillation at every visit and was observed even among patients already receiving antithrombotic therapy.[8] A potential explanation advanced by the investiga-tors of that study is the modest blood pressure reduction observed with dronedarone therapy, because even small reductions in blood pressure have been reported to significantly reduce stroke.

The biggest concern with dronedarone is its potential risk in patients with severe and/or acute heart failure. The Antiarrhythmic Trial with Drone-darone in Moderate-to-Severe Congestive Heart Failure Evaluating Morbidity Decrease (ANDROMEDA) study compared dronedarone with placebo in patients with or without a history of atrial fibrillation but with severe left ventricular dysfunction who were hospitalized for worsening heart failure at the time of randomization. The study was prematurely terminated by the Data Safety and Monitoring Board after enrolling 627 patients (the study planned to include 1000 patients) because of increased mortality in the active treatment group (8.1%) compared with the placebo group (3.8%).[9] Most of the mortality events occurred within the first 90 days of treat-ment. On the other hand, 20% of the patients in the ATHENA trial had a history of heart failure and were in New York Heart Association Class II or III at baseline, and subgroup analysis did not indicate an increased risk from dronedarone for the primary outcome for those patients, nor for patients with a left ventricular ejection fraction of

less than 35%. The main difference between the ANDROMEDA population and the heart failure patients in ATHENA appears to be the acuteness of the heart failure. Thus, dronedarone is not rec-ommended for patients with acute or recently worsening heart failure, and the FDA has ordered a boxed warning on the label in this regard. Caution should also be exercised when using dronedarone in patients with chronic heart failure.

Side effects and tolerability In these medium-term follow-up trials outlined, dronedarone did not exhibit pulmonary or thyroid toxicity, support-ing the concept of changes being made to the amiodarone molecule. Regarding side effects, bradycardia, QT prolongation, diarrhea, nausea, and rash occurred significantly more frequently among patients taking dronedarone than among patients taking placebo.[7] Only one case of torsade de pointes ventricular tachycardia was noted out of 3282 patients treated with dronedarone.

Comparative efficacy There was only one trial conducted that compared dronedarone with another antiarrhythmic drug. The Efficacy and Safety of Dronedarone versus Amiodarone for the Maintenance of Sinus Rhythm in Patients with AF (DIONYSOS) randomized 504 patients with persistent atrial fibrillation to dronedarone 400 mg twice a day or amiodarone 600 mg daily for 28 days, followed by 200 mg a day. Preliminary results showed that the composite primary end point of atrial fibrillation recurrence or study drug discontinuation for intolerance or lack of efficacy occurred significantly less frequently in the amio-darone treatment group than in the dronedarone group (55.3% vs 73.9%, $P = .001$) after a mean follow-up of 7 months.[2,10] In terms of side effects, gastrointestinal side effects (diarrhea) were more common in the dronedarone group, whereas cardiac adverse effects such as bradycardia or QT prolongation as well as thyroid, skin, ocular, and neurologic side effects were less common in this group.

EMERGING ANTIARRHYTHMIC DRUG THERAPY
Vernakalant

One of the main disadvantages of repolarization-delaying (Class III) antiarrhythmic agents to be used for the treatment of atrial fibrillation is the unwanted effect of QT prolongation and risk of torsade de pointes ventricular tachyarrhythmia. A novel concept for antiarrhythmic drugs is atrially selective potassium channel blockade, which is based on the observation that a major repolarizing current in atrial myocardium, the ultrarapid potassium current (I_{Kur}) (as well as the acetylcholine activated potassium current), is little expressed in the ventricular myocardium. Vernakalant (RSD1235) is the most developed example of a relatively atrially selective antiarrhythmic agent. Its intravenous form has completed phase 3 studies, although a further study is ongoing (ACT V, ClinicalTrials.gov Identifier: NCT00989001), which will need to be completed before application for approval by the FDA will be submitted. Vernakalant is also bioavailable by oral administration. A dose-ranging study of an oral formulation of vernakalant to assess its safety and efficacy in prevention of recurrent atrial fibrillation in patients requiring cardioversion has been completed but not yet reported (ClinicalTrials.gov Identifier: NCT00526136). Vernakalant mainly blocks the ultrarapid potassium channel but also blocks other ion currents such as the transient outward current and the inward sodium current. In healthy adults, intravenous vernakalant hydrochloride, 4 mg/kg over 10 min followed by 1 mg/kg/h for 35 min, prolonged atrial effective refractory period by a mean of 25 milliseconds without significantly prolonging the ventricular effective refractory period.[11] There was a small but significant prolongation of atrioventricular nodal refractoriness, and the sinus node recovery time also increased.

Three randomized, placebo-controlled, medium-sized studies involving 150 to 416 patients with paroxysmal or persistent atrial fibrillation or flutter, called the Atrial Arrhythmia Conversion Trials (ACT), assessed the efficacy and safety of intravenous vernakalant in various clinical settings.[12–14] One of those studies included patients with atrial fibrillation or flutter following open heart surgery,[13] whereas the other 2 studies involved patients presenting with recent onset atrial fibrillation of 3 hours' to 7 days' duration. In the 3 completed studies, vernakalant, 3 mg/kg intravenously, with a possible additional 2 mg/kg intravenous dose, had a conversion rate of approximately 50% with a median time to conversion of about 10 minutes compared with a 4% to 14% conversion rate with placebo. vernakalant was most effective for atrial fibrillation of less than 3 days' duration (conversion efficacy of 70%–80%), while only converting 8% of patients with atrial fibrillation of longer than a week. It was also relatively ineffective in patients with atrial flutter, with a conversion rate of less than 10%. Vernakalant was well tolerated, the most common side effects being dysgeusia and nausea. Less ventricular arrhythmia occurred than in the placebo group (9.0% vs 17.4%), with no torsade de pointes ventricular tachycardia reported.

Celivarone

Celivarone (SSR149744C) is a noniodinated benzofuran derivative similar to dronedarone, with multiple channel–blocking properties. A phase 2 dose-ranging study in 673 patients showed a borderline efficacy of preventing recurrence of atrial fibrillation at 90 days by celivarone 50 mg a day orally (recurrence rate 52% in the 50-mg celivarone group vs 67% in the placebo group, $P = .055$).[15] A pilot study of 153 patients with an implantable defibrillator receiving celivarone 100 mg or 300 mg once daily or placebo showed that celivarone 300 mg a day reduces appropriate ICD therapy by 46% compared with placebo (ClinicalTrials.gov Identifier: NCT00232297). At present, celivarone is being investigated in the prevention of ICD therapies for ventricular arrhythmias in a larger-scale study (ClinicalTrials.gov Identifier: NCT00993382).

Ranolazine

Ranolazine, like amiodarone, was developed as an antianginal agent, but later it was found to have blocking effects on multiple ion channels including the late sodium current, both the rapidly activating and the slowly activating delayed-rectifier potassium currents, and the L-type calcium current.[16] The use-dependent blockade of sodium channels by ranolazine is atrially selective in an animal model, which would make it particularly useful in the treatment of atrial fibrillation.[17] The Metabolic Efficiency with Ranolazine for Less Ischemia in Non ST-Elevation Acute Coronary Syndrome Thrombolysis in Myocardial Infarction 36 (MERLIN-TIMI36) large randomized trial showed a significant decrease in the incidence of new-onset atrial fibrillation, supraventricular tachycardia, and ventricular tachycardia in patients with acute coronary syndrome.[18] The effect of ranolazine on arrhythmias and microvolt T-wave alternans is currently being investigated in patients with significant left ventricular dysfunction (ClinicalTrials.gov Identifier: NCT00998218).

Other Agents

Approximately a half dozen other antiarrhythmic drugs are at various stages of clinical investigation, but the journey to approval is long and uncertain. Recently, the further development of 2 drugs, azimilide and tedisamil, was halted despite completed phase 2 and phase 3 clinical trials showing moderate efficacy.

New Mechanisms of Action to Treat Arrhythmias

Gap junction modulators

Gap junctions are a critical part of cell-to-cell electrical coupling. Connexin40 is expressed in atrial myocardium, connexin43 is present in both the atrial and ventricular myocardium, and connexin45 is expressed in connective tissue. Alteration of gap junction kinetics, which can occur during ischemia or acidosis, or a change in the distribution of gap junctions slows conduction and can be arrhythmogenic.[19] Rotigaptide (ZP123), a peptide analogue of a gap junction protein, improves conduction and suppresses atrial fibrillation in the setting of acute ischemia in an animal model but not in a model of congestive heart failure or a model of atrial remodeling due to atrial tachypacing.[20] In a dog model of atrial fibrillation, rotigaptide reduced the inducibility and duration of atrial fibrillation only in subjects without extensive atrial remodeling.[21]

However, rotigaptide and other peptide analogues have poor oral bioavailability because of poor absorption and presystemic degradation, which is a significant obstacle for their potential use as an oral antiarrhythmic drug. A phase 2 study looking at the acute effect of rotigaptide on the inducibility of ventricular tachyarrhythmia in patients with coronary artery disease has been completed (ClinicalTrials.gov Identifier: NCT00137332).

Upstream Therapy: Primary Prevention of Atrial Fibrillation

Because controlling atrial fibrillation is difficult once it has developed, research has also focused on the primary prevention of atrial fibrillation. The so-called upstream therapy is directed toward the underlying substrate, which is atrial remodeling.[22] Mechanisms such as electrical remodeling, oxidative stress, tissue inflammation, and fibrosis contribute to the atrial changes that favor the occurrence and maintenance of atrial fibrillation.

Renin-Angiotensin System Antagonists

Substudies of multiple randomized, double-blind, placebo-controlled trials showed a reduction in the incidence of new atrial fibrillation by an angiotensin-converting enzyme (ACE) inhibitor as compared with placebo in patients with left ventricular dysfunction. In the Trandolapril Cardiac Evaluation (TRACE) trial, trandolapril reduced the relative risk of developing atrial fibrillation over a follow-up period of 2.4 years by 55% (2.8% vs 5.3%), while enalapril treatment was associated with a 72%

relative risk reduction (5.4% vs 24%) over a follow-up period of 2.9 years in the Studies Of Left Ventricular Dysfunction (SOLVD) trial.[23,24] Similar findings were reported in the Valsartan Heart Failure Trial (Val-HeFT) (with valsartan) and the *Candesartan* in Heart failure Assessment of Reduction in Mortality and morbidity (CHARM) trial (with candesartan). The Losartan Intervention For Endpoint reduction (LIFE) trial, which compared losartan with atenolol for the treatment of hypertension with left ventricular hypertrophy, showed a lower incidence of atrial fibrillation in the angiotensin receptor blocker (ARB) arm despite there being no difference in the blood pressure control.[25] However, other studies (CAPP, STOP-2) did not demonstrate a reduction in new-onset atrial fibrillation with ACE inhibitor therapy as compared with therapy with β-blockers, calcium channel blockers, or diuretics in patients with hypertension. Of importance, all these trials involved patients who had an indication for an ACE inhibitor because of hypertension, previous myocardial infarction, or left ventricular dysfunction. Among patients with high cardiovascular risk (presence of coronary, peripheral, or cerebrovascular disease, or diabetes with end-organ damage) in the Telmisartan Randomized Assessment Study in ACE-intoleraNt subjects with cardiovascular Disease (TRASCEND) trial, telmisartan did not reduce the incidence of new atrial fibrillation as compared with placebo (6.3% vs 6.4%, $P = .83$), while there was no difference between telmisartan and ramipril in the development of new-onset atrial fibrillation in a similar patient population in the ONgoing Telmisartan Alone and in combination with Ramipril Global Endpoint Trial (ONTARGET).[26,27]

In terms of secondary prophylaxis of atrial fibrillation, irbesartan added to amiodarone was better than amiodarone alone in maintaining sinus rhythm during a 2-month follow-up in patients with persistent atrial fibrillation following electrical cardioversion.[28] In a small study of 62 patients with lone atrial fibrillation and no hypertension or any other indication for an ACE inhibitor, ramipril, as compared with placebo, was associated with a lower incidence of Holter documented atrial fibrillation recurrence.[29] On the other hand, treatment with an ACE inhibitor or an ARB was not associated with a reduced recurrence of atrial fibrillation during a short-term follow-up in the Atrial Fibrillation Follow-up Investigation of Rhythm Management (AFFIRM) trial in patients without left ventricular dysfunction or congestive heart failure.[30]

Overall, ACE inhibitor/ARB therapy appears to have a favorable effect on preventing atrial fibrillation mainly in patients who already have an indication for that therapy (most notably, patients with heart failure).

Statins

The first study to show a reduction in new-onset atrial fibrillation with statin therapy was a moderate-size observational study of 449 patients with coronary artery disease, which suggested a 52% relative risk reduction in the development of atrial fibrillation over a 5-year follow-up.[31] Since then, a series of retrospective studies have been reported with conflicting results. In a large study of 13,783 patients with coronary artery disease, statin therapy was associated with a reduction in new-onset atrial fibrillation only in patients with congestive heart failure.[32] In the ADVANCENT Heart Failure Registry of 25,268 patients, lipid-lowering drug use (mainly statins) reduced the odds of atrial fibrillation more than ACE inhibitor/ARB therapy.[33] Secondary prevention data is even more limited. A small, retrospective study of patients with lone atrial fibrillation suggested a reduced recurrence of atrial fibrillation with statin therapy following cardioversion, while a small, prospective, open-label study of statin therapy 3 weeks before and 6 weeks after cardioversion did not reduce the recurrence of atrial fibrillation. Seven studies on prevention of the recurrence of atrial fibrillation after thoracic surgery indicate that statin therapy initiated before surgery reduces the risk of postoperative atrial fibrillation.[22]

Overall, data supporting the use of statins in the primary or secondary prevention of atrial fibrillation are limited and are obtained mainly from retrospective studies, and the results are sometimes conflicting. Just as for ACE inhibitors/ARBs, most studies involved patients who already had an indication for statin therapy.

n-3 Polyunsaturated Fatty Acids

n-3 Polyunsaturated fatty acids (PUFAs) have the potential to prevent atrial fibrillation because of their possible anti-inflammatory, antifibrotic, and antiarrhythmic effects.[34] Using surrogate measures of ventricular arrhythmogenicity (microvolt T-wave alternans, signal-averaged electrocardiogram, heart rate variability) in a small study of 44 patients with idiopathic dilated cardiomyopathy, administration of PUFAs resulted in favorable changes in those surrogate parameters compared with placebo.[35]

Fish oil, which is an important source of PUFAs, was first evaluated prospectively for the prevention of new-onset atrial fibrillation in 4815 elderly patients in the Cardiovascular Health Study.[36]

The investigators showed that consumption of tuna or other broiled or baked fish 1 to 4 times per week, as compared with intake less than once per month, was associated with a 28% lower risk of new-onset atrial fibrillation over a 12-year follow-up. However, other cohort studies did not support this finding. A small, randomized, open-label study of perioperative PUFA treatment in patients undergoing coronary bypass surgery showed a reduction in the incidence of postoperative atrial fibrillation compared with no therapy.[37] However, a recent randomized, double-blind, placebo-controlled trial did not confirm this finding.[38] A phase 3 placebo-controlled trial assessing the efficacy of PUFAs for the maintenance of sinus rhythm in patients with persistent atrial fibrillation is under way (ClinicalTrials.gov Identifier: NCT00597220).

SUMMARY

The search continues for the ideal antiarrhythmic drug with excellent efficacy and tolerability as well as very low risk of side effects. Dronedarone probably fits the low risk of side effect criterion, but has only a moderate efficacy and tolerability. The directions of research include further modification of the most effective available drug, amiodarone; the search for drugs with "target-specific" antiarrhythmic effect such as the atrially selective ion channel blockers to treat atrial fibrillation; and the exploration of potential targets above the cellular level: the gap junctions at the intercellular level and the substrate of arrhythmia at the tissue/organ level.

REFERENCES

1. Patel C, Yan GX, Kowey PR. Dronedarone. Circulation 2009;120:636–44.
2. Briefing document of the Advisory Committee Meeting of the cardiovascular and renal drugs division of the US Food and Drug Administration on Multaq. Available at: http://www.fda.gov/downloads/AdvisoryCommittees/CommitteesMeetingMaterials/Drugs/CardiovascularandRenalDrugsAdvisoryCommittee/UCM134981.pdf. Accessed November 8, 2009.
3. Tschuppert Y, Buclin T, Rothuizen LE, et al. Effect of dronedarone on renal function in healthy subjects. Br J Clin Pharmacol 2007;64:785–91.
4. Touboul P, Brugada J, Capucci A, et al. Dronedarone for prevention of atrial fibrillation: a dose-ranging study. Eur Heart J 2003;24:1481–7.
5. Singh BN, Connolly SJ, Crijns HJ, et al. Dronedarone for maintenance of sinus rhythm in atrial fibrillation or flutter. N Engl J Med 2007;357:987–99.

6. Davy JM, Herold M, Hoglund C, et al. Dronedarone for the control of ventricular rate in permanent atrial fibrillation. Am Heart J 2008;156:527–9.

7. Hohnloser SH, Crijns HJ, Eickels M, et al. Effects of dronedarone on cardiovascular events in atrial fibrillation. N Engl J Med 2009;360:668–78.

8. Connolly SJ, Crijns HJ, Torp-Pedersen C, et al. Analysis of stroke in ATHENA: a placebo-controlled, double-blind, parallel-arm trial to assess the efficacy of dronedarone 400 mg BID for the prevention of cardiovascular hospitalization or death from any cause in patients with atrial fibrillation/atrial flutter. Circulation 2009;120:1174–80.

9. Kober L, Torp-Pedersen C, McMurray JJ, et al. Increased mortality after dronedarone therapy for severe heart failure. N Engl J Med 2008;358: 2678–87.

10. Sanofi-aventis. DIONYSOS Study results showed the respective profiles of dronedarone and amiodarone. Available at: http://en.sanofi-aventis.com/binaries/20081223_dionysos_fe_en_en_tcm28-23624.pdf. Accessed December 23, 2008.

11. Dorian P, Pinter A, Mangat I, et al. The effect of vernakalant (RSD1235), an investigational antiarrhythmic agent, on atrial electrophysiology in humans. J Cardiovasc Pharmacol 2007;50:35–40.

12. Roy D, Pratt CM, Torp-Pedersen C, et al. Vernakalant hydrochloride for rapid conversion of atrial fibrillation: a phase 3, randomized, placebo-controlled trial. Circulation 2008;117:1518–25.

13. Kowey PR, Dorian P, Mitchell LB, et al. Vernakalant hydrochloride for the rapid conversion of atrial fibrillation after cardiac surgery. Circ Arrhythm Electrophysiol 2009;2:652–9.

14. Roy D, Pratt CM, Juul-Moller S, et al. Efficacy and tolerance of RSD1235 in the treatment of atrial fibrillation or atrial flutter: results of a phase III, randomized, placebo controlled, multicenter trial [abstract]. J Am Coll Cardiol 2006;47:10A.

15. Kowey PR, Aliot EM, Capucci A, et al. Placebo-controlled double-bind dose-ranging study of the efficacy and safety of SSR149744C in patients with recent atrial fibrillation/flutter [abstract]. Heart Rhythm 2007;4:S72.

16. Antzelevitch C, Belardinelli L, Zygmunt AC, et al. Electrophysiological effects of ranolazine, a novel antianginal agent with antiarrhythmic properties. Circulation 2004;110:904–10.

17. Burashnikov A, Di Diego JM, Zygmunt AC, et al. Atrium-selective sodium channel block as a strategy for suppression of atrial fibrillation. Circulation 2007; 116:1449–57.

18. Scirica BM, Morrow DA, Hod H, et al. Effect of ranolazine, an antianginal agent with novel electrophysiological properties, on the incidence of arrhythmias in patients with non ST-segment elevation acute coronary syndrome. Circulation 2007;116:1647–52.

19. Gutstein DE, Morley GE, Tamaddon H, et al. Conduction slowing and sudden arrhythmic death in mice with cardiac restricted inactivation of connexin43. Circ Res 2001;88:333–9.

20. Shiroshita-Takeshita A, Sakabe M, Haugan K, et al. Model-dependent effects of the gap junction conduction enhancing antiarrhythmic peptide rotigaptide on experimental atrial fibrillation in dogs. Circulation 2007;115:310–8.

21. Laurent G, Leong-Poi H, Mangat I, et al. Effects of chronic gap junction conduction-enhancing antiarrhythmic peptide GAP-134 administration on experimental atrial fibrillation in dogs. Circ Arrhythm Electrophysiol 2009;2:171–8.

22. Dorian P, Singh BN. Upstream therapies to prevent atrial fibrillation. Eur Heart J Suppl 2008;10:H11–31.

23. Pedersen OD, Bagger H, Kober L, et al. Trandolapril reduces the incidence of atrial fibrillation after acute myocardial infarction in patients with left ventricular dysfunction. Circulation 1999;100:376–80.

24. Vermes E, Tardif JC, Bourassa MG, et al. Enalapril decreases the incidence of atrial fibrillation in patients with ventricular dysfunction: insight from the Studies of Left Ventricular Dysfunction (SOLVD) trials. Circulation 2003;107:2926–31.

25. Wachtell K, Lehto M, Gerdts E, et al. Angiotensin II receptor blockade reduces new onset atrial fibrillation and subsequent stroke compared to atenolol. J Am Coll Cardiol 2005;45:712–9.

26. Yusuf S, Teo KK, Pogue J, et al. Telmisartan, ramipril, or both in patients at high risk for vascular events. N Engl J Med 2008;358:1547–59.

27. Yusuf S, Teo KK, Anderson C, et al. Effects of the angiotensin-receptor blocker telmisartan on cardiovascular events in high-risk patients intolerant to angiotensin-converting enzyme inhibitors: a randomized controlled trial. Lancet 2008;372:1174–83.

28. Madrid AH, Escobar C, Rebollo JM, et al. Angiotensin receptor blocker as adjunctive therapy for rhythm control in atrial fibrillation: results of the Irbesartan-Amiodarone trial. Card Electrophysiol Rev 2003;7:243–6.

29. Belluzzi F, Sernesi L, Preti P, et al. Prevention of recurrent lone atrial fibrillation by the angiotensin-II converting enzyme inhibitor ramipril in normotensive patients. J Am Coll Cardiol 2009;53:24–9.

30. Murray KT, Rottman JN, Arbogast PG, et al. Inhibition of angiotensin II signaling and recurrence of atrial fibrillation in AFFIRM. Heart Rhythm 2004;1:669–75.

31. Young-Xu Y, Jabbour S, Goldberg R, et al. Usefulness of statin drugs in protecting against atrial fibrillation in patients with coronary artery disease. Am J Cardiol 2003;92:1379–83.

32. Adabag AS, David B, Nelson DB, et al. Effects of statin therapy on preventing atrial fibrillation in coronary disease and heart failure. Am Heart J 2007;154:1140–5.

33. Hanna IR, Heeke B, Bush H, et al. Lipid-lowering drug use is associated with reduced prevalence of atrial fibrillation in patients with left ventricular systolic dysfunction. Heart Rhythm 2006;3:881–6.

34. Laurent G, Moe G, Hu X, et al. Long chain n-3 polyunsaturated fatty acids reduce atrial vulnerability in a novel canine pacing model. Cardiovasc Res 2008;77:89–97.

35. Nodari S, Metra M, Milesi G, et al. The role of n-3 PUFAs in preventing the arrhythmic risk in patients with idiopathic dilated cardiomyopathy. Cardiovasc Drugs Ther 2009;23:5–15.

36. Mozaffarian D, Psaty BM, Rimm EB, et al. Fish intake and risk of incident atrial fibrillation. Circulation 2004;110:368–73.

37. Calo L, Biancone L, Colivicchi F, et al. N-3 fatty acids for the prevention of atrial fibrillation after coronary artery bypass surgery. J Am Coll Cardiol 2005;45:1723–8.

38. Saravanan P, Bridgewater B, West LA, et al. Omega-3 fatty acid supplementation does not reduce risk of atrial fibrillation after coronary artery bypass surgery. Circ Arrhythm Electrophysiol 2010;3:46–53.

Principles of Anticoagulation and New Therapeutic Agents in Atrial Fibrillation

Pamela S.N. Goldman, DO,
Michael D. Ezekowitz, MB, ChB, DPhil, FRCP*

KEYWORDS

• Anticoagulation • Atrial fibrillation • Warfarin

Anticoagulation is effective in patients with atrial fibrillation (AF) and atrial flutter, to reduce the risk of thromboembolism. In this article, principles of anticoagulation are discussed. The principles of anticoagulation for both AF and atrial flutter are similar because the location and nature of the arrhythmias are similar. AF is the most common cardiac arrhythmia[1] in the general population and increases with age, placing the elderly population at increased risk. Approximately 2 million people in the United States are affected by AF, and the prevalence is expected to exceed 10 million by the year 2050.[1] About 15% of all strokes can be attributed to AF, and patients with this condition have a 5-fold greater risk of having a stroke than the general population.[2] Warfarin is known to reduce stroke risk by 68% in patients with AF and is the most effective agent for this indication, although it is not without risk.[3] Therefore, starting warfarin therapy requires a balanced decision regarding embolic and bleeding risks.[4,5]

RISK STRATIFICATION FOR EMBOLIC RISK IN PATIENTS WITH AF

Stratification for stroke risk in patients with nonvalvular AF can be performed using both clinical and echocardiographic parameters.[4] The rates of thromboembolism can be predicted using either single risk factors, such as age, or a combination of risk factors included in validated risk models. The embolic risk seems equivalent in both chronic and paroxysmal AFs.[6–8]

Clinical Parameters

The need for anticoagulation can be determined by 3 schemas. These schemas include the Atrial Fibrillation Investigators (AFI) scheme that has pooled data from 5 randomized stroke prevention trials in patients with nonvalvular or nonrheumatic AF, including the Boston Area Anticoagulation Trial for Atrial Fibrillation (BAATAF),[5] Veteran Affairs Stroke Prevention in Nonrheumatic Atrial Fibrillation (SPINAF),[9] Atrial Fibrillation, Aspirin, and Anticoagulation Study (AFASAK),[10] Canadian Atrial Fibrillation Anticoagulation Study,[11] and Stroke Prevention in Atrial Fibrillation Study (SPAF),[6] the SPAF III trial scheme, and the most accurate predictor of stroke, the CHADS2 scoring.

The pooled data of the AFI, which was the first risk stratification system developed, identified 4 independent risk factors: history of stroke or transient ischemic attack (TIA), age greater than 65 years (**Fig. 1**), diabetes mellitus, and history of systemic hypertension (**Box 1**).[12]

SPAF III trial on nonvalvular AF (**Table 1**) identified the following risk factors for embolism in AF:

> Women older than 75 years
> History of stroke or TIA
> Impaired left ventricular (LV) systolic function (clinical heart failure in the last 3 months or fractional shortening <25% on transthoracic echocardiography [TTE]).

From the AFI and SPAF III Models, the CHADS2 score was derived and is the most widely used

Lankenau Institute for Medical Research, Clinical Research Center, 100 Lancaster Avenue, Wynnewood, PA 19096, USA
* Corresponding author.
E-mail address: ezekowitzm@mlhs.org

Card Electrophysiol Clin 2 (2010) 479–492
doi:10.1016/j.ccep.2010.08.003
1877-9182/10/$ — see front matter © 2010 Published by Elsevier Inc.

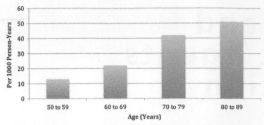

Fig. 1. AFI scheme risk by age range (regardless of sex). (*Data from* Frost L, Engholm G, Johnsen S, et al. Incident stroke after discharge from hospital with a diagnosis of atrial fibrillation. Am J Med 2000:108:36–40; with permission.)

clinical model. The CHADS2 score (**Table 2**) indicates that the risk of stroke is increased when certain comorbidities are present in patients with AF. Following is the stroke rate per 100 patient-years without antithrombotic therapy (**Table 3**) for each 1-point increase: 1.9 for a score of 0, 2.8 for 1 point, 4.0 for 2 points, 5.9 for 3 points, 8.5 for 4 points, 12.5 for 5 points, and 18.2 for 6 points.[13]

CHADS2 includes the following risk factors:

Congestive heart failure (any history), 1 point
Hypertension (history), 1 point
Age greater than 75 years, 1 point
Diabetes mellitus, 1 point
Secondary prevention in patients with ischemic stroke, TIA (with or without systemic embolic event), 2 points.

In 2009, the Birmingham research group performed further analysis on the Euro Heart Survey

---

Box 1
AFI scheme: independent risk factors for increased stroke rates

Age (see **Fig. 1**)

Diabetes

History of cerebrovascular accident or TIA

Peripheral atherosclerosis

Secondary Risk Factors

Hypertension

Hospital diagnosis of AF[a]

Ischemic heart disease (men only)

Heart failure (men only)

[a] Stroke risk highest in first 12 months after diagnosis.
Data from Frost L, Engholm G, Johnsen S, et al. Incident stroke after discharge from hospital with a diagnosis of atrial fibrillation. Am J Med 2000:108:36–40; with permission.

Table 1
SPAF III scheme

SPAF III Risk Stratification for Primary Prevention of Stroke

Risk Stratification	Rate of Stroke Per Year (%)
High risk	7.1
Moderate risk	2.6
Low risk	0.9

SPAF III Independent Risk Factors for Stroke

Risk Factor	Relative Risk, P value
Women	1.6, P = .01
Age	2.0/decade, P<.001
History of hypertension	1.8, P<.001
Systolic blood pressure >160 mm Hg	2.3, P<.001
Prior stroke or TIA	2.9, P<.001
Estrogen hormone replacement therapy (risk of ischemic stroke)	3.2, P = .007
Diabetes mellitus	1.9, P = .02

SPAF III Reduced Stroke Risk

Reduced Stroke Risk	Relative Risk, P value
≥14 Alcohol-containing drinks per week	0.4, P = .04

Data from Hart RG, Pearce LA, McBride R, et al. Factors associated with ischemic stroke during aspirin therapy in atrial fibrillation. Stroke 1999;30:1223–9; with permission.

on Atrial Fibrillation and identified additional risk factors for stroke, which is known as the 2009 Birmingham schema. The Birmingham group divided the stroke-risk groups into definitive risk, which includes history of stroke or TIA and/or age greater

---

Table 2
CHADS2 scoring

	Risk Factor	Point Value
C	Congestive heart failure	1
H	Hypertension	1
A	Age>75 y	1
D	Diabetes mellitus	1
S2	Stroke or TIA, with or without systemic embolic event	2

Data from Gage BF, Waterman AD, Shannon W, et al. Validation of clinical classification schemes for predicting stroke: results from the National Registry of Atrial Fibrillation. JAMA 2001;285(22):2864–70; with permission.

Table 3
Stroke rate without antithrombotic therapy

CHADS2 Points	Stroke Rate (Per 100 Patient-Years)
0	1.9
1	2.8
2	4.0
3	5.9
4	8.5
5	12.5
6	18.2

Data from Gage BF, Waterman AD, Shannon W, et al. Validation of clinical classification schemes for predicting stroke: results from the National Registry of Atrial Fibrillation. JAMA 2001;285(22):2864−70; with permission.

than 75 years, and combination risk, including hypertension, heart failure, diabetes, age 65 to 74 years, female gender, and vascular disease. The new schema is CHA_2DS_2-VASc (**Table 4**).[14]

Transthoracic Echocardiography[15]

A pooled analysis of 3 anticoagulation trials, BAATAF, SPINAF, and SPAF I, found the following:

- LV systolic function diagnosed by TTE was an independent risk factor for stroke in patients with AF. The relative risk of stroke was 2.5 times higher for those with

Table 4
CHA_2DS_2-VASc schema (2009 Birmingham schema)

	Risk Factor	Point Value
C	Congestive heart failure[c]	1
H	Hypertension[c]	1
A_2	Age>75 y[b]	2
D	Diabetes mellitus[c]	1
S_2	Stroke or TIA ± systemic embolic event[b]	2
V	Vascular disease[a,c]	1
A	Age 65−74 y[c]	1
Sc	Sex category, female[c]	1

[a] Vascular disease includes myocardial infarction, peripheral arterial disease, or aortic plaque.
[b] Definitive risk factors.
[c] Combination risk factors.
Data from Lip GY, Nieuwlaat R, Pisters R, et al. Refining clinical risk stratification for predicting stroke and thromboembolism in atrial fibrillation using a novel risk factor-based approach: the Euro Heart Survey on atrial fibrillation. Chest 2010;137:263−72; with permission.

moderate to severe LV dysfunction compared with patients with mildly abnormal or normal LV function.

- Among 163 patients categorized as low risk based on clinical criteria, 10 had moderate to severe LV dysfunction and a stroke rate of 9.3% per year. By comparison, the stroke rate was lower at 4.4% per year in 728 of the 847 patients at high risk for stroke based on clinical criteria and who had normal or mildly abnormal LV function on TTE.

- LA dimension was not a predictor of stroke in the pooled analysis possibly because of the effect of mitral regurgitation and mitral stenosis. In contrast, the SPAF investigators found that the LA dimension, that is, diameter greater than 2.5 cm/m^2 was an independent predictor of thromboembolism.

- Findings on TTE often changed the risk group based on clinical criteria alone. Among patients placed in a low-risk group clinically, 38% were judged to be at high risk when TTE data were included in the categorization.

Transesophageal Echocardiography

Transesophageal echocardiography (TEE) is not recommended in patients with AF purely for risk stratification. TEE may be useful in some patients before cardioversion to document the presence of a LA appendage clot that may lead to stroke after the procedure.

Recommended Risk Model

CHADS2 score, derived from SPAF and AFI schemes, is considered the easiest to implement and the most clinically useful model for risk stratification of patients with AF.

RECOMMENDATIONS FOR ANTITHROMBOTIC THERAPY IN AF

Antithrombotic therapy with antiplatelets or anticoagulants is recommended for most patients with AF. Anticoagulant therapy is preferred, except in the lowest-risk patients. The decision to use antithrombotic therapy is best made with an appreciation of both embolic and bleeding risks.[4]

The decision to use either aspirin (antiplatelet) or warfarin (anticoagulant) is based on the challenging assessment of the benefit in preventing thromboembolism and the risk of bleeding related to antithrombotic therapy. Recommendations for antithrombotic therapy have been published by American College of Cardiology (ACC)/American

Heart Association (AHA)/European Society of Cardiology (ESC) and American College of Chest Physicians. Both aspirin and warfarin can significantly reduce the risk of stroke, but warfarin is 3 times more effective.[6–12,16,17]

The 2006 ACC/AHA/ESC guidelines recommend treatment with an anticoagulant if CHADS2 score is greater than or equal to 2. The risk of thromboembolism based on CHADS2 scoring is listed below and recommended for use by non-specialists as an initial assessment of stroke risk.[18]

- Patients with a CHADS2 score of 0 are at very low risk for stroke (1.9% in the absence of warfarin) and can be managed with aspirin therapy alone (81 mg or 325 mg daily); patients who are younger than 60 years with no risk factors (lone AF) are at very low risk, as low as 1.2% per year, and may require no therapy at all.
- Patients with a CHADS2 score of 1 or 2 are at intermediate risk (2.8%–4% per year) and would benefit from anticoagulant therapy in the absence of contraindications.
- Patients with a CHADS2 score of 3 or more are at high risk (≥4.5%) and should be managed with anticoagulant therapy in the absence of contraindications.

The 2010 ESC Guidelines recommend the use of the CHA_2DS_2-VASc score to determine the rate of stroke, taking into consideration major and non-major stroke risk factors and recommend the following anticoagulant therapy based on this latest scheme:[18a]

- Patients with a CHA_2DS_2-VASc score of 0 are at very low risk for stroke (0% adjusted stroke rate per year) and can be managed with aspirin therapy alone (75 mg to 325 mg daily) or no therapy at all (preferred).
- Patients with a CHA_2DS_2-VASc score of 1 have one non-major risk factor (1.3% adjusted stroke rate per year) and would benefit from aspirin or anticoagulant therapy (preferred).
- Patients with a CHA_2DS_2-VASc score of 2 or more are at higher risk for stroke (2.2% to 15.2% for a score of 9) and should be managed with anticoagulant therapy in the absence of contraindications.

It should be noted that patients with paroxysmal AF should be managed in the same way as those with persistent AF.[13,19,20] Most patients with paroxysmal AF have recurrent episodes of AF,[21] most of which are not detected by the patient.

The Atrial Fibrillation Follow-up Investigation of Rhythm Management (AFFIRM) and Rate Control versus electrical cardioversion for Persistent Atrial Fibrillation (RACE) trials demonstrated that most strokes occur when the international normalized ratio (INR) was subtherapeutic, irrespective of whether the patient had AF or sinus rhythm.[22,23]

Recommendations for Antithrombotic Therapy in Cardioversion

Patients undergoing cardioversion require anticoagulation for the prevention of thromboembolic complications associated with the procedure due to stunning of the LA appendage. The risk of thromboembolism is greatest within 3 to 10 days after cardioversion, with 80% of events occurring within this time frame.[24] Class I recommendations from the 2006 ACC/AHA/ESC guidelines include anticoagulation to an INR of 2 to 3 at least 3 weeks before and 4 weeks after cardioversion. Unfractionated heparin is administered to an activated partial thromboplastin time of 1.5 to 2 times the normal range before emergent cardioversion, and oral anticoagulant therapy is continued for 4 weeks after the procedure. The Anticoagulation in Cardioversion using Enoxaparin (ACE) trial evaluated the use of enoxaparin (low-molecular-weight heparin [LMWH]) for preventing thromboembolism, although limited evidence is available for the use of LMWH in cardioversion (evidence level C).[25] Patients with hemodynamic instability and AF should have cardioversion performed as soon as clinically indicated. Anticoagulation is recommended.

Warfarin

Patients with intermediate to high risk for embolic stroke should be treated with warfarin with a goal to keep the INR from 2 to 3. In high-risk patients, such as those with prior thromboembolism, rheumatic heart disease, or prosthetic heart valves, a higher range of INR may be necessary. Overall, warfarin reduces the risk of stroke by 62% to 69%, with the degree of benefit depending on baseline risk. The greatest benefit of warfarin therapy is in patients who maintain a therapeutic INR. Despite the benefit, warfarin therapy continues to be underused,[17,18,22,23,26–30] and even when it is appropriately started, it is often discontinued.[29] When warfarin is prescribed, maintaining the target INR is often not achieved, and the failure to achieve therapeutic INR is associated with worse outcomes. In most clinical trials evaluating the benefit of warfarin, as much as 25% of patients were subtherapeutic in spite of using a warfarin nomogram and frequent monitoring. All strokes in major trials occurred when INR values were subtherapeutic or when subjects stopped using warfarin.[22,23] Challenges with warfarin include many endogenous and exogenous interactions including, but not limited to, altered bowel flora, foods containing vitamin K that require dietary adjustment, medications competing for binding sites within the liver, and the frequent adjustments in dose relying on patient compliance and understanding.

Aspirin and Aspirin with Clopidogrel[31,32]

The Atrial fibrillation Clopidogrel Trial with Irbesartan for prevention of Vascular Events (ACTIVE) program is a set of 3 randomized controlled trials, namely, ACTIVE I, ACTIVE A, and ACTIVE W, comparing aspirin and clopidogrel (antiplatelet therapy) with an oral anticoagulant (vitamin K antagonist [VKA]/warfarin) in the prevention of strokes and vascular events. The ACTIVE W trial compared antiplatelet therapy with oral anticoagulant therapy. Oral anticoagulants proved to be superior in the prevention of vascular events compared with aspirin and clopidogrel, with a 45% increase in events with aspirin and clopidogrel (annual event rates, 3.93% vs 5.64%; $P<.001$). Because of the superiority of the oral anticoagulation therapy, the study was stopped early. ACTIVE I compared blood pressure monitoring with irbesartan and placebo, and ACTIVE A evaluated clopidogrel and aspirin versus aspirin alone for protection against vascular events in patients who were unsuitable for VKA therapy. For patients unable to take oral anticoagulants, the results suggested a reduction in stroke rates with the addition of clopidogrel to aspirin-alone therapy.

NEW ANTICOAGULANT AGENTS

Several agents are being developed to overcome the inadequacies of warfarin (**Table 5**). Although the clinical efficacy of warfarin is undeniable, new compounds are being developed to overcome the side effect profiles and be more user friendly. New agents are being developed using a similar mechanism of action as warfarin and others with novel mechanisms of action that will act on the coagulation cascade at other sites. Two novel compounds in clinical development that are farthest along in the clinical trial process are the direct thrombin inhibitor (DTI) dabigatran and the factor X inhibitor rivaroxaban. Other compounds in earlier phases of development are apixaban, a factor Xa (FXa) inhibitor; factor IX inhibitors; tissue factor inhibitors; and ATI-5923, a novel

VKA with a more stable metabolism and less drug-drug interactions than warfarin. This review discusses the mechanism of action, pharmacologic profile, and phase of development of each agent. **Fig. 2** illustrates the coagulation pathway and the point of action of each anticoagulant. **Table 5** summarizes the mechanism of action, pharmacokinetic profile, and phase of development of each agent. **Table 6** emphasizes the metabolism and benefits and interactions of each new therapy.

VKA

ATI-5923 (tecarfarin)

ATI-5923 (tecarfarin), like warfarin, is a selective noncompetitive inhibitor of vitamin K epoxide reductase. ATI-5923 is not metabolized by cytochrome P450 (CYP), which allows it to produce a more consistent response than other VKAs that compete for the binding site, resulting in varied response.[33,34]

In 2007, a phase 2, open-label, multicenter, genotype-guided, dose-finding study of ATI-5923 in patients with AF (www.clinicaltrials.gov; NCT00431782) was completed. The primary endpoints of this study were duration in therapeutic range, time to reach therapeutic range, and time to achieve stable dose when compared with retrospective warfarin therapy. The study results indicate that patients on tecarfarin had a 71.4% mean time in therapeutic range.[35] Further study is needed.

DTIs

Thrombin converts fibrinogen to fibrin and is active in the final stage of the coagulation cascade (see **Fig. 2**). DTIs can neutralize thrombin by occupying its catalytic binding sites, fibrinogen-binding sites, or both.[36] DTIs have a predictable mechanism of anticoagulation because they are not metabolized by the CYP system, and their binding to plasma proteins and cellular elements is limited. Unlike warfarin, DTIs have a broad therapeutic window and do not require frequent laboratory monitoring and dose adjustments. DTIs inhibit thrombin in both its inactive fluid phase and its stabilized fibrin-bound state and neutralize further progression of thrombus growth.[19] The prevention of clot propagation is another advantage that DTIs exhibit over warfarin. To date, two oral DTIs, ximelagatran and dabigatran, have been studied extensively in clinical trials. Ximelagatran, a compound developed by AstraZeneca (London, UK), had reached phase 3 development. However, the Food and Drug Administration (FDA) suspended the

Table 5
Anticoagulant Summary

Agent (Manufacturer)	Mechanism and Site of Action	Route of Administration	Characteristics	Phase of Development[a]
Warfarin	VKA (factors II, VII, IX, X)	PO	CYP metabolism; narrow therapeutic range	Established therapy
ATI-5923 (ARYx)	Novel VKA (factors II, VII, IX, X)	PO	Not metabolized by CYP2C9; more consistent response	Phase 2 complete
Ximelagatran (AstraZeneca)	DTI	PO	Blocks catalytic activity of thrombin, prevents clot propagation	Phase 3 complete; suspended by FDA due to liver toxicity
Dabigatran etexilate (Boehringer Ingelheim)	DTI	PO	Pro-drug; inactivates both fibrin-bound and unbound thrombin	Approved by US FDA October 2010
Rivaroxaban (Bayer/JNJ/Ortho-McNeil)	FXa inhibitor	PO	Inhibits free and clot-bound FXa, prothrombinase	Phase 3 ongoing
Apixaban (BMS/Pfizer)	FXa inhibitor	PO	Inhibits free and prothrombinase FXa	Phase 3 ongoing
Betrixaban (Merck/Portola)	FXa inhibitor	PO	No renal excretion; antidote developed	Phase 2 complete
Edoxaban (Daiichi Sankyo)	FXa inhibitor	PO	Direct and highly specific inhibitor	Phase 3 ongoing
Idraparinux (Sanofi-Aventis)	FXa inhibitor	SQ	Synthetic analogue of an active pentasaccharide sequence found in unfractionated heparin	Phase 3; terminated
LY517717 (Lilly)	FXa inhibitor	PO	Hepatobiliary metabolism/fecal excretion	Phase 2
YM150 813893 AVE-3247 EMD-503982 KFA-1982	Various	PO	Various	Various stages
TTP889 Antibody (Trans Tech Pharma)	Factor IXa inhibition	PO	Competitive inhibitor of factor IX binding to platelet surface membrane	Phase 2; not tested in patients with AF
TF Inhibitors	TF inhibition at the initiation site	IV	Monoclonal antibody	Preclinical models

Abbreviations: CYP, cytochrome P450; DTI, direct thrombin inhibitor; FDA, Food and Drug Administration; FXa, factor Xa; IV, intravenous; Pgp, P-glycoprotein; PO, per os; SQ, subcutaneous; TF, tissue factor.
  [a] As of publication date.

development of ximelagatran due to severe liver toxicity. Dabigatran, developed by Boehringer Ingelheim (Ingelheim, Germany), was approved as Pradaxa by the US FDA in October 2010.

Ximelagatran

Ximelagatran is an oral prodrug of melagatran and functions by blocking the catalytic activity of thrombin. It has 20% oral bioavailability and

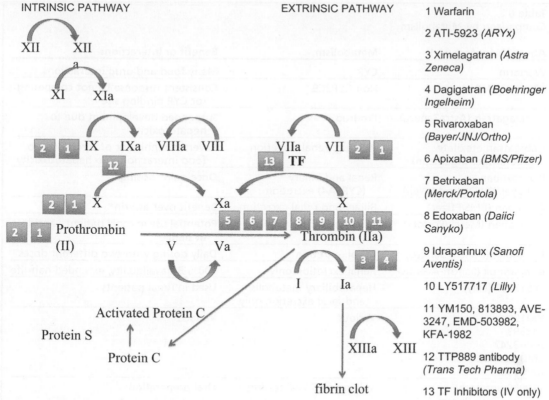

Fig. 2. Coagulation cascade. IV, intravenous; TF, tissue factor.

a half-life of 5 hours. Ximelagatran (36 mg twice a day) was compared with dose-adjusted warfarin in patients with AF in the Stroke Prevention using an ORal Thrombin Inhibitor in Atrial Fibrillation III and V (SPORTIF III and SPORTIF V) trials. Ximelagatran was as clinically efficacious as dose-adjusted warfarin in the prevention of stroke and systemic embolism in both the studies (1.6% vs 2.3% annually; 95% CI, 0.73–1.3; $P = .98$), and it was associated with a lower rate of hemorrhage than warfarin (1.9% vs 2.5% annually; risk ratio 0.76; 95% CI, 0.56–1.03; $P = .07$). However, treatment with ximelagatran was associated with statistically significant increases in transaminase levels compared with warfarin and resulted in 3 cases of fatal hepatotoxicity, and the FDA permanently suspended ximelagatran development.[37]

Dabigatran
Dabigatran is an oral prodrug of dabigatran etexilate. It is a potent, competitive, and reversible inhibitor of thrombin. Like ximelagatran, dabigatran offers the advantage of producing a predictable anticoagulant response. It has no known food interactions and minimal drug interactions due to P-glycoprotein-mediated absorption.

No dose change is required for P-gp inhibitors (i.e., quinidine, ketoconazole, verapamil, amiodarone, clarithromycin,) and P-gp inducers are to be avoided (i.e., rifampin). Dabigatran has not demonstrated the hepatotoxic potential observed with ximelagatran. Dabigatran has a rapid onset of action, an oral bioavailability of 6%, and a half-life of between 14 and 17 hours. It is excreted predominantly by the kidneys (80%) and is administered twice daily.[38]

Dabigatran was first evaluated in patients with AF in the Prevention of Embolic and ThROmbotic events in patients with persistent atrial fibrillation (PETRO) study.[39] This study was a phase 2, randomized, 3-month comparison of dabigatran (50, 150, and 300 mg twice a day) with dose-adjusted warfarin (INR 2-3) or aspirin conducted in 502 patients with AF and at least 1 additional risk factor for stroke. The study found major bleeding events in the highest dose group (300 mg) who concurrently took aspirin (aspirin use stopped during the study) and thromboembolic events in the lowest dose group (50 mg).[40] Patients from 2 of the dabigatran arms (150 mg twice a day and 300 mg daily; n = 361) of the PETRO study are being followed up in the PETROExtension (PETRO-Ex)

Table 6
Comparison by Metabolism

Agent (Manufacturer)	Metabolism	Benefit or Interactions
Warfarin	CYP	Many food and drug interactions
ATI-5923 (ARYx)	Non-CYP2C9	Consistent response by not competing for CYP binding site
Ximelagatran (AstraZeneca)	Prodrug	Suspended development due to hepatotoxicity
Dabigatran etexilate (Boehringer Ingelheim)	Prodrug; renal excretion	Reversible inhibitor of thrombin, no food interactions, no hepatotoxicity
Rivaroxaban (Bayer/JNJ/Ortho-McNeil)	Renal and biliary (CYP3A4) excretion	Once-daily dosing
Apixaban (BMS/Pfizer)	Biliary and renal excretion	Benefit over aspirin*
Betrixaban (Merck/Portola)	Biliary metabolism only	Potential use in renal patients; antidote available
Edoxaban (Daiichi Sankyo)	Renal excretion	Daily dosing with two different doses
Idraparinux (Sanofi-Aventis)	Renal excretion only	100% Bioavailability, extended half-life
LY517717 (Lilly)	Hepatobiliary metabolism and fecal excretion only	Used in renal patients
YM150 813893 AVE-3247 EMD-503982 KFA-1982	Various	Various
TTP889 antibody (Trans Tech Pharma)	Still in preclinical testing	Oral preparation
Tissue factor inhibitors	Poor oral bioavailablilty	IV

Abbreviations: CYP, cytochrome P450; IV, intravenous.

* As reported at the ESC 2010 Congress in Stockholm, Sweden 8/31/10. AVERROES trial terminated early: apixaban associated with "important" relative risk reduction for stroke and systemic embolism in AF. Available at http://www.escardio.org/about/press/press-releases/esc10-stockholm/Pages/AVERROES-trial.aspx. Accessed 10/31/10.

trial (www.clinicaltrials.gov; NCT00157248; maximum follow-up of 28 months).[41] The PETRO-Ex study is only assessing patients on dabigatran and is not comparing dabigatran to warfarin.

The Randomized Evaluation of Long-term Anticoagulant Therapy (RE-LY) trial showed promising results for dabigatran. In this trial, 18,113 patients with AF and at least 1 risk factor for stroke were assigned in an unblinded fashion to dose-adjusted warfarin or in a blinded fashion to fixed dosages of dabigatran, 110 mg or 150 mg twice daily. Results showed that 110 mg of dabigatran was noninferior to warfarin in preventing stroke and systemic embolism with a lower rate of major hemorrhage, whereas 150 mg of dabigatran was associated with lower rates of stroke and systemic embolism and similar rate of major hemorrhage but a much lower rate of hemorrhagic stroke as compared with warfarin.[42] There was a higher incidence over the duration of the trial of dyspepsia and gastritis-like symptoms in the 150 mg dabigatran group compared to warfarin (35% versus 24%). The risk of myocardial infarction was higher in those on dabigatran over the course of the trial compared to warfarin (1.5% versus 1.1%).[42a] On October 19, 2010, the FDA unanimously approved dabigatran (Pradaxa) for use in stroke prevention in AF. Two doses have been approved: 150 mg BID for creatinine clearance (CrCl) greater than 30, and 75 mg BID for CrCl between 15 and 30.[42a]

FXa Inhibitors

FXa is common to both the intrinsic and extrinsic pathways of the coagulation cascade. In vitro studies have shown that FXa activates clotting over a wide concentration range, and therefore FXa inhibitors, like DTIs, would also have a wide therapeutic window without dose-adjustment requirements. Proponents of FXa inhibitors argue that greater upstream inhibition of the coagulation cascade (see **Fig. 2**) and hence an amplified anticoagulation response theoretically result in fewer hemorrhagic outcomes because of facilitated hemostasis by virtue of "thrombin sparing" and more controlled anticoagulation.[43] However, no preclinical or clinical studies have been conducted to substantiate this hypothesis. Several FXa inhibitors are in various phases of development. These oral agents include rivaroxaban, apixaban, betrixaban, and edoxaban. The subcutaneous (SQ) agent idraparinux was being evaluated in a phase 3 trial that was eventually stopped.

Rivaroxaban

Rivaroxaban inhibits both free and clot-bound FXa as well as prothrombinase.[44,45] It is administered as a fixed once-daily dose and achieves peak plasma concentrations within 4 hours of oral administration, with a terminal half-life ranging from 5 to 9 hours in young healthy subjects and up to 12 hours in the elderly (>75 years).[46,47] It has 80% oral bioavailability and a dual excretion via both the biliary (34%) and renal (66%) routes. Rivaroxaban demonstrated predictable dose-proportional pharmacokinetics and pharmacodynamics in phase 1 studies and its dosing was not influenced by gender and body weight. Its absorption was moderately increased by coadministration of food, and it has potent interactions with the CYP3A4 inhibitors such as macrolide antibiotics and ketoconazole.[48,49]

Rivaroxaban is being compared with warfarin in the Rivaroxaban Once Daily Oral Direct Factor Xa Inhibition Compared with Vitamin K Antagonism for Prevention of Stroke and Embolism Trial in Atrial Fibrillation (ROCKET-AF) study (www.clinicaltrials.gov; NCT00494871). ROCKET-AF is a phase 3 double-blind study comparing rivaroxaban (20 mg once daily) to warfarin in patients with nonvalvular AF and at least one other risk factor for stroke. The study aims to recruit 14,000 patients worldwide. Rivaroxaban has not had smaller phase 2 comparisons to warfarin for the indication of AF, and dose assignment in the ROCKET-AF study is based on non-AF study results.

Apixaban

Apixaban is a derivative of razaxaban, a direct FXa inhibitor with selectivity for both free and prothrombinase-bound FXa.[50,51] Its mechanism of action is similar to rivaroxaban, and it has 50% to 85% oral bioavailability[51a] with greater hepatobiliary than renal excretion (25% renal and 75% hepatobiliary)and a half-life of 12 hours. A phase 2 double-blinded comparison of apixaban with warfarin for the prevention of venous thromboembolism (VTE) in patients undergoing total knee replacement has been completed, and this study compared 6 doses (5, 10, or 20 mg daily or in divided doses twice daily) of apixaban with open-label enoxaparin or warfarin for 10 to 14 days in 1217 patients.[20] At the lowest apixaban dose tested (5 mg daily or 2.5 mg twice a day), the primary outcome rates of apixaban were lower than those of enoxaparin and warfarin (9.0% and 11.3% vs 15.6% and 26.6%; $P = .09$. There was no significant difference in outcomes with either dosing regimen). Also, bleeding outcomes and increase in hepatic transaminases levels were similar in apixaban and warfarin.

Phase 2 studies are now being conducted, which compare apixaban to warfarin for the treatment of deep venous thrombosis (www.clinicaltrials.gov; NCT00252005) as well as unstable angina and myocardial infarction (www.clinicaltrials.gov; NCT00313300) and for the prevention of thromboembolic events in patients with advanced metastatic disease (www.clinicaltrials.gov; NCT00320255). In addition, apixaban is being compared with warfarin for the prevention of stroke and systemic embolism in patients with nonvalvular AF and at least one risk factor for stroke in the Apixaban for Reduction In STroke and Other ThromboemboLic Events in Atrial Fibrillation (ARISTOTLE) study (www.clinicaltrials.gov; NCT00412984). This phase 3, randomized, double-blind, parallel-arm study is expected to enroll 15,000 patients. The ARISTOTLE study compares twice daily dosage of apixaban (5 mg) with warfarin.

Betrixaban

Betrixaban is distinct from other FXa inhibitors in that it is not cleared by the kidneys, allowing it to have potential use in renal dysfunction. Also, it is being developed with an antidote. A multinational phase 2 study in patients with AF and at least 1 other risk factor for stroke compared 3 doses of betrixaban (40, 60, or 80 mg daily) to warfarin therapy. The study showed that there were fewer major bleeds or clinically relevant nonmajor bleeding with low-dose betrixaban compared with warfarin and similar bleeding rates with the two higher doses compared with warfarin.[52]

Edoxaban

Edoxaban is a direct and highly specific inhibitor of FXa, primarily cleared by the kidneys. The phase 2 study compared 30 mg and 60 mg twice daily dosing, 30 mg and 60 mg daily dosing, and warfarin. The group that was administered 60 mg twice a day was terminated early because of significantly higher incidences of bleeding events compared with warfarin (10.6% vs 3.2%). The incidence of bleeding events with the daily-dosing groups of 30 mg (3%) and 60 mg (3.8%) remained comparable to warfarin (3.2%). A multinational, double-blind, double-dummy, phase 3 study in patients with AF, called the Effective Anticoagulation with Factor Xa Next Generation in Atrial Fibrillation (ENGAGE-AF TIMI 48) study compares prevention of stroke and systemic embolic events in warfarin and two dosages of edoxaban (30 mg and 60 mg daily). The study will continue for a 2-year period.[53]

Idraparinux and biotinylated idraparinux

Idraparinux is a synthetic analogue of the active synthetic pentasaccharide sequence contained in unfractionated heparin. Idraparinux has a high affinity for antithrombin III and an extended half-life of up to 80 hours.[54] The bioavailability of idraparinux is 100% after SQ injection, and it has 100% renal excretion. Several phase 1 and phase 2 studies of idraparinux have been completed and include trials on the prevention of VTE and AF. The Atrial fibrillation trial of Monitored, Adjusted Dose vitamin K antagonist, comparing Efficacy and safety with Unadjusted SanOrg 34006/idraparinux (AMADEUS) study was a phase 3 open-label trial that compared idraparinux (2.5 mg SQ once weekly) with dose-adjusted warfarin (INR 2.0–3.0, target 2.5) in patients with AF and at least one additional risk factor. The study comprised 4576 patients but recruitment was stopped because of increased bleeding in the idraparinux arm (19.7% vs 11.3%; $P<.001$) compared with the warfarin arm. Despite this outcome, there was no difference in mortality between the treatment groups, and idraparinux established noninferiority to warfarin with respect to the composite endpoint of stroke and non-CNS systemic embolism (0.9% with idraparinux vs 1.3% with warfarin; $P = .007$).[55] Results from the AMADEUS trial also showed an increased propensity for bleeding with decreasing renal function and increasing age. These safety issues have led to the search for suitable modifications of the compound. As a result, biotinylated idraparinux (SSR126517E) has been developed. This compound has a strong affinity for avidin, which is its neutralizing agent. The pharmacologic and pharmacokinetic profile of biotinylated idraparinux is otherwise similar to idraparinux. Biotinylated idraparinux is being compared with warfarin in the Biotinylated idraparinux once a week in Randomized trial EvALuatIng the Stroke prevention in AF (BOREALIS-AF) study. This is a multicenter, randomized, double-blind, noninferiority study comparing biotinylated idraparinux (starting dosage of 3 mg SQ weekly is adjusted after 7 doses to age and creatinine clearance) to warfarin (INR 2–3) for a follow-up period of 2 years. The study was then terminated.

Other factor X inhibitors

LY517717, YM150, 813893, AVE-3247, EMD-503982, and KFA-1982 are oral anticoagulants in clinical development for the prevention of thromboembolism in patients with VTE after total knee and hip replacement and in patients with AF. Phase 2 evaluation of LY517717 (being developed by Lilly [Eli Lilly and Company, Indianapolis, IN, USA]) has recently been completed, in which it was compared with enoxaparin for the prevention of VTE in patients undergoing total hip and total knee replacement and was found to be of comparable efficacy and safety at three dosages (100, 125, and 150 mg daily; $P<.001$).[56] LY517717 has an elimination half-life of 25 hours and is unique from other agents in this group by virtue of almost 100% hepatobiliary metabolism and fecal excretion. Therefore, it is of particular use in patients with renal insufficiency.[57]

Factor IX Inhibitors

Factor IX occupies a pivotal role in the coagulation cascade by serving as a conduit between tissue-factor–bearing cells and platelets. Selective inhibition of this critical interaction between activated factor IX and platelets may effectively diffuse further clot propagation.[58] In addition, factor IX is activated when conjugated with factor VIII, and both the factors collectively activate factor X via the contact activation process. Studies suggest that factor X activation by the factor IXa/VIIIa pathway is more efficient and potent than the alternative tissue factor/factor VIIa–mediated extrinsic pathway.[59]

The first factor IX inhibitor to be developed was an antibody to factor IXai that was a competitive inhibitor of factor IX binding to platelet surface membrane.[60] Since then, numerous preclinical and phase 1 studies have been completed on various intravenous infusions ranging from humanized monoclonal antibodies against factor IX to RNA aptamers directed against factor IX binding sites.[61,62] TTP889 (Trans Tech Pharma, High Point, NC, USA) is the only oral agent that has undergone extensive preclinical testing and was found to be as equally efficacious as heparin without a significant effect on bleeding.[63] TTP889 has recently been compared with placebo for long-term prevention of VTE in patients undergoing total hip replacement in the Factor IX Inhibition in Thrombosis prevention Trial (FIXIT; www.clinicaltrials.gov; NCT00119457). This trial was a phase 2 proof-of-concept study that failed to demonstrate the superiority of TTP889 over placebo for VTE prevention (VTE events 32.1% vs 28.2% in placebo; $P = .58$).[64] TTP889 has not

Table 7
Clinical Trial Summary[a]

Agent (Manufacturer)	Clinical Trial	Comparison
ATI-5923 (ARYx)	Phase 2	Time in therapeutic range vs warfarin
Ximelagatran (AstraZeneca)	SPORTIF III SPORTIF V	Stroke prevention vs warfarin
Dabigatran (Boehringer Ingelheim)	PETRO PETRO-Ex RE-LY RELY-ABLE	Stroke prevention vs warfarin Study drug only Noninferiority to warfarin Study drug only
Rivaroxaban (Bayer/JNJ/Ortho-McNeil)	ROCKET-AF	Stroke prevention vs warfarin
Apixaban (BMS/Pfizer)	ARISTOTLE	Stroke prevention vs warfarin
Betrixaban (Merck/Portola)	Phase 2	3 doses tested compared to warfarin
Edoxaban (Daiichi Sankyo)	ENGAGE-AF TIMI 48	Stroke prevention vs warfarin
Idraparinux (Sanofi-Aventis)	AMADEUS BOREALIS-AF	Stroke prevention vs warfarin
LY517717 (Lilly)	Phase 2	VTE prevention after knee and hip replacement surgery
YM150 813893 AVE-3247 EMD-503982 KFA-1982	Various	Various
TTP889 antibody (Trans Tech Pharma)	FIXIT	Proof of concept of the drug over placebo, failed
Tissue factor inhibitors	Preclinical models	Human suitability and bioavailability

Abbreviations: RELY-ABLE, Long term multi-center extension of dabigatran treatment in patients with atrial fibrillation who completed the RE-LY trial and a cluster randomised trial to assess the effect of a knowledge translation intervention on patient outcomes.
[a] As of publication date.

yet been tested in patients with AF, and to date there is no information on further testing in VTE-prevention studies (**Table 7**).

Tissue Factor Inhibitors

Tissue factor activation is the primary step in the initiation and sequential amplification of proteolytic activity that leads to thrombus formation.[65] Inhibiting coagulation at this stage is thought to require less potency because of amplified serine protease inhibition, leading to fewer hemorrhagic complications when compared with other stages of anticoagulation.[66] In addition, inhibition of coexistent neointimal proliferation is an additional advantage that tissue factor inhibition might offer.[67]

The first monoclonal antibody directed at tissue factor (AP-1) was developed at Yale University.[67] Several other monoclonal antibodies to tissue factor have been tested in preclinical models.[67,68]

To date, no oral agents are suitable for human testing, although the recombinant nematode anticoagulant protein c2 has shown potential as an intravenous agent for VTE prophylaxis after orthopedic procedures and percutaneous coronary intervention.[69,70] The primary reason is either low oral bioavailability via gastrointestinal absorption of any inactive prodrug or decreased plasma activity of agents that have good oral bioavailability.[71]

SUMMARY

Although warfarin is effective in preventing thromboembolism in patients with AF, it is very difficult to keep warfarin in therapeutic range and it has multiple interactions. Because the effects of warfarin vary, the risk of stroke is high whenever INR is subtherapeutic. For this reason, many agents are being developed to replace warfarin as an effective anticoagulant for stroke prevention in patients with AF. Dabigatran has been approved by the US FDA and can be used in a fixed dose of 150 mg BID for patients with a CrCl greater than 30 and at a dose of 75 mg BID for patients whose CrCl is between 15 and 30.

REFERENCES

1. Miyasaka Y, Barnes ME, Gersh BJ, et al. Secular trends in incidence of atrial fibrillation in Olmsted County, Minnesota, 1980 to 2000, and implications on the projections for future prevalence. Circulation 2006;114:119–25.

2. Kannel WB, Abbott RD, Savage DD, et al. Epidemiologic features of chronic atrial fibrillation: the Framingham Study. N Engl J Med 1982;306:1018–22.

3. Hart RG, Pearce LA, Aguilar MI. Meta-analysis: antithrombotic therapy to prevent stroke in patients who have nonvalvular atrial fibrillation. Ann Intern Med 2007;146:857–67.

4. Rockson SG, Albers GW. Comparing the guidelines: anticoagulation therapy to optimize stroke prevention in patients with atrial fibrillation. J Am Coll Cardiol 2004;43:929.

5. Ezekowitz MD, Falk RH. The increasing need for anticoagulant therapy to prevent stroke in patients with atrial fibrillation. Mayo Clin Proc 2004;79:904.

6. The Boston Area Anticoagulation Trial for Atrial Fibrillation Investigators. The effect of low-dose warfarin on the risk of stroke in patients with nonrheumatic atrial fibrillation. N Engl J Med 1990;323:1505.

7. Stroke Prevention in Atrial Fibrillation Investigators. Stroke prevention in atrial fibrillation study: final results. Circulation 1991;84:527.

8. Hart RG, Pearce LA, Rothbart RM, et al. Stroke with intermittent atrial fibrillation: incidence and predictors during aspirin therapy. Stroke Prevention in Atrial Fibrillation Investigators. J Am Coll Cardiol 2000;35:183.

9. Ezekowitz MD, Bridgers SL, James KE, et al. Warfarin in the prevention of stroke associated with nonrheumatic atrial fibrillation. N Engl J Med 1992; 327:1406.

10. Petersen P, Boysen G, Godtfredsen J, et al. Placebo-controlled, randomized trial of warfarin and aspirin for prevention of thromboembolic complications in chronic atrial fibrillation. The Copenhagen AFASAK study. Lancet 1989;1:175.

11. Connolly SJ, Laupacis A, Gent M, et al. Canadian Atrial Fibrillation Anticoagulation (CAFA) study. J Am Coll Cardiol 1991;18:349.

12. Risk factors for stroke and efficacy of antithrombotic therapy in atrial fibrillation. Analysis of pooled data from five randomized controlled trials. Arch Intern Med 1994;154:1449.

13. Gage BF, Waterman AD, Shannon W, et al. Validation of clinical classification schemes for predicting stroke: results from the National Registry of Atrial Fibrillation. JAMA 2001;285(22):2864–70.

14. Lip GY, Nieuwlaat R, Pisters R, et al. Refining clinical risk stratification for predicting stroke and thromboembolism in atrial fibrillation using a novel risk factor-based approach: the Euro Heart Survey on atrial fibrillation. Chest 2010;137:263–72.

15. Echocardiographic predictors of stroke in patients with atrial fibrillation: a prospective study of 1066 patients from 3 clinical trials. Arch Intern Med 1998;158:1316.

16. Van Walraven C, Hart RG, Singer DE, et al. Oral anticoagulants vs aspirin in nonvalvular atrial fibrillation: an individual patient meta-analysis. JAMA 2002;288:2441.

17. Cooper NJ, Sutton AJ, Lu G, et al. Mixed comparison of stroke prevention treatments in individuals with nonrheumatic atrial fibrillation. Arch Intern Med 2006;166:1269.

18. Fuster V, Ryden LE, Cannom DS, et al. ACC/AHA/ESC 2006 guidelines for the management of patients with atrial fibrillation: a report of the American College of Cardiology/American Heart Association Task Force on Practice Guidelines and the European Society of Cardiology Committee for Practice Guidelines (writing committee to revise the 2001 guidelines for the management of patients with atrial fibrillation). J Am Coll Cardiol 2006;48(4):854–906.

18a. European Heart Rhythm Association; European Association for Cardio-Thoracic Surgery, Camm AJ, Kirchhof P, Lip GY, et al. Guidelines for the management of atrial fibrillation: the Task Force for the Management of Atrial Fibrillation of the European Society of Cardiology (ESC). Eur Heart J 2010; 31(19):2369–429. Epub 2010 Aug 29.

19. Weitz JI, Leslie B, Hudoba M. Thrombin binds to soluble fibrin degradation products where it is protected from inhibition by heparin-antithrombin but susceptible to inactivation by antithrombin-independent inhibitors. Circulation 1998;97:544–52.

20. Lassen MR, Davidson BL, Gallus A, et al. The efficacy and safety of apixaban, an oral, direct factor Xa inhibitor, as thromboprophylaxis in patients following total knee replacement. J Thromb Haemost 2007;5(12):2368–75.

21. Israel CW, Gronefeld G, Ehrlich JR, et al. Long-term risk of recurrent atrial fibrillation as documented by an implantable monitoring device. Implications for optimal patient care. J Am Coll Cardiol 2004;43:47.

22. Wyse DG, Waldo AL, DiMarco JP, et al. A comparison of rate control and rhythm control in patients with atrial fibrillation. The Atrial Fibrillation Follow-up Investigation of Rhythm Management (AFFIRM) investigators. N Engl J Med 2002;347:1825.

23. Van Gelder IC, Hagens VE, Bosker HA, et al. A comparison of rate control and rhythm control in patients with recurrent persistent atrial fibrillation. N Engl J Med 2002;347:1834.

24. Khan IA. Atrial stunning: determinants and cellular mechanisms. Am Heart J 2003;145:787–94.

25. Stellbrink C, Nixdorff U, Hofmann T, et al. Safety and efficacy of enoxaparin compared with unfractionated heparin and oral anticoagulants for prevention of thromboembolic complications in cardioversion of nonvalvular atrial fibrillation: the Anticoagulation in Cardioversion using Enoxaparin (ACE) trial. Circulation 2004;109:997–1003.

26. Glazer NL, Dublin S, Smith NL, et al. Newly detected atrial fibrillation and compliance with antithrombotic guidelines. Arch Intern Med 2007;167:246.

27. Mant J, Hobbs FD, Fletcher K, et al. Warfarin versus aspirin for stroke prevention in an elderly community population with atrial fibrillation (the Birmingham Atrial Fibrillation Treatment of the Aged Study, BAFTA): a randomised controlled trial. Lancet 2007;370:493.

28. Hylek EM, Evans-Molina C, Shea C, et al. Major hemorrhage and tolerability of warfarin in the first year of therapy among elderly patients with atrial fibrillation. Circulation 2007;115:2689.

29. Go AS, Hylek EM, Borowsky LH, et al. Warfarin use among ambulatory patients with nonvalvular atrial fibrillation: the anticoagulation and risk factors in atrial fibrillation (ATRIA) study. Ann Intern Med 1999;131:927.

30. Gage BF, Boechler M, Doggette AL, et al. Adverse outcomes and predictors of underuse of antithrombotic therapy in Medicare beneficiaries with chronic atrial fibrillation. Stroke 2000;31:822.

31. ACTIVE Writing Group of the ACTIVE Investigators, Connolly S, Pogue J, Hart R, Pfeffer M, Hohnloser S, Chrolavicius S, Pfeffer M, Hohnloser S, Yusuf S. Clopidogrel plus aspirin versus oral anticoagulation for atrial fibrillation in the Atrial fibrillation Clopidogrel Trial with Irbesartan for prevention of Vascular Events (ACTIVE W): a randomised controlled trial. Lancet 2006;367(9526):1903–12.

32. The ACTIVE Investigators. Effect of clopidogrel added to aspirin in patients with atrial fibrillation. N Engl J Med 2009;360(20):2066–78.

33. Available at: http://www.aryx.com/wt/page/ati5923. Accessed March 10, 2010.

34. Carlquist JF, Horne BD, Muhlestein JB, et al. Genotypes of the cytochrome p450 isoform, CYP2C9, and the vitamin K epoxide reductase complex subunit 1 conjointly determine stable warfarin dose: a prospective study. J Thromb Thrombolysis 2006;22:191–7.

35. Ellis DJ, Usman MH, Milner PG, et al. The first evaluation of a novel vitamin K antagonist, tecarfarin (ATI-5923), in patients with atrial fibrillation. Circulation 2009;120(12):1024–6.

36. Bates SM, Weitz JI. The mechanism of action of thrombin inhibitors. J Invasive Cardiol 2000;12(Suppl F):27F–32F.

37. Kaul S, Diamond GA, Weintraub WS. Trials and tribulations of non-inferiority: the ximelagatran experience. J Am Coll Cardiol 2005;46:1986–95.

38. Mungall D. BIBR-1048 Boehringer Ingelheim. Curr Opin Investig Drugs 2002;3:905–7.

39. Wallentin L, Ezekowitz M, Simmers TA, et al. On behalf of PETRO-investigators. Safety and efficacy of a new oral direct thrombin inhibitor dabigatran in atrial fibrillation: a dose finding trial with comparison to warfarin. Eur Heart J 2005;26 (Suppl):482.

40. Ezekowitz MD, Reilly PA, Nehmiz G, et al. Dabigatran with or without concomitant aspirin compared with warfarin alone in patients with nonvalvular atrial fibrillation (PETRO Study). Am J Cardiol 2007;100(9):1419–26.

41. The Petro-Ex Investigators. Safety and efficacy of extended exposure to several doses of a new oral direct thrombin inhibitor dabigatran etexilate in atrial fibrillation [abstract 5]. Cerebrovasc Dis 2006;21(Suppl 4):2.

42. Connolly SJ, Ezekowitz MD, Yusuf S, et al. Dabigatran versus warfarin in patients with atrial fibrillation. N Engl J Med 2009;361(12):1200–2.

42a. Pradaxa [package insert]. Ridgefield, CT: Boehringer Ingelheim Pharmaceuticals, Inc.; 2010.

43. Bauer KA. New anticoagulants: anti IIa vs anti Xa—is one better? J Thromb Thrombolysis 2006;21(1):67–72.

44. Perzborn E, Strassburger J, Wilmen A, et al. In vitro and in vivo studies of the novel antithrombotic agent BAY 59-7939—an oral, direct Factor Xa inhibitor. J Thromb Haemost 2005;3(3):514–21.

45. Mueck W, Becka M, Kubitza D, et al. Population model of the pharmacokinetics and pharmacodynamics of rivaroxaban—an oral, direct factor xa inhibitor—in healthy subjects. Int J Clin Pharmacol Ther 2007;45(6):335–44.

46. Kubitza D, Becka M, Wensing G, et al. Safety, pharmacodynamics, and pharmacokinetics of BAY 59-7939—an oral, direct factor Xa inhibitor—after multiple dosing in healthy male subjects. Eur J Clin Pharmacol 2005;61(12):873–80.

47. Kubitza D, Becka M, Mueck W, et al. The effect of extreme age, and gender, on the pharmacology and tolerability of rivaroxaban—an oral, direct factor Xa inhibitor [abstract 905]. Blood 2006;108.

48. Kubitza D, Becka M, Zuehlsdorf M, et al. Body weight has limited influence on the safety, tolerability, pharmacokinetics, or pharmacodynamics of rivaroxaban (BAY 59-7939) in healthy subjects. J Clin Pharmacol 2007;47(2):218–26.

49. Kubitza D, Becka M, Zuehlsdorf M, et al. Effect of food, an antacid, and the H2 antagonist ranitidine on the absorption of BAY 59-7939 (rivaroxaban), an oral, direct Factor Xa inhibitor, in healthy subjects. J Clin Pharmacol 2006;46:549–58.

50. Pinto DJ, Orwat MJ, Koch S, et al. Discovery of 1-(4-methoxyphenyl)-7-oxo-6-(4-(2-oxopiperidin-1-yl) phenyl)-4,5,6,7-tetrahydro-1H-pyrazolo[3,4-c]pyridine-3-carboxamide (apixaban, BMS-562247), a highly potent, selective, efficacious, and orally bioavailable inhibitor of blood coagulation factor Xa. J Med Chem 2007;50(22):5339–56.

51. He K, He B, Grace JE, et al. Preclinical pharmacokinetics and metabolism of apixaban, a potent and selective Factor Xa inhibitor [abstract 910]. Blood 2006;108:273.

51a. Hirsh J, O'Donnell M, Eikelboom JW. Beyond unfractionated heparin and warfarin: current and future advances. Circulation 2007;116(5):552–60.

52. Ezekowitz M. A randomized clinical trial of three doses of a long-acting oral direct factor Xa inhibitor betrixaban in patients with atrial fibrillation. Presented at the ACC 2010 conference. Atlanta, GA. March 15, 2010.

53. Weitz J. Randomized, parallel group, multicenter, multinational study evaluating safety of DU-176b compared with warfarin in subjects with non-valvular atrial fibrillation. Presented at the annual meeting of the American Society of Hematology. San Franscisco, CA, December 7, 2008.

54. Koopman MM, Buller HR, (Academic Medical Center, Amsterdam, The Netherlands). Short- and long-acting synthetic pentasaccharides (minisymposium). J Intern Med 2003;254:335–42.

55. Idraparinux shows encouraging results in the prevention of thromboembolic events in patients with atrial fibrillation. July 11, Paris: Sanofi-Aventis; 2007.

56. Agnelli G, Haas S, Ginsberg JS, et al. A phase II study of the oral factor Xa inhibitor LY517717 for the prevention of venous thromboembolism after hip or knee replacement. J Thromb Haemost 2007;5:746–53.

57. Agnelli G, Haas SK, Krueger KA, et al. A phase II study of the safety and efficacy of a novel oral FXa inhibitor (LY-517717) for the prevention of venous thromboembolism following TKR or THR [abstract]. Blood 2005;106:278.

58. Neels JG, van Den Berg BM, Mertens K, et al. Activation of factor IX zymogen results in exposure of a binding site for low-density lipoprotein receptor-related protein. Blood 2000;96:3459–65.

59. Lawson JH, Mann KG. Cooperative activation of human factor IX by the human extrinsic pathway of blood coagulation. J Biol Chem 1991;266:11317–27.

60. Ahmad SS, Rawala-Sheikh R, Walsh PN. Platelet receptor occupancy with factor IXa promotes factor X activation. J Biol Chem 1989;264: 20012–6.

61. Chow FS, Benincosa LJ, Sheth SB, et al. Pharmacokinetic and pharmacodynamic modeling of humanized anti-factor IX antibody (SB 249417) in humans. Clin Pharmacol Ther 2002;71:235–45.

62. Dyke CK, Steinhubl SR, Kleiman NS, et al. First-in-human experience of an antidote-controlled anticoagulant using RNA aptamer technology: a phase 1a pharmacodynamic evaluation of a drug-antidote pair for the controlled regulation of factor IXa activity. Circulation 2006;114:2490–7.

63. Rothlein R, Shen JM, Naser N, et al. TTP889, a novel orally active partial inhibitor of FIXa inhibits clotting in two A/V shunt models without prolonging bleeding times [abstract]. Blood 2005;106:1886.

64. Eriksson BI, Dahl OE, Lassen MR, et al. The FIXIT Study Group, Partial factor IXa inhibition with TTP889 for prevention of venous thromboembolism: an exploratory study. J Thromb Haemost 2008;6:457–63.

65. Ragni M, Cirillo P, Pascucci I, et al. Monoclonal antibody against tissue factor shortens tissue plasminogen activator lysis time and prevents reocclusion in a rabbit model of carotid artery thrombosis. Circulation 1996;93:1913–8.

66. Himber J, Kirchhofer D, Riederer M, et al. Dissociation of antithrombotic effect and bleeding time prolongation in rabbits by inhibiting tissue factor function. Thromb Haemost 1997;78:1142–9.

67. Pawashe A, Golino P, Ambrosio G, et al. A monoclonal antibody against rabbit tissue factor inhibits thrombus formation in stenotic injured rabbit carotid arteries. Circ Res 1994;74:56–63.

68. Szalony JA, Suleymanov OD, Salyers AK, et al. Administration of a small molecule tissue factor/factor VIIa inhibitor in a non-human primate thrombosis model of venous thrombosis: effects on thrombus formation and bleeding time. Thromb Res 2003;112:167–74.

69. Lee A, Agnelli G, Buller H, et al. Dose-response study of recombinant factor VIIa/tissue factor inhibitor recombinant nematode anticoagulant protein c2 in prevention of postoperative venous thromboembolism in patients undergoing total knee replacement. Circulation 2001;104:74–8.

70. Giugliano RP, Wiviott SD, Stone PH, et al. Recombinant nematode anticoagulant protein c2 in patients with non-ST-segment elevation acute coronary syndrome: the ANTHEM-TIMI-32 trial. J Am Coll Cardiol 2007;49:2398–407.

71. Shirk RA, Vlasuk GP. Inhibitors of factor VIIa/tissue factor. Arterioscler Thromb Vasc Biol 2007;27: 1895–900.

Index

Note: Page numbers of article titles are in **boldface** type.

Card Electrophysiol Clin 2 (2010) 493–498
doi:10.1016/S1877-9182(10)00127-9

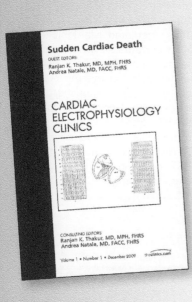
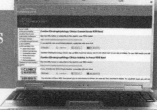

Printed and bound by CPI Group (UK) Ltd, Croydon, CR0 4YY

03/10/2024

01040354-0017